Acetylcholine Synthesis in Neurons

ACETYLCHOLINE SYNTHESIS IN NEURONS

S. Tuček

Head, Department of Neuromuscular Physiology, and Deputy Director, Institute of Physiology, Czechoslovak Academy of Sciences, Prague

LONDON
CHAPMAN AND HALL

A Halsted Press Book
John Wiley & Sons, New York

First published 1978
by Chapman and Hall Ltd
11 New Fetter Lane, London EC4P 4EE

Typeset by C. Josée Utteridge-Faivre and printed in Great Britain at the University Printing House, Cambridge

ISBN 0 412 15030 1

Distributed in the U.S.A. by Halsted Press, a Division of John Wiley & Sons, Inc., New York

Library of Congress Cataloging in Publication Data

Tuček, S.
Acetylcholine synthesis in neurons.

'A Halsted Press book.'
Bibliography: p.
1. Acetylcholine–Metabolism. 2. Neurons.
I. Title.
QP921.A25T83 599′.01′88 77-19346
ISBN 0-470-26304-0

TO DANA

Contents

Preface

The investigation of the cholinergic mechanisms in the nervous system has been developing rapidly during the last four decades, and the rate of progress in the field seems to accelerate all the time. In the studies of the synthesis of acetylcholine, the most important steps forward have stemmed from the discovery of choline acetyltransferase, acetylcoenzyme A, and of axonal transport; from the introduction of subcellular fractionation techniques and of radioisotopic methods into research on cholinergic synapses; and from the realization that the electric organ of fish is an extremely valuable source of information, not only about the biophysical basis, but also about the biochemical and ultrastructural basis of cholinergic transmission. Although, in recent years, cholinergic mechanisms have been analysed in several excellent books and symposia (Heilbronn and Winter, 1970; Fardeau *et al.*, 1973; Michelson and Zeimal, 1973; Waser, 1975; Goldberg and Hanin, 1976; Zaimis, 1976), none of them gave to the topic of acetylcholine synthesis the degree of attention which, in my opinion, it deserves. It is my hope that this volume, which discusses the cellular aspects of the synthesis of acetylcholine in the nervous system, will, despite its imperfections, be a useful addition to the existing books on cholinergic transmission.

S. Tuček

Acknowledgements

It is my pleasant duty to thank my colleagues all over the world who have helped me to write this book by sending reprints of their articles; they are too numerous to be mentioned here individually. I am especially grateful to all colleagues who sent me their scientific papers before their publication; among them were H. Banns, E.A. Barnard, J.P. Blass, P. Boksa, A.M. Burt, D.L. Cheney, B. Collier, E. Costa, M.F. Diebler, M.J. Dowdall, Y. Dunant, J. Ekström, D.M. Fambrough, A.L. Goldberg, E. Giacobini, C. Hebb, D. Ilson, M. Israël, P. Kása, P.A. Lavoie, B. Lesbats, S. Lovat, R. Manaranche, S.P. Mann, R. Massarelli, R.E. McCaman, P.L. McGeer, R. Miledi, P.C. Molenaar, Y. Morot-Gaudry, R.L. Polak, G. Pilar, J. Rossier, G. Racagni, V.K. Singh, J.H. Schwartz, M. Trabucchi, V.P. Whittaker, J.M. Wright, H. Zimmermann, G. Zsilla and many others to whom I apologize for the imperfection of my memory. Drs M. Frizell, P. Lefresne, S.P. Mann, G.L.A. Reijnierse and J. Rossier very kindly sent me their dissertations and Drs B. Ansell, D. Malthe-Sørenssen, H.G. Mautner and R. Roskoski were most helpful in answering my questions on controversial points. My thanks are also due to the authors and the copyright holders of the illustrations for permission to use illustrations, to Mrs B. Buchtová for her invaluable secretarial help, and to Dr Ruth Payne for advice on many linguistic problems. I cannot adequately express the extent of my gratitude to Dr Ann Silver for her comments on the style and scientific content of the book. I am also greatly indebted to Dr Catherine O. Hebb for her long lasting interest in my experimental work.

Abbreviations

Acetyl–CoA	acetylcoenzyme A
ACh	acetylcholine
AChE	acetylcholinesterase
ADP	adenosine diphosphate
AMP	adenosine monophosphate
ATP	adenosine triphosphate
CDP	cytidine diphosphate
Ch	choline
ChAc	choline acetyltransferase
ChE	cholinesterase
CoA	coenzyme A
d.p.m.	disintegrations per minute
HMG–CoA	3-hydroxy-3-methylglutaryl–coenzyme A
GABA	γ-aminobutyric acid
K_{eq}	equilibrium constant
K_m	Michaelis constant
MW	molecular weight
p	probability of the null hypothesis
P_i	inorganic phosphate
PP_i	inorganic pyrophosphate
S.E.M.	standard error of the mean
V_{max}	maximal velocity of enzymatic reaction (at saturating concentrations of the substrates)
v/v	volume/volume
w/v	weight/volume

1 Introduction

Acetylcholine (ACh) serves as the transmitter of nerve impulses at cholinergic synapses. In man and homoiothermic animals, it effects transmission from motor nerves to skeletal muscle, from preganglionic parasympathetic and sympathetic fibres to neurons in the autonomic ganglia and adrenal medulla, from postganglionic parasympathetic fibres to the heart, and from postganglionic parasympathetic and some postganglionic sympathetic fibres to the glandular and smooth muscle cells. ACh is also the transmitter at some synapses in the central nervous system. A certain (but varying) quantity of ACh is released from the presynaptic nerve ending by each impulse. The released ACh diffuses in the synaptic gap and reacts with the cholinergic receptor protein, located in the postsynaptic membrane. The reaction with the receptor starts the chain of events resulting in the excitation or inhibition of the postganglionic cell.

Repeated nerve impulses, with the repeated release of ACh from the nerve endings, would exhaust the store of useable ACh and block the transmission at cholinergic synapses (with catastrophic consequences for the organism), if the cholinergic neurons were incapable of ensuring the synthesis of sufficient amounts of new ACh. The substrates for the biosynthesis of ACh are acetylcoenzyme A (acetyl–CoA) and choline. The synthesis is catalysed by the enzyme choline acetyltransferase (ChAc; acetyl–CoA: choline-*O*-acetyltransferase, EC2.3.1.6). The synthesis proceeds according to the equation:

$$\text{choline} + \text{acetylcoenzyme A} = \text{acetylcholine} + \text{coenzyme A}$$

It is evident that, in order to synthesize ACh, the nerve ending needs the presence of three substances–ChAc, choline, and acetyl–CoA. Only one of these substances, acetyl–CoA, is produced directly in the nerve ending. Choline is probably obtained from the extracellular fluid and ChAc is supplied from the cell bodies of cholinergic neurons by the mechanism of axonal transport.

This book represents an attempt to summarize the present understanding of the synthesis of ACh in cholinergic neurons and particularly in the presynaptic endings of their axons. Attention is paid mainly to:

(a) basic data on the properties of ChAc, on the methods of measuring its activity, and on the ChAc catalysed reaction;
(b) the transport of ChAc and ACh from neuronal cell bodies to the presynaptic endings of their axons;
(c) the synthesis of acetyl–CoA in the nervous tissue and its supply for the synthesis of ACh;
(d) the biosynthesis of choline and its supply for the synthesis of ACh;
(e) the organization of the synthesis of ACh in the presynaptic nerve endings and its control;
(f) changes of ACh synthesis and ChAc activity in the neurons occurring under some physiological and pathological conditions.

In general, this book attempts to analyse the synthesis of ACh at the level of single cells, rather than at that of the whole nervous system. Consequently, the problem of ACh turnover in the brain has not been included; this particular topic has been well covered in recent reviews by Hanin and Costa (1976) and Cheney and Costa (1977).

2 Choline acetyltransferase

2.1 INTRODUCTION

Nachmansohn and Machado (1943) were the first to observe the synthesis of ACh in cell-free tissue extracts. They ascribed the synthesis to the activity of an enzyme for which they proposed the name choline acetylase. The substrates for the synthesis were acetate, choline and ATP. Later work showed that the synthesis of ACh requires the presence of a heat-stable, diffusible cofactor (Nachmansohn and Berman, 1946; Feldberg and Mann, 1946); this has proved to be identical with the cofactor used in other acetylation reactions and has been termed coenzyme A (CoA; see Lipmann, 1954). It has become clear that the synthesis of ACh in the system used by Nachmansohn and Machado (1943) was based on the activity of two enzymes, one producing acetyl–CoA from acetate and CoA (see Chapter 4), the other transferring the acetyl groups from acetyl–CoA to choline. The term choline acetylase (ChAc) has been retained specifically for the enzyme responsible for this transfer (Korey *et al.*, 1951).

ChAc is able to use acetyl–CoA supplied by several different enzymes (Korkes *et al.*, 1952), but the presence of CoA is essential for the synthesis of ACh in such a coupled enzymatic system (Balfour and Hebb, 1952). More complete information about the first exciting years of the investigation of ChAc is given by Nachmansohn (1959) in his monograph. A new name for ChAc – choline acetyltransferase (acetyl–CoA:choline-*O*-acetyltransferase, EC 2.3.1.6) was recommended by the Enzyme Commission of the International Union of Biochemistry in 1961. Literature on ChAc has been reviewed by, among others, Hebb (1963, 1972), Hardegg (1966), Artenie (1968), Haubrich (1976) and Rossier (1977a).

2.2 CHOLINE ACETYLTRANSFERASE AS A PROTEIN

ChAc is a globular protein with an apparent radius of 3.39 nm (Rossier, 1976c) and a comparatively high positive surface charge (Potter *et al.*, 1968; Fonnum, 1970b; Fonnum and Malthe-Sørenssen, 1972, 1973). Its molecular weight has been measured mainly by gel filtration and sedimentation analysis; the results of these measurements are summarized in Table 2.1. The molecular weight of ChAc in mammalian nervous tissue is most probably close to 68 000 daltons, but the molecular weight of placental ChAc seems to be lower. The molecules of ChAc tend to associate as dimers and heavier aggregates, particularly under the influence of ammonium sulphate precipitation and other purification procedures (Chao and Wolfgram, 1974; Banns, 1976; Rossier, 1976c). Thiol groups of the enzyme play an important role in the aggregation (Polsky and Shuster, 1976b; Rossier, 1976c), which is not necessarily accompanied by loss of enzymatic activity and is reversible. Although difficult to prove, it appears unlikely that ChAc dimers or aggregates exist *in vivo*. Squid ChAc contains subunits with molecular weights of approximately 37 000 and 56 000 daltons, possibly composed of still smaller subunits with a molecular weight of 18 000 (Polsky and Shuster, 1976b). It has been suggested that mammalian ChAc is also composed of small, enzymatically active subunits, either identical (Chao, 1975) or non-identical (Chao and Wolfgram, 1973); these suggestions require further examination. An attempt to investigate the amino acid composition of ChAc (Chao, 1975) may have been premature in view of the high degree of purity necessary for material used for this purpose.

Many attempts have been made to isolate ChAc from tissue homogenates, but complete separation of ChAc from other proteins has not been achieved. The methods used and the problems encountered in studies aimed at the purification of ChAc are clearly described in Rossier's (1977a) review. Preparations with the highest specific activities have been obtained from squid optic lobes. Using such a source, Husain and Mautner (1973) purified ChAc to a specific activity of 67 μmol ACh synthesized/mg protein/min and Polsky and Shuster (1976a) achieved a specific activity of 58 μmol/mg protein/min. The activity of ChAc in mammalian tissues, relative to their protein content, is much lower than in squid optic lobes and the specific activity of the preparations of purified ChAc obtained from them is also lower. High degrees of purification have been described by Rossier (1976a–ChAc from rat brain, 20 μmol/mg protein/min), Ryan and McClure (1976–ChAc from bovine caudate nuclei, more than 16 μmol/mg protein/min), Malthe-Sørenssen *et al.* (1973–ChAc from rat brain, 4 μmol/mg protein/min), Malthe-Sørenssen (1976b–ChAc from bovine caudate nuclei, 2.5 μmol/mg protein/min), and Morris (1966–ChAc from human placenta, 2.4 μmol/mg protein/min). Judging from the amount of impurities in his preparation of highly purified ChAc from rat brain, Rossier (1975) estimates that completely pure preparations of mammalian ChAc should have a specific activity of about 100 μmol ACh synthesized/mg protein/min.

Much evidence has recently been provided about the presence of multiple

Table 2.1 Molecular weight of choline acetyltransferase

Source	Method of measurement	Molecular weight (daltons)	Related observations	References
Rat brain	Sedimentation analysis	67 000		Bull *et al.* (1964)
Human placenta	Sedimentation analysis	59 000		Bull *et al.* (1964)
Rat cerebral cortex	Gel filtration	50 000		Potter *et al.* (1968)
Lactobacillus plantarum	Gel filtration	70 000	Activity also in fractions corresponding to MW of 35 000–70 000	White and Cavallito (1970b)
Bovine caudate nuclei	Gel filtration	100 000 or more		White and Cavallito (1970b)
Bovine caudate nuclei	Gel filtration	65 000		Glover and Potter (1971)
Human basal ganglia	Gel filtration	62 000	Dimers or aggregates with higher MW	White and Wu (1973b)
Bovine caudate nuclei	Gel filtration	120 000	Subunits with MW of 51 000 and 69 000	Chao and Wolfgram (1973)
Bovine caudate nuclei	Gel filtration	60 000–1 500 000		Chao and Wolfgram (1974)
Bovine caudate nuclei	Polyacrylamide gel electrophoresis	60 000–67 000		Eng *et al.* (1974)
Squid head ganglia	Gel filtration	120 000; 125 000; 200 000		Husain and Mautner, (1973)
Bovine caudate nuclei	Gel filtration	87 000	Possibly subunits with MW of 14 700	Chao (1975)
	Sedimentation analysis	88 000		

Table 2.1 Molecular weight of choline acetyltransferase (*continued*)

Source	Method of measurement	Molecular weight (daltons)	Related observations	References
Human striatum	Polyacrylamide gel electrophoresis	67 000		Singh *et al.* (1975)
Rat brain	Gel filtration	60 000–65 000		Wenthold and Mahler (1975)
Squid head ganglia	Gel filtration and sedimentation analysis	35 000–300 000	Subunits with MW of 37 000 and 56 000	Polsky and Shuster (1976b)
Human placenta	Gel filtration Sedimentation analysis	58 000–60 000 62 000	Aggregates with MW of up to 1 900 000; peaks with MW of 69 000 and 76 000	Banns (1976)
Rat brain	Calculation from biophysical constants obtained by sedimentation analysis and gel filtration	68 000	Dimers with MW of 136 000 and aggregates with MW $> 400\,000$	Rossier (1976c)
Human striatum	Gel filtration	67 000		Singh and McGeer, (1977)

molecular forms of ChAc in some species. The existence of multiple forms of ChAc was suggested by observations on the distribution of ChAc during electrophoresis (Rentsch, 1961) and was inferred from the analysis of the activating effect of salts on squid ChAc (Prempeh *et al.*, 1972). A clear demonstration that ChAc does exist in multiple forms was provided by isoelectric focusing (Malthe-Sørenssen and Fonnum, 1972). In experiments with isoelectric focusing, a pH gradient is formed in a carrier medium under the influence of an electric field. The components of a mixture of proteins separate on the pH gradient as a result of the fact that individual proteins accumulate in the regions which correspond to their isoelectric points. The isoelectric focusing technique has shown three molecular forms of ChAc in the brain of rat (Malthe-Sørenssen and Fonnum, 1972; Fonnum and Malthe-Sørenssen, 1973), ox (Malthe-Sørenssen, 1975), mouse, monkey (Malthe-Sørenssen, 1976a) and man (White and Wu, 1973b). Two forms have been found in the brain of cat, but only one in the brain of guinea-pig, pigeon (Malthe-Sørenssen and Fonnum, 1972) and rabbit (White and Wu, 1973b; Malthe-Sørenssen, 1976a). The electric organ of *Torpedo* (Malthe-Sørenssen, 1976a) and the nervous tissue of the cockroach and horse-shoe crab (Emson *et al.*, 1974) similarly possess only one form. Different molecular forms of ChAc have also been isolated by chromatography of human brain ChAc (Singh *et al.*, 1975), bovine brain ChAc (Malthe-Sørenssen, 1975, 1976a) and squid ChAc (Hussain and Mautner, 1973; Polsky and Shuster, 1976a,b) on cellulose phosphate, sulphopropyl–Sephadex or CM–Sephadex columns and by polyacrylamide gel electrophoresis.

In some cases, differences between various samples of ChAc separated by isoelectric focusing or chromatography, are caused by the aggregation of ChAc subunits or molecules. Relations between apparent molecular weight (as indicated by gel filtration) and isoelectric fractions have been clearly demonstrated by Polsky and Shuster (1976a). Changes in the extent of aggregation may have been responsible for the interconversion of different isoelectric forms sometimes observed when the procedure of isoelectric focusing was repeated (White and Wu, 1973b; Polsky and Shuster, 1976a). Some of the ChAc 'forms' described in the literature may have been based on the association of ChAc molecules with other proteins. Most multiple forms of ChAc, however, are stable during repeated isolation procedures and can be separated under conditions preventing enzyme–protein interactions, e.g. in the presence of 3 M urea (Fonnum and Malthe-Sørenssen, 1972; Malthe-Sørenssen, 1975, 1976a); it is therefore unlikely that their existence is based on the formation of molecular aggregates. At the same time, a conspicuous feature of the multiple molecular forms of ChAc is their close chemical similarity. Different molecular forms of ChAc isolated from bovine, mouse and monkey brain have the same molecular weight within each species and do not differ in their affinity to choline (Malthe-Sørenssen, 1975, 1976a). Molecular forms of squid ChAc, isolated chromatographically, are indistinguishable immunologically (Polsky and Shuster, 1976b). Available evidence does not allow a conclusion about the biochemical or biophysical basis of the differences between the multiple forms of ChAc. One of the possibilities is, of course, that they are true isoenzymes, i.e. different proteins, coded by different genes. In view of the similarities between them, it seems difficult to accept this possibility without more evidence.

Several successful attempts to produce antibodies against ChAc have been reported. It appears to be easier to stimulate the production of antibodies against ChAc using partially purified enzyme from human (Singh and McGeer, 1974a,b) or bovine brain (Eng *et al.*, 1974; Malthe-Sørenssen, 1975) or from squid head ganglia (Polsky and Shuster, 1976b) than from the brain of rat (Rossier *et al.*, 1973a,b; Malthe-Sørenssen *et al.*, 1973; Rossier, 1976b) or mouse (Shuster and O'Toole, 1974). No monospecific antisera against ChAc have yet been prepared (Rossier, 1977a); this is understandable, since no entirely pure ChAc has been available for immunization. Antisera against ChAc inhibit, but do not entirely block its enzymatic activity; some activity is retained by the precipitated enzyme–antibody complexes (Rossier, 1976b). Antibodies against rat brain ChAc react also with ChAc from other organs of the rat and with ChAc from all vertebrate species tested (including the enzyme from *Torpedo* electric organ). They do not react with ChAc from squid optic lobe and, conversely, antibodies against squid optic lobe ChAc do not react with rat brain ChAc (Rossier, 1977a).

2.3 CHOLINE ACETYLTRANSFERASE AS AN ENZYME

ChAc catalyses the reversible transfer of acetyl groups from acetyl–CoA to choline. The stoichiometry of the ChAc catalysed reaction is described by structural formulae in Fig. 2.1. The equilibrium of the reaction favours the synthesis of ACh. Published values for the equilibrium constant,

$$K_{eq} = \frac{[\text{ACh}] \times [\text{CoA}]}{[\text{choline}] \times [\text{acetyl–CoA}]}$$

based on measurements at 37°–38°C, are surprisingly variable. In Schuberth's (1966) experiments with placental ChAc, K_{eq} was equal to 145 in the presence of 0.3 M NaCl, but to 5100 in the absence of NaCl. Potter *et al.* (1968) calculated the value of K_{eq} for brain ChAc as 514, and Glover and Potter (1971) as only 41. The last value matches best the available information on the free energy of hydrolysis of acetyl–CoA and ACh. Data on the free energy of hydrolysis of acetyl–CoA at pH 7.0 vary in the range −7.2 to −8.9 kcal/mol (review Holldorf, 1964; Guynn *et al.*, 1973). The free energy of hydrolysis of ACh at pH 7.0 equals −6.5 kcal/mol (Jencks *et al.*, 1960) or −6.0 kcal/mol (Gerstein and Jencks, 1964). It is evident from these values that the ChAc-catalysed reaction is slightly exergonic. The relation between the free energy change (ΔG_o) and the equilibrium constant (K_{eq}) of a reaction is given by the equation

$$\Delta G_o = -RT \ln K_{eq}$$

(Morris, 1968), where R is the gas constant and T the temperature. According to this

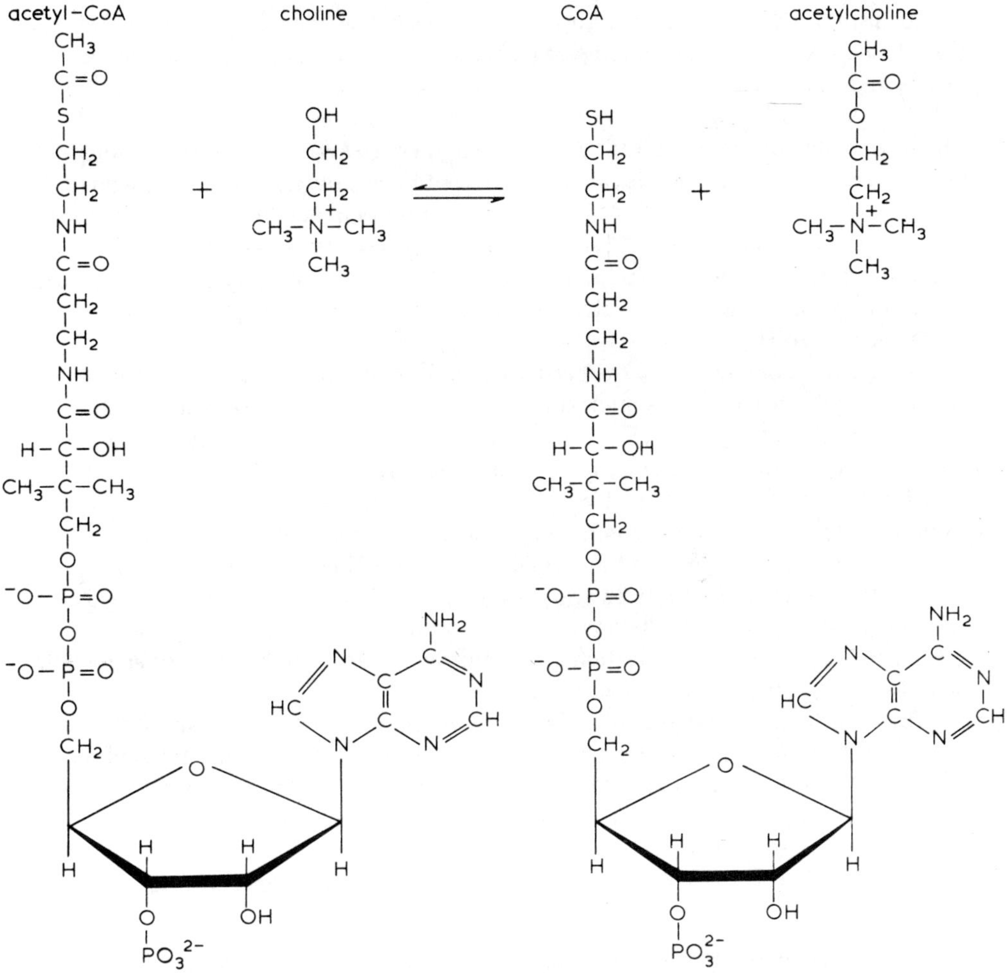

Fig. 2.1 The reaction for the biosynthesis of ACh: acetyl—CoA + choline ⇌ CoA + ACh.

equation, the difference of –2.4 kcal/mol between the free energy of hydrolysis of acetyl—CoA and of ACh corresponds to $K_{eq} = 49$. The value of the equilibrium constant of the reaction catalysed by ChAc is important particularly in considering the mechanism of control of ACh synthesis in the nerve cell *in vivo.* The discussion of this mechanism in Chapter 6 will be based on the value of 41, as found by Glover and Potter (1971).

In spite of much effort, comparatively little is known about the structure of the active centre of ChAc and the nature of its catalytically active groups. Most attention has been concentrated on the role of imidazole and sulphydryl groups in the mechanism of the ChAc catalysed reaction. The view that the imidazole group of histidine plays a part in the binding of reactants to the enzyme, first advanced by White and Cavallito (1970a), is now receiving general acceptance. It is supported by observations that ChAc is inactivated by photo-oxidation in the presence of methylene blue or rose bengal (Currier and Mautner, 1974) and by ethoxyformic anhydride; in the latter case, it can be reactivated by hydroxylamine and protected by acetyl–CoA (Roskoski, 1974c). ChAc immobilized on mercuribenzoate sepharose gel can bind the label from [^{14}C] acetyl–CoA, but loses this ability when its histidine residues are masked with diethylpyrocarbonate. It is therefore likely that the imidazole group of histidine is directly involved in the binding of the acetyl group (Malthe-Sørenssen, 1976b).

Although it does not prove the participation of imidazole in the mechanism of the ChAc catalysed reaction, it is interesting to note here that imidazole increases the stability of ChAc on storage (Severin and Artenie, 1968) and its activity during incubation (Severin and Artenie, 1968; White and Cavallito, 1970a; but cf. Severin and Popova, 1965, and Chao and Wolgram, 1974). It may also be relevant that ACh is produced non-enzymatically in the presence of acetylimidazole and choline (Severin and Popova, 1965) and that imidazole itself is able to catalyse the non-enzymatic synthesis of ACh from acetyl–CoA and choline (Burt and Silver, 1973a). This raises the question of whether the reported increase of ChAc activity by imidazole was due to true activation of the enzyme, or to a combination of enzymatic and non-enzymatic synthesis of ACh.

The evidence regarding the role of sulphydryl groups in the mechanism of the ChAc catalysed reaction is complicated and controversial. It has been estimated that the molecule of ChAc contains at least 8 sulphydryl groups (Severin and Artenie, 1967). Their presence has been successfully exploited in attempts to purify ChAc by binding it to organomercurial sepharose (Husain and Mautner, 1973; Chao and Wolfgram, 1973). The main arguments in support of the importance of thiol groups in the activity of ChAc are these:

(a) ChAc is inhibited by compounds known to react with sulphydryl groups. The activity of squid ChAc is reduced by 60% or more by iodoacetate 5×10^{-3} M, *p*-chloromercuribenzoate 1×10^{-5} M, iodosobenzoate 1×10^{-4} M and $CuSO_4$ 5×10^{-6} M (Berman-Reisberg, 1957). The various thiol reagents do, however, differ in their inhibitory potency. For example, bovine brain ChAc is inhibited by 78% in the presence of 2, 2′-dithiopyridine 10^{-7} M but it is not inhibited by iodoacetate and iodoacetamide even at a concentration of 10^{-3} M (Mannervik and Sörbo, 1970).

(b) Acetyl–CoA and, to some extent, ACh protect ChAc against the inhibition by thiol reagents (Roskoski, 1974a; but cf. Mannervik and Sörbo, 1970).

(c) The binding of ChAc to mercurisepharose gel can be prevented by pre-incubating the enzyme with acetyl–CoA (Malthe-Sørenssen, 1976b).

(d) ChAc has been described as forming an acetylated complex with the acetyl group of acetyl–CoA or ACh (Roskoski, 1973) and with the bromoacetyl group of bromoacetyl–CoA or bromoacetylcholine (Roskoski, 1974b). The acetyl and bromoacetyl groups appeared to be connected with the enzyme by thioester bonds. No formation of acetyl–enzyme complex has been found, however, by other investigators following Roskoski's (1973) procedure (Currier and Mautner, 1974; Malthe-Sørenssen, 1976b). Since Roskoski was using ChAc of low purity, the acetyl groups were probably bound to proteins other than ChAc (Malthe-Sørenssen, 1976b).

It has been shown recently (Currier and Mautner, 1976) that the thiol reagent, methane thiolsulphonate, inhibits ChAc not so much by reacting with enzymic thiol groups, but by reacting with CoA and producing a new potent inhibitor. Notwithstanding this finding, most thiol reagents are likely to inhibit ChAc by a direct action on the enzyme. It should be remembered, however, that the inhibitory effect of a thiol reagent on an enzyme does not prove that the sulphydryl groups of the enzyme are directly involved in the mechanism of enzymatic reaction. Even though the inhibitor may be acting on sulphydryl groups outside the active centre, or on catalytically inactive sulphydryl groups in the area of the active centre, the activity of the enzyme will be inhibited if the binding of the inhibitor to the sulphydryl groups brings about significant conformational changes of the whole enzyme molecule or steric hindrance in the area of the active centre. The observation by Malthe-Sørenssen (1976b) that ChAc inhibited by 5, 5′-dithio-bis(2-nitrobenzoate) is partly reactivated when the thionitrobenzoate derivative is cleaved by KCN treatment to thiocyanate derivative indicates, on one hand, that ChAc activity is not absolutely dependent on the presence of free sulphydryl groups, and, on the other, that steric interference is an important factor in the action of thiol reagents on ChAc. In view of all the available evidence, it appears most likely that the thiol groups of ChAc do not participate directly in the binding of reaction substrates, intermediates or products, but that at least one thiol group is present in the area of the active centre.

The problem of the binding sites for choline and for coenzyme A in the active centre of ChAc is still entirely open and the only information about their characteristics can be inferred from data on the substrate specificity and on the inhibitors of ChAc. Choline probably binds to an anionic site similar to that in the active centre of acetylcholinesterase (see review by Main, 1976). The binding of CoA and acetyl–CoA depends on the presence of the nucleotide moiety in the molecule of CoA (the pantothenic part of CoA being unimportant for the binding) and occurs at a hydrophobic site of ChAc, similar to the 'nucleotide fold' described in several nucleotide metabolizing enzymes (Rossier, 1977b).

The affinity of ChAc for acetyl–CoA is much higher than for choline. In experiments with ChAc from bovine caudate nuclei, the Michaelis constants (K_m) for acetyl–CoA and choline were not dependent on the concentration of the second substrate; the K_m for acetyl–CoA was 10 μM, and for choline, 0.75 mM (Glover and Potter, 1971). In experiments with the enzyme from human, rabbit and rat brain and from human and rabbit peripheral nerves, the K_m for one substrate was dependent on the concentration of the other substrate. Interpolated values of K_m for acetyl–CoA at a saturating concentration of choline were in the range 7–18 μM; the values of K_m for choline at a saturating concentration of acetyl–CoA were

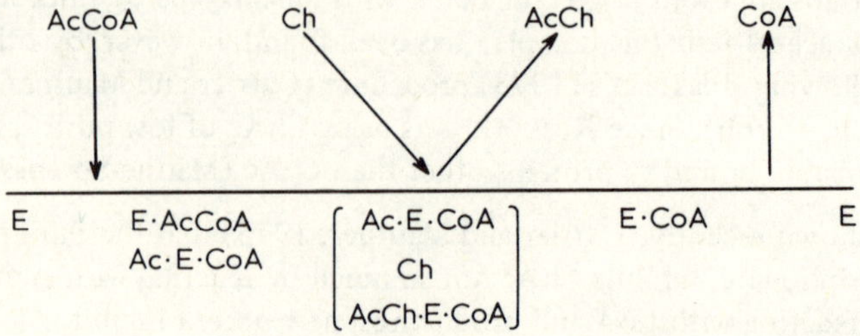

Fig. 2.2 The most likely course of the enzymatic reaction catalysed by ChAc, described in Cleland's (1963) shorthand notation. During ACh biosynthesis, the reaction proceeds from left to right. Abbreviations: E = enzyme, Ac = acetyl, Ch = choline, CoA = coenzyme A. The dots represent the binding between the enzyme and the substrate, intermediary product or product. See text for further explanations and for discussion of other proposed mechanisms of ChAc catalysed reaction.

0.41–1.20 mM (White and Wu, 1973a).

Both reaction products, ACh and CoA, have an inhibitory effect on ChAc. Most investigators have found ACh to be a competitive inhibitor towards choline and non-competitive towards acetyl–CoA, and CoA to be a competitive inhibitor towards acetyl–CoA and non-competitive towards choline (White and Cavallito, 1970a; Morris *et al.*, 1971; Sastry and Henderson, 1972; White and Wu, 1973). Whereas Kaita and Goldberg (1969) also classify the inhibitory effect of ACh as competitive towards choline and non-competitive towards acetyl–CoA, Glover and Potter (1971) describe it as non-competitive towards choline and uncompetitive towards acetyl–CoA; an inhibitor is deemed uncompetitive if it causes a change of both V_{max} and K_m. The inhibitory constants, K_i, found with ChAc from different samples of nervous tissue are for CoA (as a competitive inhibitor towards acetyl–CoA) in the range 5.5–20 μM, and for ACh (as a competitive inhibitor towards choline) in the range 27–$>$100mM (White and Wu, 1973a).

The mechanism of the ChAc catalysed reaction has been investigated kinetically along the lines generally accepted in enzymology (Cleland, 1963, 1970). The reaction is of the sequential ordered type: i.e. a reaction in which all substrates are first bound to the enzyme in an obligatory order and the products are released, again in an obligatory order, only after the last substrate had been bound. Most studies (White and Cavallito, 1970a; Morris *et al.*, 1971; Sastry and Henderson, 1972; White and Wu, 1973a; Emson *et al.*, 1974a) indicate that the reaction proceeds according to the so-called Theorell–Chance mechanism. This is a particular case of the sequential ordered reaction, in which the concentration of the central complex (substrates-enzyme-products) approaches zero – immediately after the last substrate binds to the enzyme, the first product is released. The leading substrate, binding to the enzyme first, is acetyl–CoA; choline binds next. The first product released is ACh, followed by CoA. Fig. 2.2 gives a schematic description of the reaction using the shorthand notation by

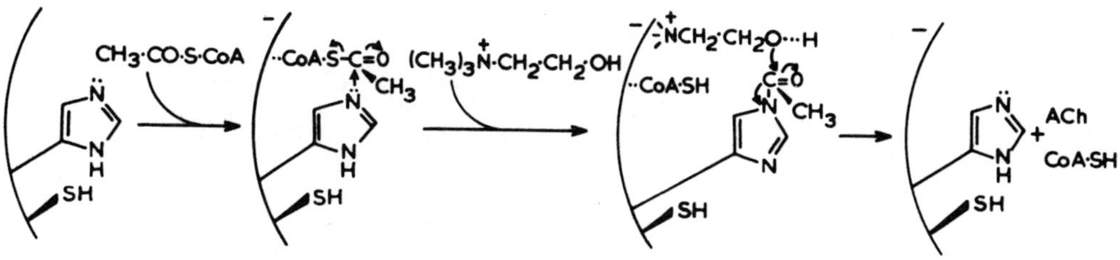

Fig. 2.3 Mechanism of the reaction catalysed by ChAc, as visualized by Malthe-Sørenssen (1976b). See text for explanation.

Cleland (1963) and is based on the assumption that the acetyl group becomes directly bound to the enzyme.

Mechanisms other than the Theorell–Chance type have been proposed for ChAc in two investigations. Glover and Potter (1971), working with bovine striatal ChAc, concluded that the reaction is of an ordinary sequential ordered type, while Schuberth (1966), working with placental ChAc, proposed that the enzyme catalyses a ping pong type reaction. In such reactions the binding of the first substrate is followed by the release of the first product, and only then by the binding of the second substrate and the release of the second product. The ping pong type mechanism is incompatible with the results of isotope exchange experiments (Morris and Grewaal, 1971) and, moreover, Schuberth's (1966) experimental data can also be explained by the Theorell–Chance mechanism (see Sastry and Henderson, 1972). A schematic drawing of the events probably occurring in the active centre of ChAc is given in Fig. 2.3 taken from Malthe-Sørenssen (1976b). The scheme shows the binding of acetyl–CoA to the active centre, the nucleophilic attack of imidazole on acetyl–CoA, the formation of acetylated imidazole, the binding of choline to an anionic site, the transfer of the acetyl group to choline and the release of both products.

The specificity of ChAc towards substrates is comparatively wide. The enzyme can transfer the acyl groups not only from acetyl–CoA, but also from several other derivatives of CoA, e.g. propionyl–CoA (Berman *et al.*, 1953; Gardiner and Whittaker, 1954; Berry and Whittaker, 1959; Potter and Glover, 1971; Rossier, 1977b) and butyryl–CoA (Rossier, 1977b). The affinity of ChAc for acetyl–CoA, propionyl–CoA and butyryl–CoA is about the same, but the rate of acyl transfer decreases considerably with increasing acyl chain length (Rossier, 1977b). ChAc also effects the transfer of acetyl groups from acetylethenoCoA (Rossier, 1977b), acetyl-dephospho-CoA (Banns *et al.*, 1977) and acetylpantetheine (Berman-Reisberg, 1957; Banns *et al.*, 1977). The K_m for acetyl-dephosphoCoA is about twice, and that for acetyl-pantetheine fifteen times, that for acetyl–CoA (Banns *et al.*, 1977).

In addition to choline, many molecules of similar structure may serve as acceptors of ChAc-transferred acyl groups. The analogue of choline in which one methyl group has been replaced by an ethyl group (monoethylcholine) is acetylated very efficiently; the acetylation of diethylcholine is much slower and that of triethylcholine is

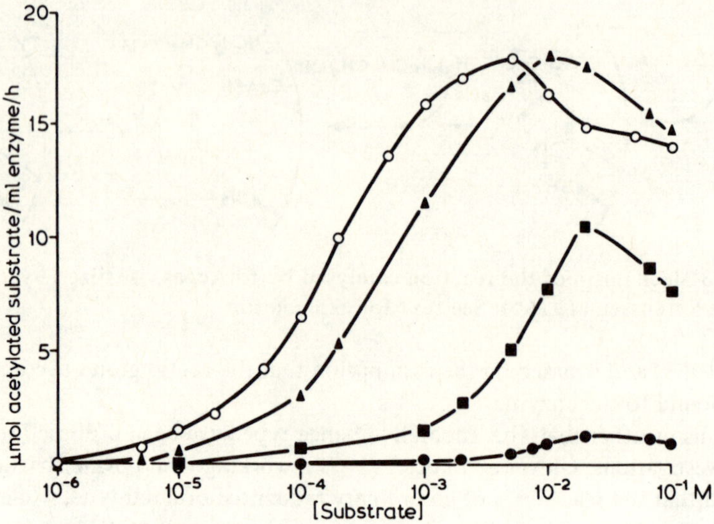

Fig. 2.4 Acetylation of choline analogues by ChAc from bovine caudate nuclei. Abscissa: molar concentration of substrate. Ordinate: initial reaction rate expressed in μmoles of acetylated substrate/ml enzyme solution/h. ○, choline; ▲, 'monoethylcholine' (choline analogue in which one methyl group has been replaced by an ethyl group); ■, 'diethylcholine'; ●, 'triethylcholine' (after Hemsworth and Smith, 1970).

extremely slow (Hemsworth and Morris, 1964; Hemsworth and Smith, 1970; Baker and Dowdall, 1976; see Fig. 2.4). The action of ChAc is very seriously affected if the hydroxyethyl group of choline is modified by elongation or side chain substitution; e.g., soluble ChAc does not acetylate homocholine, an analogue in which the hydroxyethyl group of choline has been replaced by a hydroxypropyl group (Burgen *et al.*, 1956; Dauterman and Mehrotra, 1963; Currier and Mautner, 1974; Collier *et al.*, 1977). Slow rates of acetylation have been described for *N*-methyl and *N*-ethyl derivatives of aminoethanol (Potter and Glover, 1971), pyrrolcholine (Baker and Dowdall, 1976), polymethylene-bis-(hydroxyethyl)dimethyl ammonium compounds (Burgen *et al.*, 1956; Hemsworth, 1976), and for compounds in which the *n*-propyl or *n*-butyl group has been substituted for one methyl group of choline (Dauterman and Mehrotra, 1963). It may be that the specificity of ChAc for some substrates is not the same when the enzyme is in solution *in vitro* as when it is *in situ* in the nerve terminals. This interesting possibility has been raised by the experiments with homocholine, a compound which is not acetylated by solubilized ChAc, but is acetylated in unbroken synaptosomes (Collier *et al.*, 1977).

Of all substrates tested, only choline, acetyl–CoA and propionyl–CoA are likely to play a role *in vivo*; the suggestion that propionyl–CoA is possibly important is based on the observation that propionylcholine is a normal chemical constituent of the spleen (Gardiner and Whittaker, 1954).

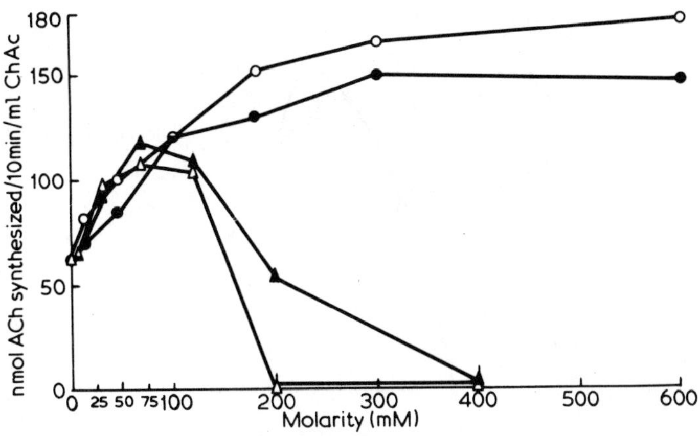

Fig. 2.5 The influence of ions on the activity of ChAc from rabbit brain. The incubation medium contained NaCl (open circles), KCl (filled circles), $MgCl_2$ (open triangles) or $CaCl_2$ (filled triangles) in the concentrations given on the abscissa. Enzymatic activity, expressed in nmoles ACh synthesized by 1 ml of the enzyme preparation during 10 min, is given on the ordinate (after Morris and Tuček, 1966).

The activity of ChAc is greatly influenced by the presence of ions in the incubation medium. It is low when the ionic strength of the medium is low and increases with increasing ionic strength (McCaman and Hunt, 1965; Morris and Tuček, 1966; Schuberth, 1966; Prince, 1967, 1971; Potter *et al.*, 1968; Prince and Hide, 1971; Prempeh *et al.*, 1972; Chao and Wolfgram, 1974; Emson *et al.*, 1974; Kuczenski *et al.*, 1975; Spantidakis *et al.*, 1976; Singh and McGeer, 1977). The activity of ChAc increases in the same way when the concentrations of NaCl, KCl, $MgCl_2$ or $CaCl_2$ in the medium increase from 0–100 mM (Morris and Tuček, 1966); an inhibition occurs at higher concentrations of $MgCl_2$ or $CaCl_2$ (Morris and Tuček, 1966; Potter *et al.*, 1968; see Fig. 2.5). Very high concentrations of Na^+ cause an inhibition of ChAc in the presence of low concentrations of choline (Mann and Hebb, 1975).

Data concerning the activating effect of different inorganic anions on ChAc are controversial. Rossier (1977a) and Spantidakis *et al.* (1976) found considerable differences between the degree of activation brought about by different anions (in the presence of Na^+), with Cl^- being the most effective. On the other hand, Potter *et al.*, (1968) observed that several anions (Br^-, I^-, acetate$^-$, HCO_3^-, SO_4^{2-}, all in the presence of K^+) activated ChAc to about the same degree as Cl^-. The reason for this discrepancy in experimental observations is not clear; it may, however, be important that a low background concentration of tris chloride was present in all samples during Potter's experiments. The mechanism of action of inorganic ions on the activity of ChAc has yet to be elucidated. Under the influence of some factors, for example, ageing of the enzyme or some purification procedures, ChAc becomes less sensitive to the activating effect of the salts. Prince and his co-workers

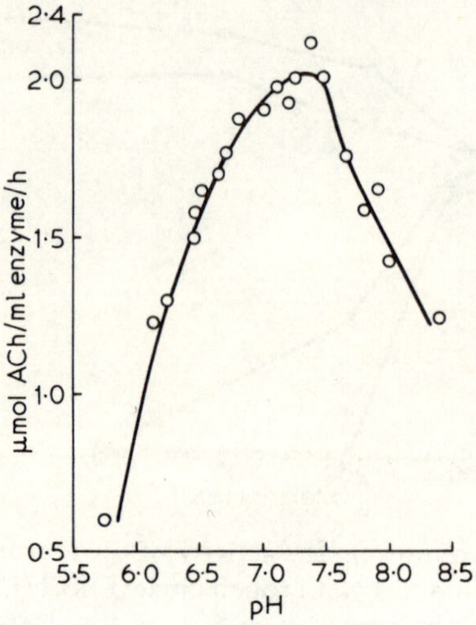

Fig. 2.6 pH dependence of ChAc from rabbit brain (after Morris and Tuček, 1966).

(Prince and Hide, 1971; Prempeh *et al.*, 1972) assume that ChAc exists in several forms which differ in their dependence on salts, and that the form which is highly active at high ionic strength may be converted to the form active at low ionic strength. The optimal pH for brain ChAc activity has been found to be 7.4 (McCaman and Hunt, 1965; Morris and Tuček, 1966; see Fig. 2.6), 7.0 (Chao and Wolfgram, 1973), 7.5–10.0 (Glover and Potter, 1971), or 7.9 (Singh and McGeer, 1977).

One of the properties of ChAc which is important in experimental work is its stability. There are contradictory reports on its *post mortem* stability in unfrozen tissues. On the one hand, McGeer and McGeer (1976) found that ChAc activity was not changed in rats kept at 4°C for 8 h after death and Hebb and Silver (1956) observed no change of ChAc activity in the pig brain kept 6 h at room temperature and an additional 42 h at 3–5°C. On the other hand, Bird and Iversen (1974) and Fahn and Côté (1976) described losses of ChAc activity due to storage at room temperature. During storage at −20°C, ChAc activity in short segments of peripheral nerves does not change for at least 1–2 days (Tuček, 1974); activity in pieces of placental tissue does not change for weeks (Morris, 1966); and in homogenates and subcellular fractions of the brain, prepared in 0.32M sucrose, ChAc activity remains stable for months (Tuček, unpublished). Problems involving the stability do occur, however, during attempts to purify the enzyme. They are particularly serious with the enzyme from cephalopod ganglia. Readers planning to work with purified ChAc will find excellent advice on how to overcome the instability of the mammalian enzyme in the paper by Rossier (1977a), and of squid enzyme in the papers by Polsky and Shuster (1976a,b). Acetyl–CoA and CoA stabilize ChAc from squid ganglia against heat inactivation and reactivate the enzyme after an inactivation. Apparently both substances help to preserve the active structure of the enzyme (Prince and Hide, 1971; Prempeh *et al.*, 1972). Choline and ACh do not have a stabilizing and reactivating action.

Data which would permit the evaluation of the stability and the lifespan of ChAc in living cells are scarce. The enzyme does not turn over rapidly. In experiments with isolated nerve segments *in vivo*, all enzyme was retained after 22 h (Tuček, 1975). On the basis of data on ChAc transport to the tongue, Fonnum *et al.* (1973) estimate the half-life of ChAc at 16–21 days. Wenthold and Mahler (1975) investigated the half-life of ChAc in the rat brain by means of a double labelling technique; they arrived at a value of 5.2 days, but there is uncertainty whether their preparation of ChAc was sufficiently pure to permit valid conclusions.

2.4 DISTRIBUTION OF CHOLINE ACETYLTRANSFERASE IN THE BODY

ChAc is present mainly in the nervous tissue. It is difficult to be absolutely certain whether it is localized exclusively in cholinergic neurons, or whether it is also present in nerve cells using transmitters other than ACh. Most workers in the field of synaptic biochemistry would probably support the view that the presence of ChAc is specific for cholinergic neurons. Such an assumption corresponds to Dale's (1935) view that each neuron produces, and uses at all its presynaptic endings, a single transmitter. Nachmansohn's (1959) hypothesis that the synthesis and hydrolysis of ACh are involved in the mechanism of nerve impulse conduction in the nerve cells and their processes (i.e. extrasynaptically) requires that ACh be synthesized in all neurons. The hypothesis is based on indirect evidence and has not been accepted by most physiologists (Dale, 1953; Hebb, 1963), although a detailed critical evaluation of all Nachmansohn's arguments has never apparently been published. Direct experimental examination of the question whether the presence of ChAc is specific for cholinergic neurons encounters many obstacles:

(1) it is frequently more difficult to prove the complete absence of a substance from some cells than to prove its presence;
(2) it is very hard to obtain isolated nerve cells which are quite pure, i.e. not contaminated by neuropil or synaptic boutons of other neurons;
(3) the transmitter released from presynaptic endings is known with certainty in the case of only a few neurons;
(4) the presence of several putative transmitters together in one cell does not prove that the cell uses all of them for synaptic transmission.

In spite of these difficulties, recent studies on isolated neurons and cell cultures have provided much important evidence. Studies of ACh synthesis in neurons isolated directly from the body have been performed on cells from invertebrate animals, where the isolation and identification of neurons is easier than in vertebrates. Extremely large differences among the abilities of various neurons to synthesize ACh have been revealed in most studies. In the abdominal ganglion of *Aplysia californica* some neurons synthesize more than 500 pmol/h, whereas no synthesis is measurable in others (i.e the synthesis is less than 2 pmol/h; McCaman and Dewhurst, 1970). According to Giller and Schwartz (1971), only 3 out of 30 identified neurons in this ganglion are able to synthesize ACh. In the lobster nervous system, the distribution of ChAc parallels that of sensory neural elements (Hildebrand *et al.*, 1974). Neurons which very actively synthesize ACh show very little synthesis of serotonin and vice versa. This is apparent from observations on the neurons of *Aplysia* (Eisenstadt *et al.*, 1973; Weinreich *et al.*, 1973), leech (Coggeshall *et al.*, 1972) and snail (Emson and Fonnum, 1974). Snail neurons have, however, been found which contain both ChAc and aromatic acid decarboxylase, i.e. the enzyme responsible for the production of serotonin (Hanley *et al.*, 1974), and both ACh and serotonin (Brownstein *et al.*, 1974; Cottrell, 1976). It has yet to be clarified whether such neurons not only contain both substances, but also release and use both as their transmitters.

Big differences in the ability of various neural cells to synthesize different transmitters are also evident from experiments with cloned cell cultures from mammalian brain tumors. Working with murine neuroblastoma, Amano *et al.* (1972) isolated cell clones which had a high activity of either tyrosine hydroxylase (participating in the synthesis of catecholamines), or ChAc, or cell clones in which the activities of both ChAc and tyrosine hydroxylase were low; no clone had a high activity of both enzymes simultaneously. Prasad *et al.* (1973) revealed similar differences between the clones from murine neuroblastoma, but they also isolated a clone with cells containing both ChAc and tyrosine hydroxylase. Cloned and recloned neurons from brain tumors of rats differed very much in their ability to synthesize ACh, γ-aminobutyric acid and dopamine, but some neurons apparently were enzymatically equipped for the synthesis of two or three putative transmitters (Schubert *et al.*, 1974; Kimes *et al.*, 1974). These cells made no synaptic contacts. It has been suggested that neurons become specialized for the synthesis of a single transmitter only after the establishment of functional interactions with other neurons (Schubert *et al.*, 1974; Kimes *et al.*, 1974). The importance of interactions with other types of cells for the expression of a neuron's genetic ability to produce ChAc or other transmitter-synthesizing enzymes has been clearly shown in studies of the development of cholinergic properties in sympathetic neurons *in vitro* (Patterson and Chun, 1974; Nurse and O'Lague, 1975; Patterson *et al.*, 1976; Ko *et al.*, 1976; Johnson *et al.*, 1976; Furshpan *et al.*, 1976). Simultaneous presence of ChAc and tyrosine hydroxylase has been discovered in some subclones of a noradrenergic pheochromocytoma cell line (Greene and Rein, 1977).

In the light of experiments on freshly isolated neurons and on neurons cultivated *in vitro*, it is virtually certain that only some specific neurons are equipped with ChAc and can synthesize ACh. Most experimental data are in agreement with the principle 'one neuron – one transmitter', but some observations suggest that this principle may not be universally valid; in view of our inadequate knowledge of which substances are

Table 2.2 ChAc activity in different regions of the nervous system of the dog (Hebb and Silver, 1956)

Region	Activity (μg ACh synthesized/g acetone-dried tissue)/h
Cortical area 17	1325
Cortical area 4	3000
Cortical area 51	3750
Ammon's horn	2600
Olfactory bulb	1150
Olfactory tract	3750
Retina	570
Optic nerve	0
Superior colliculus	2 200–2 400
Inferior colliculus	1400
Thalamus	3100
Hypothalamus	2000
Caudate nucleus	13 000–13 500
Cerebellar cortex	88
Cerebellar peduncles	325
Ventral spinal roots	11 050
Dorsal spinal roots	0–25

transmitters and in which neurons, it would seem premature to draw definite conclusions on this point (Burnstock, 1976; McCaman and McCaman, 1976).

Measurements of ChAc activity in different parts of the mammalian nervous system reveal big regional differences. The reader may get an idea about the distribution of ChAc in the nervous system from data in Tables 2.2 and 2.3. Of the regions of canine brain included in Table 2.2, the caudate nucleus and the ventral spinal roots show the highest ChAc activity. No activity has been found in the optic nerve; the activity in dorsal spinal roots is either zero or extremely low. In the brain of rhesus monkey (Table 2.3), the highest activity has been discovered in the putamen; the lowest values have been found in the cerebellar cortex and corpus callosum. The regional distribution of ChAc has been described in the human brain by Hebb and Silver (1956), Bull *et al.* (1970) and McGeer and McGeer (1973, 1976) and, in simian brain, by Fahn and Côté (1968) and Yamamura *et al.* (1974).

Data on the activity of ChAc in different parts of rat brain can be found, for example, in Cheney *et al.* (1975a, 1976b). Extensive studies on the distribution of ChAc in the nuclei and tracts of individual regions of the brain have been made: in the limbic system, by Palkovits *et al.* (1974); in the brain stem, by Kobayashi *et al.* (1975); in the diencephalic nuclei, by Brownstein *et al.* (1975); in the amygdaloid complex, by Ben-Ari *et al.*, 1977; and in the hippocampal region, by Fonnum (1970a). The highest activity of ChAc in rat brain has been found in the interpeduncular nuclei (Cheney *et al.*, 1975a). The extent of regional differences in the activity of

Table 2.3 Regional distribution of ChAc in the brain of rhesus monkey (*Macaca mulatta*) (Yamamura *et al.*, 1974)

Region	Activity (nmol ACh synthesized/mg protein/h
Cerebral hemispheres	
Frontal pole	4.4
Occipital pole	3.3
Precentral gyrus	6.5
Postcentral gyrus	7.9
Cingulate gyrus	6.3
Pyriform cortex	18.6
White matter areas	
Corpus callosum	1.4
Corona radiata	3.5
Optic chiasma	3.6
Cerebral peduncles	3.2
Limbic cortex	
Amygdala	26.2
Hippocampus	13.2
Hypothalamus	13.9
Thalamus	
Anterior	14.6
Medial	23.9
Lateral	12.7
Extra-pyramidal areas	
Caudate nucleus (head)	72.8
Caudate nucleus (body)	90.0
Putamen	111.0
Globus pallidus	9.3
Midbrain	
Superior colliculi	35.2
Inferior colliculi	10.5
Raphe area	36.0
Cerebellum–lower brain stem	
Pons	9.2
Cerebellar cortex	0.8
Floor of fourth ventricle	21.4
Medulla oblongata	10.2
Inferior olivary nucleus	2.4
Pontine tegmentum	12.6
Spinal cord	
Cervical cord	8.1

ChAc in different parts of rat brain is well seen from Fig. 5.4. The activity of ChAc in different regions of the nervous system is probably a measure of the density of cholinergic neurons, axons or presynaptic terminals in these regions; data on the distribution of ChAc indicate that cholinergic cells are spread very unevenly through the central nervous system.

Under physiological conditions ChAc is probably present only in the neurons, not in the glia. This is indicated by the absence of ChAc from the optic nerve, which does contain glial cells. In a culture of cells from embryonic chick brain ChAc was found only in the neurons; it was absent from the non-neuronal population of flat cells (Peterson *et al.*, 1973). After the interruption of the peroneal nerve in rabbit, the activity of ChAc in the degenerating peripheral nerve stump decreased to below 1% of control values (Tuček, 1974). This suggests that ChAc is not present or is only very slightly active in rabbit Schwann cells. It will be shown in Chapter 7.6, however, that Schwann cells of frog nerves start to produce ACh during Wallerian degeneration. Hebb and Silver (1970) observed the synthesis of ACh in a human tumor formed by glial cells and Schubert *et al.* (1974) described the presence of ChAc in cultures of glial cells from rat brain tumors.

Very high ChAc activity has been discovered in the retina. For example, Hebb and Silver (1956) showed that the enzyme in sheep retina produced 15–17.5 mg ACh/g acetone-dried powder/h, which exceeded the value of 9.7 found in sheep caudate nuclei. The activity of ChAc in chick retina has been 22–32 mg/g acetone dried powder/h, but in canine and feline retina less than 1. The way in which ACh synthesis in the retina responds to stimulation by light suggests that it occurs either in amacrine or bipolar cells (Masland and Livingstone, 1976). The distribution of ChAc in various layers of the retina, with the highest activity in the inner plexiform layer and in the inner third of the inner nuclear layer, is consistent with this suggestion. Large interspecies differences in the activity of ChAc, paralleling interspecies differences in the density of the amacrine cells, indicate that ChAc is present in one type of amacrine cell (Ross and McDougal, 1976). It is certain that ChAc is not contained in the ganglionic cells, the axons of which form the optic nerve, but a low level of ACh synthesis has been discovered in the cones and rods of turtle retina (Lam, 1972).

Although ChAc is present in many organs, it is usually confined to the nerve fibres innervating them. The activity in several organs of rats and guinea pigs is shown in Fig. 2.7. The enzyme is not invariably connected with the nervous system, however. An extreme example of non-neural ChAc is the enzyme in bacteria (see for example Stephenson and Rowatt, 1947; White and Cavallito, 1970b) and in plants (Barlow and Dixon, 1973). In vertebrates, there is no doubt about the extra-neural localization of ChAc in human placenta, a tissue receiving no innervation (Comline, 1946; Kato, 1960; Hebb and Ratković, 1962; Schuberth, 1966; Morris, and Grewaal, 1971; Morris *et al.*, 1971; Sastry and Henderson, 1972). The concentration of ChAc in human placenta reaches the highest values between 18–24 weeks of pregnancy; the total amount increases until 34 weeks, and then decreases. At its

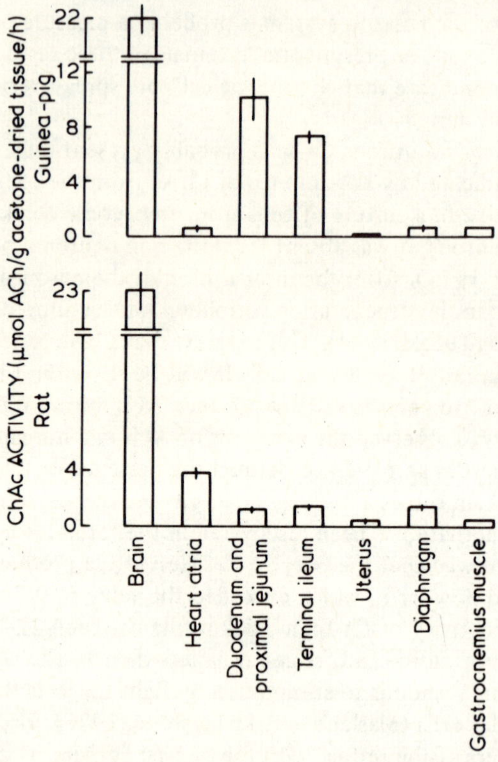

Fig. 2.7 Comparison of ChAc activity in different organs of rats and guinea pigs (after Tuček and Koudelková, 1966).

maximum, the ChAc activity/g placental tissue is about 4 times that in the caudate nuclei, one of the regions with the highest capacity for ACh synthesis in the nervous system. ChAc has also been found in the placenta of the monkeys *Maccacus rhesus* (Hebb and Ratković, 1962) and *Maccaca mulatta* (Welsch, 1977), but not in the placentae of several other mammals (Hebb and Ratković, 1962). Placental ACh is probably localized in the syncytiotrophoblast (Sastry *et al.*, 1976). Its function is not clear.

Data indicating the presence of low levels of extraneural ChAc in other tissues have to be treated with caution in view of the finding that another enzyme, carnitine acetyltransferase, is able to use choline as a poor alternative substrate and to acetylate it to ACh (White and Wu, 1973c). The affinity of carnitine acetyltransferase towards choline is so low that it would not be expected to produce any ACh under *in vivo* conditions. The presence of ACh in a tissue *in vivo* thus suggests that any synthesis of ACh measured in its homogenate *in vitro* is based on the presence of ChAc, rather than carnitine acetyltransferase. ChAc activity, together with ACh, has been found in human and bovine spermatozoa (Bishop *et al.*, 1976). It has been proposed that ChAc in the corneal epithelium is also located extraneurally (Gnädiger *et al.*, 1973), but it is difficult to reconcile this view with the loss of ACh which occurs in the cornea after denervation (Fitzgerald and Cooper, 1971). Data indicating the presence ChAc in the blood platelets (Chuang *et al.*, 1976) require additional evidence that the synthesis of ACh observed during the incubation of the platelets is not based on the activity of carnitine acetyltransferase.

Some extraneural ChAc may be present in skeletal muscles and in the heart (see Vlk and Tuček, 1961; Tuček and Vlk, 1962; Tuček, 1973a). For skeletal muscles this assumption is based on the observations of high residual ChAc activity in denervated muscles (Tuček, 1973a; Tuček *et al.*, in preparation). Although some of the residual ACh synthesizing capacity of denervated muscles may be due to the high carnitine acetyltransferase activity of the muscles, the recent finding that ACh is also present in denervated muscles, including their aneural parts (Miledi *et al.*, 1977), supports the view that ChAc does, indeed, remain in the muscles after denervation.

2.5 MEASUREMENT OF CHOLINE ACETYLTRANSFERASE ACTIVITY

Biochemical methods used for measurement of ChAc activity have been reviewed by Schuberth and Sörbo (1971), Prince (1971) and Fonnum (1976). In this Chapter, the stages of biochemical assay and the problems involved will be discussed in the following order:

(1) how to prepare the tissue;
(2) how to perform the incubation;
(3) how to measure the synthesis of products or the disappearance of substrates. The method used in the author's laboratory will be described in detail. Histochemical methods for the detection of ChAc have been described but these will be mentioned only briefly as they are still relatively undeveloped.

2.5.1 Preparation of the tissue

The activity of ChAc is generally measured in tissue homogenates and their subcellular fractions. In order to measure total ChAc activity in the tissue, it is necessary to remove the barriers preventing the solubilization and the access of reaction substrates to the enzyme. If the tissue is homogenized in isotonic saline or sucrose, the amount of ACh synthesized during incubation is less than would correspond to the total content of ChAc in the homogenate. Synthesis is increased if the homogenate is treated with ether or if a suitable detergent is included in the medium used for homogenization. Synthesis is also increased, but to a lesser degree than with a detergent, when a strongly hypotonic homogenization medium is used instead of the isotonic medium. The 'activation' of ChAc in the homogenates by

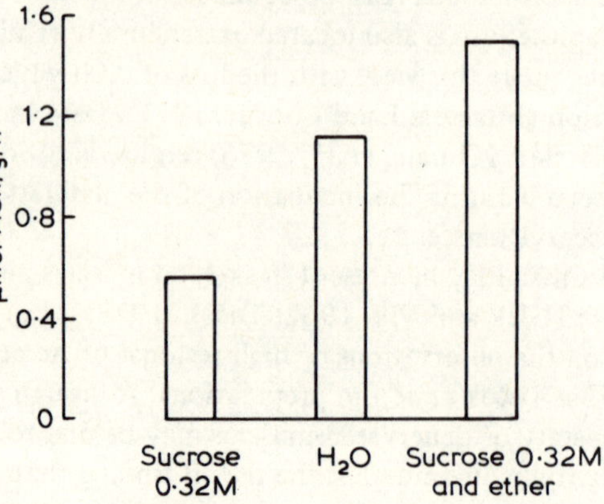

Fig. 2.8 ChAc activity in the crude mitochondrial fraction (P_2) from dog brain which has been prepared in three different ways: (1) P_2 pellet suspended in 0.32 M sucrose; (2) P_2 pellet suspended in water and thus exposed to strongly hypo-osmotic conditions; (3) P_2 pellet suspended in 0.32 M sucrose and then treated with ether. The activity is expressed in μmoles ACh per g fresh tissue (from which the P_2 fraction had been prepared) per h (based on data by Tuček, 1967d).

detergents, organic solvents, or hypotnic medium results from the disintegration of the membranes enclosing ChAc. Fig. 2.8 compares the activity of ChAc in crude mitochondrial fractions from canine brain, either suspended in isotonic sucrose or in pure water, or suspended in isotonic sucrose and treated with ether (Tuček, 1967d). The easiest way to remove permeability barriers is to add a detergent directly to the homogenization medium. This was not possible before the introduction of radioisotopic methods for measuring ChAc activity, because detergents interfered with the measurement, by bioassay, of ACh produced during incubation. When bioassay was routinely used the activity of ChAc was frequently measured in extracts from acetone dried tissues, but this method was slow and was difficult to apply to small tissue samples.

The choice of the homogenization medium may be rather arbitrary, but it should take account of the procedures to be used for the isolation of the products or substrates of the reaction and for the measurement of their concentration after the end of the incubation. Thus if bioassay is to be used, the homogenization and incubation media should not contain substances which might interfere with it; when ACh is to be extracted with sodium tetraphenylboron, potassium ions in the media should be kept to a minimum. Another point to consider is that a large proportion of ChAc will be adsorbed to tissue particles if the ionic strength of the medium is low. Pipetting errors, resulting from the unequal distribution of tissue particles in the suspension, will be reduced if the enzyme is better solubilized, as will be the case in a medium of higher ionic strength. In Fonnum's (1968) study, ChAc was released from its association with tissue particles into the bathing medium (pH 7.2) by NaCl solutions, the release increasing with NaCl concentration up to a plateau at 150 mM.

2.5.2 Incubation of choline acetyltransferase

The rules for the incubation of ChAc are similar as for other enzymes. The incubation medium must contain the substrates (i.e. acetyl–CoA and choline), a buffer and an inhibitor of ChE. Earlier studies on ChAc did not usually employ acetyl–CoA as such. Instead, the incubation medium contained CoA, a source of acetyl groups (e.g. acetate) and a surplus of enzyme (e.g. acetyl–CoA synthetase), which produced a surplus of acetyl–CoA in the course of the incubation. The use of chemically produced acetyl-CoA saves time and gives more reproducible results. In view of the known K_m of ChAc for its substrates (Section 2.3), the concentration of choline in the incubation medium should be about 10 mM and the concentration of acetyl–CoA about 0.2 mM. Some workers have suggested, however, that the concentration of acetyl–CoA should be higher; for example, a figure of 0.5 mM was proposed by Bull and Oderfeld-Nowak (1971) and by Hebb *et al.* (1975). Eserine or neostigmine are usually used as ChE inhibitors; their presence in the incubation medium is not necessary for the work with purified preparations of ChAc, uncontaminated with ChE, or in experiments using methods which are not dependent on the measurement of the amount of ACh formed during the incubation.

Earlier studies stressed the need for the presence in the incubation medium of a substance with free sulphydryl groups (e.g. cysteine). Apparently, these reagents were necessary to protect the sulphydryl groups of the coupled acetyl–CoA producing enzyme (particularly acetyl–CoA synthetase). It has been found, however, that some substances with sulphydryl groups diminish the synthesis of ACh by causing the thiolysis of acetyl–CoA (Morris, 1967). The recommendations that the incubation medium should contain NaCN (Morris, 1967) or creatine (Chao and Wolfgram, 1974) have not been generally accepted. Since ChAc is very unstable when it is in a solution in which the total protein concentration is below 1 mg/ml, it is advantageous to protect it by adding plasma albumin to the incubation medium. It is usually convenient to perform the incubation at pH 7.2–7.4.

2.5.3 Quantitative evaluation of enzyme activity

Since the reaction equilibrium of the ChAc catalysed reaction favours the synthesis of ACh, the activity of the enzyme is usually measured with the reaction proceeding in the direction of ACh formation. Quantitative evaluation of its rate can be based on the rate of disappearance of acetyl–CoA or choline or on the rate of production of ACh or CoA. Measurements of enzyme activity based on the rate of disappearance of the substrate are usually less convenient than those based on the rate of formation of the product, because the need to saturate the enzyme with the substrates requires that the change of concentration of the substrates during the incubation will be comparatively small. In view of the high K_m of ChAc for choline, the incubation is made in the presence of a high concentration of choline; hence the relative change in concentration is very small and its measurement would be extremely difficult. Acetyl–CoA is used at a much lower concentration and the change during incubation is therefore comparatively higher. This can be measured in various ways; the method of following changes of acetyl–CoA concentration spectrophotometrically from the changes in extinction at 230 nm (Berry and Whittaker, 1959) may prove particularly interesting for kinetic studies. One has to take into account, however, that the disappearance of acetyl–CoA may also be caused by its spontaneous hydrolysis, by hydrolysis caused through acetyl–CoA hydrolase, or by the utilization of acetyl–CoA in chemical reactions other than the synthesis of ACh.

The increase in the concentration of CoA can be detected by changes of the content of free sulfhydryl groups, which can be easily measured spectrophotometrically using the reaction with nitroprusside (Berman *et al.*, 1953; Berman-Reisberg, 1957), 5, 5′-dithio-bis(2-dinitrobenzoate) (Schuberth, 1966; Prince, 1967; Potter *et al.*, 1968) or 4, 4′-dithiopyridine (Chao and Wolfgram, 1972). With this approach the course of the reaction cannot be followed continuously, as the substances that react with thiol groups can be added only after the incubation has ended. The use of methods based on the measurement of thiol groups of CoA is limited by the fact that the thiol groups of tissue proteins give non-specific reactions and that CoA may also be formed from acetyl–CoA independently of the action of ChAc, as pointed out in the previous paragraph.

The most frequently used methods of assaying ChAc activity are based on the measurement of the increase of ACh content in the incubation medium during the incubation. Theoretically, one can measure the content of ACh with a number of methods, as described, for example, in Whittaker's (1963) and Hanin's (1974) reviews. Two methods have found the greatest practical application: bioassays and radiochemical assays. For information on bioassays of ACh, the reader is referred to the reviews by MacIntosh and Perry (1950) and Hebb and Silver (1970). Radiochemical assays of ChAc activity are more convenient and accurate. Within the last decade, they have almost completely replaced the use of bioassays.

When the activity of ChAc is measured radiometrically, the enzyme is incubated in the presence of a labelled ACh precursor with known specific radioactivity. At the end of the incubation, labelled ACh is isolated and its radioactivity measured. The amount of ACh formed is calculated from its total radioactivity and from the known specific radioactivity of the precursor. [^{14}C]acetyl–CoA or [^{3}H]acetyl–CoA are used as labelled precursors. They are more convenient than labelled choline, because it is easier to separate labelled ACh from labelled acetyl–CoA than from labelled choline in view of the large difference in chemical properties and electric charge between ACh and acetyl–CoA. Since Schuberth (1963) first proposed the radiometric measurement of ChAc activity, a number of methods have been described; they differ from each other mainly in the procedure used for the isolation of labelled ACh. The following methods have been used most frequently:

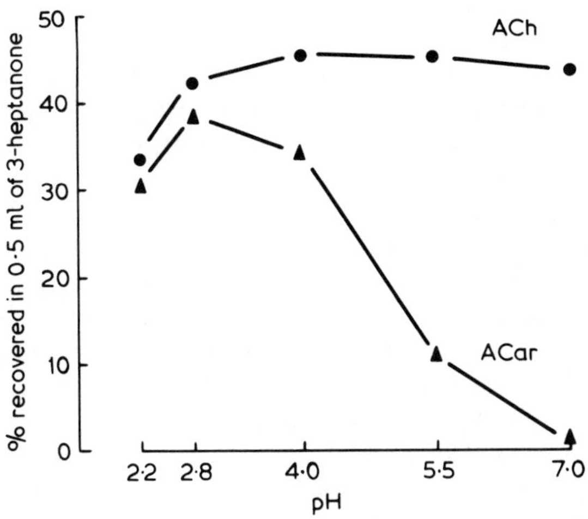

Fig. 2.9 Extraction of ACh and acetylcarnitine by sodium tetraphenylboron at different pH. 10 µl of a solution of [^{14}C] ACh or [^{14}C] acetylcarnitine were pipetted into a set of tubes. 7 ml of 10 mM buffers (HCl–NaCl for pH 2.2; citrate–phosphate for other pH values) were added, followed by 1 ml of a solution of sodium tetraphenylboron dissolved in 3-heptanone (15 mg/ml). After shaking and centrifugation, the radioactivity present in 0.5 ml of the organic layer was measured. Values on the ordinate indicate what percentage of total radioactivity originally present in the tubes was recovered in the 0.5 ml of the organic phase (out of the 1.0 ml added) transferred to the scintillation vials (after Tuček *et al.*, 1978a).

(a) Extraction of ACh with sodium tetraphenylboron. ACh and tetraphenylboron form a complex which may be extracted from the incubation medium by 3-heptanone or other organic solvents (Fonnum, 1969a,b; review Fonnum, 1976). The use of this method for measurements of ChAc activity in single neurons and with total incubation volumes as low as 1 µl has been described by, for example, Marder (1976) and Godfrey and Matschinsky (1975). A description of its application in the author's laboratory is given in Section 2.5.4. A very simplified procedure has been suggested by Fonnum (1975). One of the advantages of tetraphenylboron extraction is that, at neutral pH, acetylcarnitine is not extracted together with ACh (Fonnum, 1975; Tuček *et al.*, 1978a; Fig. 2.9).

(b) Separation of labelled ACh from labelled acetyl–CoA on ion exchange resins. The method proposed by Schrier and Shuster (1967) has been particularly widely used. In this method, acetyl–CoA is retained on a microcolumn by an anion exchanger, while ACh passes through the column directly into scintillation vials. Important improvements of the method are described by Hebb *et al.* (1975). The method is based on the assumption that all radioactivity not retained by the anion exchanger is associated with ACh. This assumption is reasonably correct in experiments with most preparations of the nervous tissue and with purified ChAc. It may lead to errors in experiments with other tissues, e.g. those containing comparatively high levels of carnitine acetyltransferase and endogenous carnitine. During incubation of a muscle homogenate, the formation of [^{14}C] ACh from [^{14}C] acetyl–CoA may be accompanied by the formation of a comparatively large amount of [^{14}C] acetylcarnitine, which is not retained by the anion exchanger and, on the principle of the method, is counted as ACh (White and Wu, 1973c). This is probably the reason for the unexpectedly high activity of ChAc described by Mahoney *et al.* (1971) in the liver. Sucrose can be acetylated by acetyl–CoA non-enzymatically and is also not retained by the anion exchanger (Hebb *et al.*, 1975). Diamond and Kennedy (1968) proposed the use of a cation exchanger instead of an anion exchanger; in their method, ACh is retained by the cation exchanger and is then eluted with acid into the scintillation vials.

(c) The separation of labelled ACh by paper electrophoresis (Potter and Murphy, 1967; Potter *et al.*, 1968; Potter, 1971; Giller and Schwartz, 1971) and thin layer chromatography (Grubić *et al.*, 1976).

Other methods are based on the extraction of labelled ACh by a solution of K_2HgI_4 in octanol (Glover and Green, 1972), precipitation of labelled ACh by reineckate (McCaman and Hunt, 1965; Buckley *et al.*, 1967a) or precipitation of labelled ACh by iodine (Goldberg *et al.*, 1969).

2.5.4 Carnitine acetyltransferase interference with assays of choline acetyltransferase activity

Carnitine acetyltransferase may interfere with ChAc activity assays in two ways (White and Wu, 1973c):

(1) by the production of labelled acetylcarnitine from endogenous carnitine and labelled acetyl–CoA used in the ChAc incubation; this interference can be easily overcome by the choice of extraction procedures which differentiate between labelled ACh and labelled acetylcarnitine (see Section 2.5.3);
(2) by the production of ACh. Choline can serve as a poor substrate for carnitine acetyltransferase and can be acetylated by it. Pigeon muscle carnitine acetyltransferase acetylates choline 25 000 times less actively than carnitine (Roskoski *et al.*, 1974). The production of ACh by carnitine acetyltransferase is therefore unlikely to interfere with ChAc activity assays except in experiments with tissues having an extremely high activity of carnitine acetyltransferase and an extremely low activity of ChAc. The degree of interference can be lessened by using low concentrations of choline. Naphthylvinylpyridine (NVP) or bromoacetylcholine might be used to determine whether the synthesis of ACh during incubation is due to the activity of ChAc or carnitine acetyltransferase, since they inhibit the former and not the latter enzyme (White and Cavallito, 1970; Roskoski *et al.*, 1974). Unfortunately, neither substance is a strong inhibitor and it is not known if their inhibitory action is the same on ChAc from different sources (Tuček *et al.*, in preparation).

2.5.5 Choline acetyltransferase activity measurements in the author's laboratory

The radiometric method used by the author is based on that proposed by Fonnum (1969b). Working instructions are given here, but these can, of course, be modified in many respects as the need arises.

(a) Homogenize the sample of tissue in an all glass homogenizer in a medium of the following composition: NaCl 200 mM, Na phosphate buffer pH 7.4, 40 mM, $MgCl_2$ 10 mM, Triton X-100 0.5%. $MgCl_2$ is not necessary for measurements of ChAc activity, but is useful when the activity of AChE is measured in the same homogenates.

(b) Transfer 35 μl aliquots of the homogenate into duplicate incubation tubes located in an ice water bath. Add 15 μl of a stock solution of the incubation medium, which is prepared by mixing 2 parts NaCl 4M, 1 part choline chloride 0.625M, 1 part eserine salicylate 10 mM, 5 parts [1-^{14}C] acetyl–CoA 2.5 mM (specific radioactivity 1.5–3 Ci/mol), 2 parts human serum albumin solution (12.5 mg/ml) and 4 parts water; the stock solution is made up in bulk in advance and is kept frozen at –20° C. After mixing with the homogenate, the final concentrations during the incubation will be: [1-^{14}C] acetyl–CoA 0.25 mM, choline chloride 12.5 mM, eserine salicylate 0.2 mM, NaCl 300 mM, Na phosphate pH 7.4, 28 mM, $MgCl_2$ 7 mM, serum albumin 0.5 mg/ml, and Triton X-100 0.35%.

(c) Start the incubation by transferring the tubes from the ice water bath to the incubator. The temperature during incubation is 38° C for mammalian and 30° C for frog enzyme. The duration of incubation must not exceed the period over which the yield of ACh increases linearly with time. Stop the incubation by transferring the tubes to the ice water bath and by adding 2 ml of an ice cold solution of Na phosphate pH 7.4, 10 mM and ACh chloride 0.2 mM.

(d) Add 1 ml of a solution of sodium tetraphenylboron in 3-heptanone (15 mg/ml) to each tube. Shake 4 min. Centrifuge to separate the organic and aqueous phases.

(e) Transfer 300 μl of the organic phase to the scintillation vials. Add 10 ml of a toluene scintillation solution (Tuček, 1973c) containing PPO 0.4% (w/v), POPOP 0.01% (w/v), Triton X-100 4% (v/v), and naphthalene 5% (w/v). Measure the radioactivity in a liquid scintillation spectrometer.

2.5.6 Histochemical determination of choline acetyltransferase

So far, two methods have been proposed for detecting the localization of ChAc in histological preparation. The first method depends on the histochemical localization of the thiol groups of the CoA formed from acetyl–CoA during ACh synthesis. The second method is based on immunofluorescence. Neither method has been widely used, because both encounter serious technical problems.

The histochemical demonstration of ChAc based on the precipitation of CoA by lead was first attempted by Burt (1969, 1971) and soon after by Kása, Mann and

Hebb (1970; Kása, 1971, 1975). With their method, tissue sections are incubated in the presence of acetyl–CoA, choline and $Pb(NO_3)_2$. The thiol groups of CoA, formed during the synthesis of ACh, react with lead to form a mercaptide of CoA and lead. The sections are then treated with ammonium or sodium sulphide; lead sulphide, which is formed from the mercaptide of CoA and Pb, is deposited at the site of enzyme activity. The precipitate of lead sulphide can be observed under the optical or electron microscope.

The method has many problems, which have been discussed by Burt and Silver (1973b). One of the difficulties arises from the fact that ChAc is not firmly connected with subcellular structures and is eluted from tissue sections into the incubation medium. In order to reduce the mobility of ChAc, fixed tissue is used and the incubation of the sections is performed in a medium of low ionic strength and low pH. Under these conditions, the enzyme is more firmly bound to subcellular structures, but its activity is low. The activity of ChAc is also decreased by the presence of lead ions. A big problem encountered during the development of this method was the production of CoA by enzymes other than ChAc. This problem has been lessened by the finding that the non-specific release of CoA thiol groups is greatly reduced by the addition of 1 mM diisopropylphosphorofluoridate to the incubation medium. In spite of this, the problem of the specificity of the method has not been solved. The specificity of the histochemical reaction cannot be checked with the use of ChAc inhibitors, since the inhibitors of ChAc known so far are not sufficiently specific and sufficiently effective in the histochemical medium. The incubation performed in the absence of added choline gives a reduced, but still positive histochemical reaction. This may be explained by the presence of endogenous sources of choline in the tissues (see Chapter 5). Some improvement of the method may be achieved by the use of the semipermeable membrane technique (Hüther and Luppa, 1976). On the whole, it seems that the histochemical method based on the localization of thiol groups of CoA is not yet able to demonstrate the presence of ChAc completely reliably, as the conditions under which the tissue is incubated and treated may lead to many artifacts.

The basic condition for the development of immunohistochemical methods of ChAc detection is the isolation of highly purified enzyme and the production of monospecific antisera against it. The first positive results with the immunofluorescence technique for the study of ChAc have been described by McGeer *et al.* (1974) and Eng *et al.* (1974). Their observations on the distribution of ChAc in microscopic preparations agree with what is known about the distribution of ChAc from studies using other methods, but the method showed only very low ChAc activity in the nerve endings (Hattori *et al.*, 1976). Although it is probable that the fluorescence observed with this method is specific for ChAc, the specificity has not been proven beyond doubt. Rossier (1975) points out that the immunohistochemical studies of ChAc performed up to 1975 were based on the use of antisera which were unlikely to be monospecific against ChAc in view of the low purity of ChAc used for immunization. This could mean that the immunofluorescence findings demonstrate the localization of proteins other than ChAc, which may possibly be present in the same neurons as ChAc.

2.6 SUMMARY

ChAc is a globular protein with a molecular weight of about 68 000 daltons. It has not been isolated in pure form. In some animal species it is present in several molecular forms which can be best separated by means of isoelectric focusing; the physico–chemical basis of the differences between various molecular forms has not been clarified.

ChAc catalyses the reaction:

$$\text{choline} + \text{acetyl–CoA} = \text{ACh} + \text{CoA}.$$

Among the various values given in the literature for the equilibrium constant of this reaction, the value of 41 appears most likely. The reaction catalysed by ChAc follows the Theorell–Chance mechanism. The sequence of events occurring at the active centre of the enzyme during the reaction of ACh synthesis is schematically shown in Fig. 2.3. One of the catalytically active groups in the active centre is imidazole. A thiol group is also present in the active centre, but it does not directly participate in the binding of reaction substrates or products. The enzyme is not strictly specific for acetyl–CoA and choline; a number of compounds with a similar structure can also serve as its substrates. The activity of ChAc is low in media with low ionic strength. The mechanism of the activating effect of ions is not clear. Unless highly purified or extremely diluted, mammalian ChAc is comparatively stable.

ChAc is present mainly in the nerve cells; under normal conditions, its presence in the glial and Schwann cells is not likely, but it can be found in them under some pathologic conditions. Not all neurons contain ChAc. Most observations support the view that the presence of ChAc is specific for cholinergic neurons, but some findings suggest that it may be present in certain neurons together with other transmitter-synthesizing enzymes. A very high ChAc activity is found in the caudate nuclei, putamen, nucleus interpeduncularis, retina, and ventral roots of the spinal cord. Extraneural ChAc is present in the placenta of some species, spermatozoa, and possibly also in skeletal muscles; insufficient or controversial evidence is available regarding its presence in the blood platelets and its partly extraneural localization in corneal epithelium.

Although ChAc activity can be measured from the rate of utilization of either of its substrates or the synthesis of either of its products, the most convenient method of its assay is based on the measurement of the production of ACh. This is best done radiochemically, using $[^{14}C]$acetyl–CoA or $[^{3}H]$acetyl–CoA as substrate and measuring the radioactivity in ACh. Labelled ACh is most conveniently separated from labelled acetyl–CoA by extraction with tetraphenylboron in 3-heptanone. Histochemical and immunofluorescence methods for detection of ChAc activity in histological preparations are promising, but are not yet sufficiently developed for routine research use.

AUTHOR'S NOTE

While the book was in press, important new data have been published. L.B. Hersh and M. Peet (*J. biol. Chem.* **252**, 4796–4802, 1977) have concluded from their kinetic analysis that the reaction catalysed by placental ChAc is based on a random binding mechanism, rather than on the Theorell–Chance mechanism. J. Rossier, Y. Spantidakis and P. Benda (*J. Neurochem.* **29**, 1007–1012, 1977) have described extensively their findings regarding the activating effect of Cl^- ions on ChAc and the strong inhibitory action of ACh on ChAc in the absence of Cl^-. D.A. Godfrey, A.D. Williams and F.M. Matschinsky (*J. Histochem. Cytochem.* **25**, 397–416, 1977) have given a detailed description of ChAc distribution in cat cochlear nuclei. D. Schubert, S. Heinemann and Y. Kidikoro (*Proc. natn. Acad. Sci. U.S.A.* **74**, 2579–2583, 1977) have described the synthesis of ACh in a clonal cell line of rat pheochromocytoma.

3 Axonal transport of choline acetyltransferase, acetylcholinesterase and acetylcholine

3.1 INTRODUCTION

Most of the ACh which is used for synaptic transmission is synthesized in the immediate vicinity of the synapses, i.e. in terminal parts of cholinergic axons. ChAc, however, which catalyses the synthesis of ACh, is produced in the bodies of the neurons and is transferred to the presynaptic nerve endings by the mechanism of axonal transport. Axonal transport also delivers to the nerve endings some, or perhaps all, of the ACh which is produced in the perikarya and the neurites of cholinergic neurons. This chapter contains introductory information on the mechanism and properties of axonal transport and a review of available data regarding the transport of ChAc and ACh. A section on axonal transport of AChE has been included in view of the fact that its transport is currently understood better than the transport of any other enzyme in the nervous system; characteristic features of the transport of other substances can be conveniently demonstrated on the basis of a comparison with the transport of AChE.

3.2 THE PHENOMENON OF AXONAL TRANSPORT

One of the characteristic features of the nerve cells is the wealth and extent of cell processes (neurites and dendrites) in comparison with the size of cell bodies. The processes of the nerve cells are independent of the cell bodies in their energy metabolism (they have their own mitochondria and can maintain electric potential on their surface membrane after being separated from the cell body), but they are not independent in the metabolism of nucleic acids and proteins. This is because the nuclei, which are the carriers of genetic information and the source of messenger RNA for the synthesis of proteins, are contained only in the bodies of the cells and, similarly the ribosomes, in which the synthesis of proteins occurs, are localized only in the cell bodies and dendrites (Peters *et al.*, 1970). Recently ribosomes have been found in myelinated axons of spinal ganglia, but these are also dendritic in nature (Zelená, 1972). Be it because of the absence of ribosomes or the lack of messenger RNA and other components necessary for the process, the synthesis of proteins in the neurites is certainly very small; the great majority, perhaps 98% (Droz, 1973), of the proteins which are produced in the nerve cells are synthesized in the perikarya. The reader is referred to the reviews by Barondes and Samson (1967), Koenig (1969) and Satake (1972) for discussion of the interesting problem of local synthesis of proteins in the axons and nerve endings.

The substances synthesized in the perikarya are delivered to the neurites and their endings by means of axonal transport. The term axonal transport will be used here to designate all mechanisms of intracellular transport of substances and organelles from the perikarya to the neurites and their presynaptic endings (proximo–distal or orthograde transport) and from the neurites and their endings towards the perikarya (disto–proximal or retrograde transport), except where the movement of substances or organelles occurs by simple diffusion or Brownian movement. Axonal transport has received an exceptional amount of attention in neurobiological research during the last twenty years and available data have been reviewed many times (Weiss, 1963, 1970; Lubińska, 1964, 1975; Barondes and Samson, 1967; Barondes, 1969; Grafstein, 1969; Zelená, 1969; Dahlström and Häggendal, 1970; Davison, 1970; Lasek, 1970, 1975; Dahlström, 1971; Mezensev and Messinova, 1971; Ochs, 1971, 1972a,b, 1974a,c; Samson, 1971; Banks and Mayor, 1972; McClure, 1972; Droz, 1973; Jeffrey and Austin, 1973; Heslop, 1975; Kerkut, 1975; Livett, 1976; Bisby, 1976).

Although the view that the body of the nerve cell represents its trophic centre and ensures the nutrition of the neurite has been repeatedly expressed since the beginning of this century (Scott, 1906; Prenant and Bouin, 1911), the concept of axonal transport acquired an experimental basis only after the study by Weiss and Hiscoe in 1948. Weiss and Hiscoe mildly compressed a nerve by a cuff and observed changes in the area of the cuff and on both sides of it. The nerve fibres became thinner in the area of the cuff and distal to it; dilatations occurred proximal to the cuff. After the cuff had been removed, the dilated fibres above the cuff became progessively thinner and regained their original size; simultaneously, the narrow fibres in the area of the cuff and distal to it became progressively wider and also regained their original size. Weiss and Hiscoe (1948) interpreted their observations to mean that the compression created an obstacle to the continuous movement of axonal contents from the perikarya to the periphery and thus caused their accumulation above the cuff. After the obstacle had been removed, the accumulated material again moved towards the periphery at a speed of approximately 1–2 mm/day. It has to be noted, however, that in later experiments described by Spencer (1972) the accumulation of the axoplasm above the site of nerve compression could be observed only in those fibres which were undergoing the process regeneration. Some experimental results from the laboratory of Ochs (1974a) also suggest that the original observations by Weiss and Hiscoe (1948) might require reinvestigation using contemporary research methods. In spite of this, the article of Weiss and Hiscoe (1948) enormously influenced the further development of the physiology of the neuron.

In the years following the publication of this article, the methods used for the investigation of axonal transport and the data regarding its properties developed rapidly. Just as the observation, that the contents of the axon accumulate proximal to the site of compression of the nerve, initiated the experimental studies of proximo–distal transport, so a similar observation, that some enzymes and cellular organelles accumulate below the site of interruption of an axon, gave rise to the idea that there is also a continuous disto–proximal (retrograde) transport of substances and organelles. The pioneering work in this direction was made by Zelená and Lubińska (1962), who observed an increase of ChE both above and below the site at which the continuity of the nerve fibres had been interrupted by crushing the nerve. The increase in the activity of the enzyme proximal to the crush could be explained by the accumulation of the enzyme being transported from the perikarya to the periphery. The increase of activity distal to the ligature was interpreted as a consequence of retrograde movement of the enzyme in the axons. As will be pointed out later in this chapter, the assumption of retrograde transport in the axons has now been confirmed in several other ways.

Axonal transport has been studied with many methods, but the following two have proved to be the most fruitful:

(a) Injection of radiolabelled precursors (amino acids as precursors of proteins, sugars as precursors of glycoproteins, phosphate as precursor of phospholipids, etc.) into the vicinity of the cell bodies, followed by an investigation of how the radioactivity incorporated into corresponding macromolecules moves away from the cell nuclei and into the nerve fibres and how it reaches the area where the fibres end. The movement of radioactivity can be followed either in the homogenates of a series of short segments of the nerve or by means of autoradiography. The sites preferentially used for injections of radioactive precursors are the ventral horns of the grey matter in the spinal cord (transport in the axons of spinal motoneurons), the fourth cerebral ventricle or the Sylvian aqueduct (transport in the axons of the motoneurons of cranial nerves and in preganglionic parasympathetic fibres), the posterior chamber of the eye (transport in the axons of retinal ganglion cells forming the optic nerve) and the spinal ganglia. The advantage of this approach is that it affords the possibility of working with intact nerves under virtually physiological conditions. The disadvantage is that the radioactive molecules, the transport of which is observed, can be characterized only in general terms (as proteins, glycoproteins, ribonucleic acids, etc), but, for technical reasons, cannot usually be accurately identified (as ChAc, tyrosine hydroxylase, etc.). Overlapping of labelled substances transported at different speeds occurs.

(b) Interruption of the nerve by a ligature and observation of changes in the content of various substances (mainly enzymes) in the segments of the nerve immediately above and immediately below the ligature. This approach is suitable mainly for the investigation of the transport of substances which are exclusive to the axons and are not present in Schwann cells. It has therefore proved particularly useful for studies of the transport of enzymes participating in the metabolism of synaptic transmitters and of the transmitters themselves. Substances transported in the axons proximo–distally accumulate immediately above the site of interruption of the nerve. The rate of accumulation is dependent on the rate of transport. If the content of a substance also increases in the segment of the nerve immediately below the ligature, the increase is frequently caused by the interruption of the disto–proximal (retrograde) transport of the substance. The advantage of this approach is that it allows the study of the transport of specified substances, for example enzymes, which are easily identified by their specific enzymatic activity. The content of such enzymes or substances in the vicinity of the ligature can be estimated biochemically or histochemically. The disadvantage of the method is that it is performed on damaged axons.

These two methods have been used both *in vivo* and *in vitro*. Other approaches to the study of axonal transport have included microcinematographic observations of the movements of cellular organelles in tissue cultures and in the nerves, injections of substances into innervated organs (e.g., muscles) followed by investigations of the presence and of the retrograde movement of the injected substances in the nerves, studies of translocations of enzymes and transmitters in nerve segments isolated by two ligature *in vivo*, investigations of drug effects on the transport, and studies of the time course of incorporation of injected substances into subcellular fractions of brain homogenates, etc.

Although the mechanisms on which axonal transport is based are not yet understood, there is no doubt about the existence of the transport both in the orthograde and in the retrograde direction. After the finding that AChE accumulated distal to the site of interruption of the nerve (Zelená and Lubińska, 1962), the existence of retrograde transport has been convincingly proved by further analysis of the translocation of AChE in interrupted nerves and in nerve segments *in vivo* (Lubińska, 1964; Lubińska *et al.*, 1964; Lubińska and Niemierko, 1971; Ranish and Ochs, 1972), by the analysis of movements of cellular organelles in interrupted axons (Zelená *et al.*, 1968; Zelená, 1969), by the demonstration of the accumulation of radioactively labelled proteins distal to ligatures (Lasek, 1967; Bray *et al.*, 1971; Edström and Hanson, 1973; Frizell and Sjöstrand, 1974c; Griffin *et al.*, 1976), by the demonstration of intra-axonal transport of some substances from the muscle into the nerve and to the motoneurons (Watson, 1968; Kristensson and Olsson, 1971; Kristensson and Sjöstrand, 1972; Griffin *et al.*, 1976) and by observations of retrograde movement of horseradish peroxidase in the axons of the central nervous system (see review by LaVail, 1975). The physiological role of the proximo–distal transport is clear – the delivery of substances produced in the perikarya for the needs of axons, nerve endings and probably also for transsynaptic delivery to neighbouring cells. The physiological role of the disto–proximal transport is less clear – perhaps it is to return surplus material which has not been utilized in the axons and their endings, or to signal information about the metabolic state of the axons, or to transfer material and information from postsynaptic cells to the cell bodies of presynaptic neurons.

The speeds of axonal transport observed in the nerves of vertebrates are in the range of 1 mm–2000 mm/day. Data from many studies are well summarized in the reviews by Lasek (1970), Jeffrey and Austin (1973) and Heslop (1975). Many experiments with radioactively labelled molecules have shown that the transport proceeds at several speeds: e.g., McEwen and Grafstein (1968) observed, in the goldfish, rates of transport of 0.4 mm/day and more than 40 mm/day; Livett *et al.* (1968), in the sympathetic nerve of cat, rates of 1 mm/day and 120 mm/day; Jakoubek *et al.* (1970), in the fish *Lebistes reticularis,* rates of 3.5 mm/day and more than 40 mm/day; Bray and Austin (1969), in chicken, rates of 2–3 mm/day and 250–300 mm/day; Karlsson and Sjöstrand (1971), in rabbit, rates of 2 mm/day, 6–12 mm/day, 40 mm/day, and 150 mm/day; Droz *et al.* (1973), in chicken, rates of 1.5–10 mm/day and 288 mm/day; Komiya and Austin (1974), in mouse, rates of 0.7 mm/day, 500 mm/day and 2000 mm/day; Willard *et al.* (1974), in rabbit, rates of 2–4 mm/day, 4–8 mm/day, 34–68 mm/day and 240 mm/day. An example of observations indicating that the transport proceeds with at least two different speeds is given in Fig. 3.1.

Measurements of the rate of transport of enzymes or transmitters from the speed at which they accumulate above a ligature also indicate different rates of transport for different substances. Very probably, all neurons have the capacity for slow transport at a rate of 1–10 mm/day and for fast transport at a higher rate. The explanation of the observations of several rates of fast transport in the same nerve is not clear. It is possible that the fast transport proceeds at several different rates in one and the same axon. The alternative possibility is that there is only one fast rate in each axon, but that this is different in different axons. Ochs (1972c) finds that the rate of the fast transport is the same in nerve fibres of a wide range of diameters. On the other hand, Lubińska (1977) demonstrated that the speed at which degenerative changes in the peripheral stump of a transected nerve spread in the proximo–distal direction is faster in thin and slower in large nerve fibres; this speed is most likely dependent on the speed of axonal transport.

The amount of material delivered by the slow transport is several times higher than that delivered by the fast transport (McEwen and Grafstein, 1968; Samson, 1971; Karlsson and Sjöstrand, 1971; Cuénod *et al.*, 1972; Singh *et al.*, 1974). The fast transport mainly conveys materials designated for building or repair of membraneous structures (synaptic vesicles, presynaptic and axolemmal plasma membrane, endoplasmic reticulum), and enzymes which are not freely dissolved in the axoplasm; the slow transport mainly delivers constituents of the axoplasm, soluble enzymes and tubulin (Grafstein *et al.*, 1970; McEwen *et al.*, 1971; Hendriclson, 1972; Cuénod *et al.*, 1972; Di Giamberardino *et al.*, 1973; Oesch *et al.*, 1973; Droz *et al.*, 1973; Sabri and Ochs, 1973; Willard *et al.*, 1974; Tuček, 1975; Hoffman and Lasek, 1975).

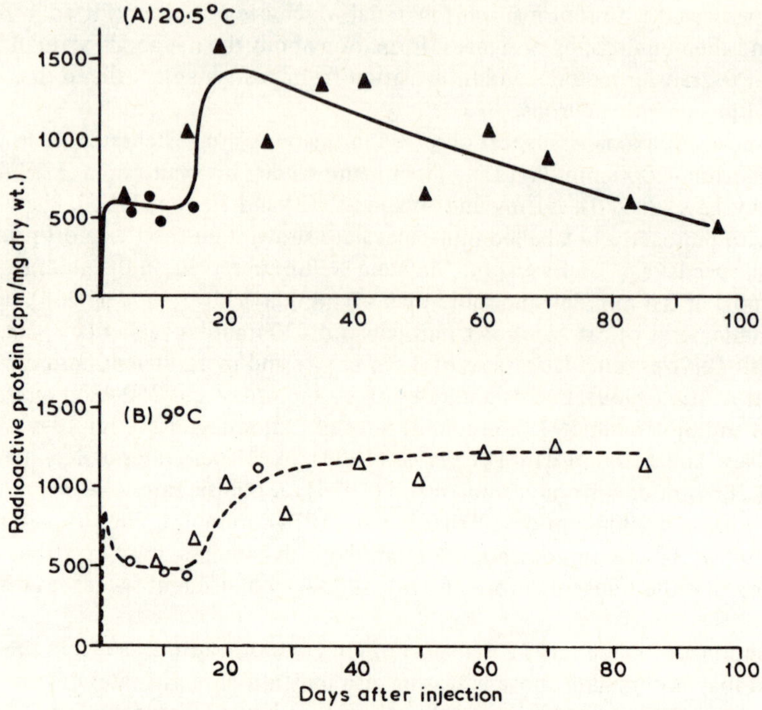

Fig. 3.1 Transport of radioactive proteins from the retina to the tectum of goldfish after intraocular injection of [^{3}H] leucine. The fish were kept at 20.5°C (A) or 9°C (B). Abscissa: days after injection. Ordinate: radioactivity in proteins (cmp/mg dry weight) in the tectum contralateral to the injected eye. The background radioactivity found in the ipsilateral tectum was subtracted. Some radioactive proteins (transported by the fast transport mechanism) reached the tectum very early, whereas other radioactive proteins (transported by the slow transport mechanism) required about two weeks to arrive at the tectum. The graph also shows that the effect of changing temperature on the rate of slow transport is very small. The scale of the graph does not reveal the effect of temperature on the fast transport (after Grafstein *et al.*, 1972).

About 80% of the slowly transported material in rat motor and cat sensory neurons is comprised of only 4–5 proteins having the same molecular weight in both species; one of these proteins is tubulin (Hoffman and Lasek, 1975). The rate of transport of mitochondria appears to be different from the speed at which they are able to move. Whereas microcinematography reveals that mitochondria make fast bidirectional movements, biochemical observations usually suggest that the accumulation of mitochondrial constituents at the ends of the axons proceeds at a slow rate (see Jeffrey and Austin, 1973).

A number of interesting hypotheses have been proposed to explain the mechanism of axonal transport. Weiss (1972a,b) interprets the slow transport (which he calls axonal flow, as opposed to the much faster intra-axonal transport) as the continuous unidirectional translocation of the axoplasmic column, mediated by peristaltic waves on the surface of the fibres, which result from the activity of the axolemma and/or Schwann cells. In this concept, the axoplasm is regarded as a semisolid gel (Weiss, 1972a; see, however, Haak *et al.*, 1976). The fast transport is explained on the assumption of streaming inside the microtubules; the propulsive force for the streaming is provided by their conformational changes (Weiss, 1970). As pointed out by Lubińska (1975), it is difficult to visualize the axoplasm moving as a cohesive body in view of the complex anatomy of the neurons. The idea of fast streaming inside the microtubules involves the problem of accounting for the fast transport of organelles which are bigger than the microtubules.

The concept of the slow flow as proposed by Weiss has been used for the interpretation of experimental results by, for example, Davison (1970) and Cuénod *et al.* (1972). Droz (1973; Droz *et al.*, 1975) assumes that the slow transport involves the proteins which are dissolved in the axoplasm or which form the subunits of the microtubules and neurofilaments, whereas the fast transport proceeds in the endoplasmic reticulum. Some authors (McEwen and Grafstein, 1968; Bray and Austin, 1969; Jeffrey and Austin, 1973) tend to explain the slow transport as a consequence of the centrifugal growth of longitudinally oriented cellular structures, mainly microtubules and neurofilaments, and the fast transport as a consequence of the movement of cellular organelles. Ochs (1974a) proposed a 'mitochondrial shuttle' hypothesis as an explanation of the slow transport. This hypothesis assumes that the slow transport of mitochondria is the result of their fast to and fro movement and that soluble proteins move in a similar way, perhaps being partly pushed by the movements of large organelles.

The hypotheses proposed to explain the mechanism of the fast transport can, with some simplification, be separated into two groups. One group of hypotheses is based on the assumption that the transport proceeds in a more or less stationary medium containing structures subserving the transport; the transported material is not moving with the axoplasm, but is moved through it. The other group of hypotheses assumes that the axoplasm itself undergoes fast movement. Several hypotheses belonging to the first group assume that the microtubules play the decisive role in the mechanism of transport. This view is based on a number of observations that the mitotic inhibitors colchicine, vinblastine and vincristine which bind to tubulin (the protein building-block of microtubules), cause the disintegration of microtubules and block axonal transport (see McClure, 1972, and Heslop, 1975, for review). It is questionable, however, whether the binding of these drugs to tubulin is the only way in which they act. This point has been critically reviewed by Lubińska (1975). According to Schmitt's (1968) hypothesis, the transported material is contained in vesicles, which move along the microtubules using a mechanism similar to that by which actin and myosin interact during muscle contraction. Ochs (1971) proposed a similar model: hypothetical transport filaments are produced in neuronal perikarya and the transported molecules and organelles are bound to them. The transport filaments move along the microtubules or neurofilaments by forming cross bridges in a similar way to actin filaments moving along the myosin filaments in the sliding filament model of muscular contraction. According to Kerkut's (1975) view, material is transported in vesicles and moved by actin and myosin filaments in the axons; actin filaments are anchored to microtubules or endoplasmic reticulum. Samson (1971) explains axonal transport as a consequence of conformational changes in a net of macromolecular polyelectrolytes to which the transported material becomes temporarily attached: in this hypothesis the microtubules provide the skeleton on which the net of polyelectrolytes is fixed.

Although the involvement of microtubules in axonal transport proved to be an extremely attractive idea, experimentally there is little to support it except for the effects of antimitotic drugs, and even this support is equivocal (see Byers, 1974; Lubińska, 1975). More direct experimental evidence has been obtained to support the involvement of the smooth endoplasmic reticulum. It has been shown, first in slightly compressed (Droz *et al.*, 1975) and later in normal ciliary ganglia and their preganglionic fibres (Markov *et al.*, 1976), that in electron microscopic autoradiographs the rapidly transported material in the axons is preferentially associated with the tubules of the smooth endoplasmic reticulum.

The fast movement of axoplasm forms the basis of transport in Lubińska's (1964) concept, according to which some layers of the axoplasm are moving cellulifugally and other layers cellulipetally. Closely related to this idea is the notion of microstreams proposed by Gross (1975). In his concept, the axoplasm has a low viscosity and is streaming only in the immediate vicinity of the microtubules. The moving force responsible for streaming is the vectorial hydrolysis of ATP proceeding on the surface of the microtubules and the transported material is moving together with the axoplasm. The speed of transport depends on the position of the transported compound or particle in the microstream (the speed of the stream first increases and then decreases with the distance from the surface of the microtubule) and on transition of transported material from the streaming to the stationary axoplasm and vice versa.

Some hypotheses clearly distinguish between the mechanisms assumed to operate in the slow transport and the fast transport. Several hypotheses, however, might be grouped together under the name of 'unitary views', since they assume that the mechanism underlying the slow and the fast transport is the same. Samson (1971) pointed out that the net of macromolecular polyelectrolytes in his transport model might be responsible for both the slow and the fast movement of transported material. In the model proposed by Gross (1975) the transport is also expected to proceed at a continuum of transport velocities; slow velocities will be expected for molecules penetrating easily into the more viscous and stationary layers of the axoplasm. Finally, Ochs (1975) also suggests that his transport filament model, originally proposed to explain the fast transport, can explain the slow transport as well, assuming that the slowly transported material is less firmly bound to the transport filaments. It is not clear, however, how to reconcile the 'unitary' models with data indicating qualitative differences between the slow and the fast transport, particulaly with that on their different sensitivity to temperature (Grafstein *et al.*, 1972) and to mitotic poisons, and with the measurements indicating clear-cut differences (rather than continuous transitions) between different rates of transport.

This account of hypotheses which try to explain the mechanism of axonal transport reveals an extremely wide diversity of views, reflecting our inadequate understanding of this basic phenomenon in the life of neurons. A few positive findings concerning some properties of axonal transport will now be added. In experiments *in vitro*, the fast transport is dependent on the supply of oxygen and on the formation of ATP (Ochs and Ranish, 1970; Ochs and Hollingsworth, 1971); *in vivo*, it is arrested under conditions of ischaemia (Tuček *et al.*, 1975, 1978b). Fast transport of proteins already present in the axons continues after the synthesis of new proteins in the cell bodies has been inhibited (see Burešová and Tuček (1977) for references). The fast transport is not dependent on the preservation of the continuity between the axon and the perikaryon (Lubińska *et al.*, 1964; Dahlström, 1967a; Jankowska *et al.*, 1969; Ochs and Hollingsworth, 1971; Lubińska and Niemierko, 1971). In contrast, the slow transport is very much reduced or blocked after the separation of the axon from the perikaryon (Fig. 3.6; Tuček, 1975; Frizell *et al.*, 1975; McLean *et al.*, 1976). The speed of axonal transport is not altered by changes in impulse activity (Jankowska *et al.*, 1969; Lux *et al.*, 1970).

3.3 AXONAL TRANSPORT OF ACETYLCHOLINESTERASE

Acetylcholinesterase (AChE, EC 3.1.1.7) in peripheral nerves of several (not necessarily all) mammalian species is located only in the axons, not in Schwann cells (Tewari and Bourne, 1960; Koelle, 1963; Silver, 1974). Its transport can thus be studied in suitable species by observing the changes in its activity in the vicinity of sites in which the continuity of the nerve had been interrupted by a ligature, cut or crush. Following the observation that the histochemically detectable activity of AChE increases both proximal and distal to a nerve crush (Zelená and Lubińska, 1962), axonal transport of AChE has been thoroughly investigated, particularly in a series of studies by Lubinska *et al.* (1963a,b, 1964; Niemierko and Lubińska, 1967). The most systematic investigation of the axonal transport of AChE has been made by Lubińska and Niemierko (1971); their main results are described below.

When the dog peroneal nerve is cut and the activity of AChE in short segments of the nerve proximal and distal to the lesion is investigated at intervals during the next 22 h, it is found that the activity of AChE increases steeply in the last 3 mm of the central nerve stump and also shows a definite rise in the first 3 mm of the peripheral nerve stump (Fig. 3.2). In experiments in which the peroneal nerve was transected simultaneously in two places several cm apart, the activity of AChE increased above and below both the proximal and the distal cut (Fig. 3.3). At the

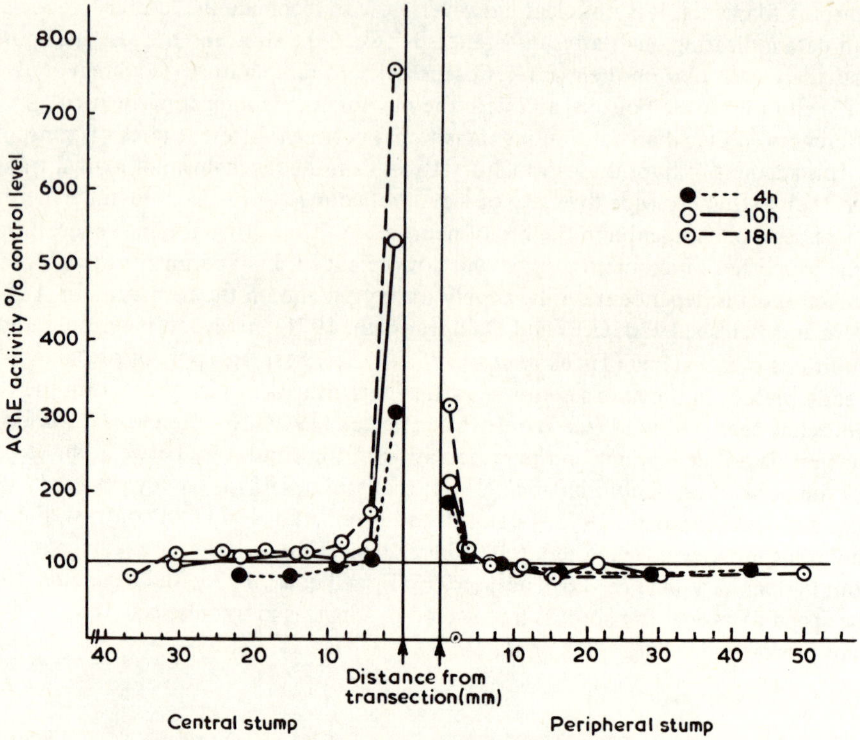

Fig. 3.2 The distribution of AChE at the end of the central stump and at the beginning of the peripheral stump of the peroneal nerve in dog. Enzyme activity is expressed as a percentage of control values. ●, 4 h after nerve section; ○, 10 h after nerve section; ⊙, 18 h after nerve section. The distance from the site of the nerve section is given on the abscissa (after Lubińska and Niemierko, 1971).

beginning, the activity of AChE increased at the same rate above the distal cut as above the proximal cut, but after a certain time the activity above the distal cut no longer increased, although the activity above the proximal cut continued to rise. The longer the distance between the proximal and distal cuts, the longer the period during which the increase in activity above the distal cut continued. Initially, the increase of AChE activity below the proximal and the distal cuts also proceeded in a similar way, but after a certain time the increase at the proximal end of the isolated segment stopped, although it continued at the proximal end of the peripheral nerve stump (i.e. below the distal cut). The total AChE activity in the isolated nerve segment did not change: the increase at the ends of the segment was the consequence of the translocation of the enzyme and was equalled by a decrease in its middle part (Lubińska and Niemierko, 1971).

The observations on movement of AChE in isolated nerve segments over short

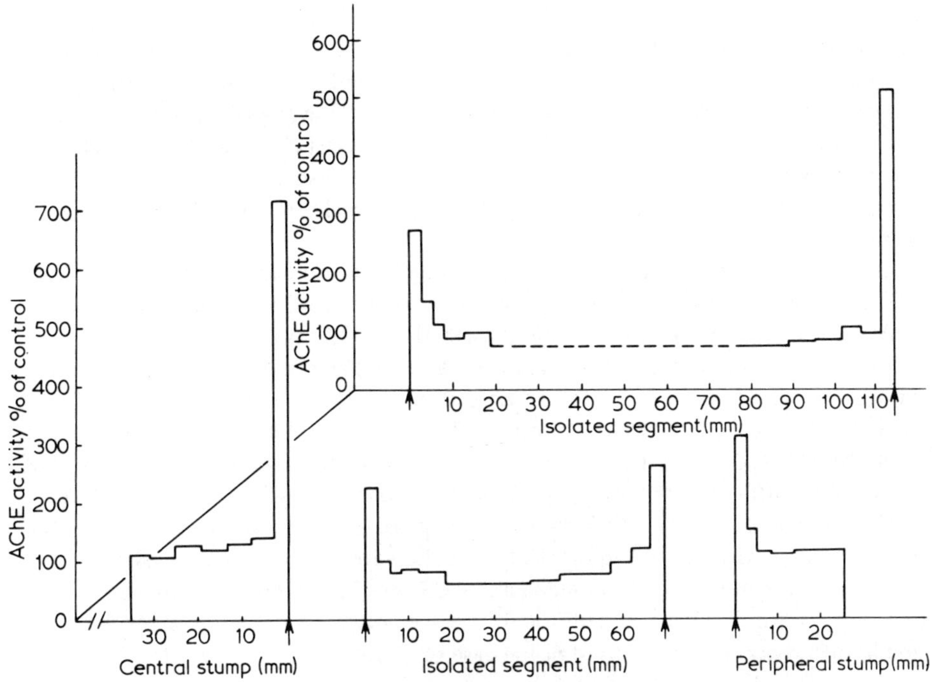

Fig. 3.3 The distribution of the activity of AChE in dog peroneal nerve 22 h after the nerve had been interrupted at 2 sites simultaneously. The lower part of the graph shows the distribution of enzyme activity at the end of the central stump, in the isolated middle segment, and at the beginning of the peripheral stump. The upper part of the graph demonstrates the distribution of AChE in a much longer isolated segment of the contralateral peroneal nerve in the same dog. Enzyme activity is expressed as percentage of control values. The distance from the site of interruption (in isolated segments – from their proximal end) is shown on the abscissa. Note that the accumulation of the enzyme at the ends of the isolated segment is higher when the segment is longer (after Lubińska and Niemierko, 1971).

time periods after their preparation indicate that the proximo–distal transport of AChE is not affected by the separation of the axons from neuronal bodies. This accords well with the findings in studies of fast axonal transport of radioactively labelled proteins: their transport is not changed after the separation of the axons from the perikarya (Ochs and Ranish, 1970; Ochs and Hollingsworth, 1971). The accumulation of AChE at the distal end of the isolated segment stops, however, after a time which is directly proportional to the length of the segment. Apparently the accumulation (and the transport) ceases when all enzymes transportable proximo–distally reached the distal end of the segment. The analysis of their observations led Lubińska and Niemierko (1971) to the conclusion that, in the peroneal nerve of the dog, 10% of the total content of AChE is transported by the fast axonal transport proximo–distally and 5% disto–proximally. The rest of the enzyme either does not move, or is moved by slow transport. The rate of transport was calculated from data on the accumulation of AChE in the vicinity of the interruption of the nerve and from the data on the proportion of the enzyme which was transported in one or other direction; the calculated rates were 250 mm/day in the proximo–distal and 134 mm/day in the disto–proximal direction (Lubińska and Niemierko, 1971).

On the basis of similar experiments and using similar reasoning, Ranish and Ochs (1972) arrived at the conclusion that, in cat sciatic nerve, 10% of the total content of AChE is moving proximo–distally at a speed of 431 mm/day and 5% disto–proximally at a speed of 220 mm/day. The value of 431 mm/day, calculated as the rate of orthograde transport, is remarkably close to the value of 410 mm/day, found to be the rate of the fast axonal transport of radioactively labelled proteins in intact cat nerves (Ochs, 1972c). Fonnum *et al.* (1973) calculated that in the vagus nerve of rabbits 4.7% of the total content of AChE moves proximo–distally at a speed of 425 mm/day and 3.8% of AChE moves disto–proximally at a speed of 123 mm/day. In experiments with rabbit hypoglossal nerve, however, they arrived at values of 11.2% and 73 mm/day for orthograde and 4.9% and 73 mm/day for retrograde transport. It is difficult to explain the difference between these two nerves, but a similar difference has been found in the case of ChAc (Fonnum *et al.*, 1973; see Section 3.4). It might be suggested that the hypoglossal nerve contains most of its AChE in somatic motor nerve fibres whereas in the vagus nerve AChE is contained mainly in preganglionic parasympathetic fibres. In rabbit peroneal nerve, however, in which AChE is contained mainly in somatic motor nerve fibres just as in the hypoglossal nerve, the rate of proximo–distal transport of AChE is 480 mm/day, with 5% of enzyme moving in this direction (Tuček, 1975).

Axonal transport of AChE in both directions may also be observed in nerves *in vitro* (Jankowska *et al.*, 1969). In frog nerves kept *in vitro* at 22°C, the enzyme is transported proximo–distally at a speed of 99 mm/day and disto–proximally at 19 mm/day; about 12% of the total amount of AChE in the nerve is moving in each direction (Partlow *et al.*, 1972).

In the axons, AChE is mainly located at two sites:

(1) in axonal membranes;
(2) associated with the tubules and vesicles of the endoplasmic reticulum (Kása, 1968; Silver, 1974). The increase of AChE activity in the vicinity of the site of nerve interruption is connected with the accumulation of intra-axonal tubules and vesicles; the activity of axolemmal AChE is not changed (Kása, 1968).

3.4 AXONAL TRANSPORT OF CHOLINE ACETYLTRANSFERASE

The transport of enzyme from the site of its synthesis in the perikaryon to the nerve endings is particularly important in the case of ChAc, because ChAc has a synaptic function and its distribution in the neuron corresponds to this function. It is evident, mainly from studies using subcellular fractionation of brain homogenates, that the enzyme is preferentially localized in presynaptic nerve endings (Hebb and Whittaker, 1958; Whittaker, 1965; Tuček, 1966a,b, 1967a,b). ChAc was one of the first enzymes for which the assumption of proximo–distal transport in the axons was made; the assumption was based on the observation that, after the sheep cervical sympathetic chain had been cut, the activity of ChAc increased proximal to the site of transection, whereas distally the activity decreased to values close to zero (Hebb and Waites, 1956). An increase in the activity of ChAc has also been found above the site of interruption of the goat sciatic nerve (Hebb and Silver, 1961), but more detailed analyses of the transport of ChAc did not begin until about 10 years after these pioneering observations, when the introduction of radiochemical methods facilitated the assay of ChAc in small tissue samples.

To date, the investigations of axonal transport of ChAc have been based on measurements of changes of its activity in the vicinity of sites of nerve interruption. The regularly observed increase of ChAc activity at the end of the central stump of interrupted nerves is generally explained as a consequence of proximo–distal transport. The changes in the activity or distribution of ChAc which appear in the peripheral nerve stump during the first day after the interruption of the nerve are most probably caused by the fact that, distal to the site of interruption, axonal transport still continues. The peripheral changes occurring from the second or third day are, however, caused by the Wallerian degeneration of the nerve and will be discussed later (Chapter 7.6). Changes in the distribution of ChAc in the peripheral nerve stump are relevant to two questions:

(1) Is the transport of ChAc dependent on the connection between the axon and the perikaryon?
(2) In addition to the proximo–distal transport, is there also disto–proximal transport of ChAc in the axons?

3.4.1 Accumulation of choline acetyltransferase proximal to the site of nerve interruption

The activity of ChAc proximal to the site of interruption of a nerve increases comparatively slowly. On this point, there is good accord between observations on frog sciatic nerve (Partlow *et al.*, 1972), the nerve innervating the electric organ of the fish *Torpedo marmorata* (Heilbronn and Pettersson, 1973), rat sciatic nerve (Saunders *et al.*, 1973; Wooten and Coyle, 1973; Kása *et al.*, 1973; Oesch *et al.*, 1973), cat sciatic nerve (Carlsson *et al.*, 1971a), rabbit hypoglossal nerve (Frizell *et al.*, 1970; Sjöstrand *et al.*, 1970; Fonnum *et al.*, 1973) and peroneal nerve (Tuček, 1975). On

Table 3.1 Rates of proximo–distal transport of ChAc*

Preparation	Rate of transport (mm/day)	References
Frog sciatic nerve	0.34	Partlow *et al.* (1972)
Rat sciatic nerve	3	Saunders *et al.* (1973)
	2.9	Wooten and Coyle (1973)
	5.5	Oesch *et al.* (1973)
Cat sciatic nerve	10.8	Carlsson *et al.* (1971a)
Rabbit hypoglossal nerve	6	Frizell *et al.* (1970)
	3	Fonnum *et al.* (1973)
Rabbit peroneal nerve	4	Tuček (1975)
Rabbit vagal nerve	17	Frizell *et al.* (1970)
	13	Fonnum *et al.* (1973)
Mouse sciatic nerve		
(normal mouse)	1.9	Jablecki and Brimijoin (1974)
(mouse with muscular) dystrophy)	0.9	Jablecki and Brimijoin (1974)

* Values in the Table have been calculated from the rates of ChAc accumulation proximal to the ligature or transection of the nerve on the assumption that the accumulation is due to the proximo–distal transport of all the enzyme present in the nerve.

the assumption that the accumulation of ChAc above the ligature or interruption is due to the proximo–distal transport of all the enzyme present in the nerve, the rate of accumulation can be taken to correspond with the rate of proximo–distal transport of ChAc. Values of the rate of proximo–distal transport, calculated on this basis, are summarized in Table 3.1. Most of them are in the range 1–10 mm/day; a somewhat higher rate of transport was calculated for the vagal nerve of the rabbit: 17 mm/day (Frizell *et al.*, 1970) and 13 mm/day (Fonnum *et al.*, 1973). Early observations that the accumulation of ChAc proximal to the site of interruption of the nerve proceeds at the same rate as that of AChE (Frizell *et al.*, 1970; Sjöstrand *et al.*, 1970) have not been confirmed by later studies; AChE accumulates at a much faster rate (Kása *et al.*, 1973; Partlow *et al.*, 1972), and this is also true in experiments on rabbits (Tuček, 1975), the species in which the investigation by Frizell *et al.* had been performed. As may be seen in Fig. 3.4, the ChAc activity found in the last 8 mm of the central stump of the rabbit peroneal nerve 22 h after ligation is increased by 51%, whereas the activity of AChE is raised by 285%. If the increases of enzyme activities at the end of the central nerve stump were caused by the proximo–distal transport of all ChAc and AChE present in the axons, they would correspond to a rate of transport of 4 mm/day in the case of ChAc and 22 mm/day in the case of AChE (Tuček, 1975).

The activity of ChAc does not increase at the extreme end of the central nerve stump, but, according to experiments on rabbit peroneal nerve, at a distance of

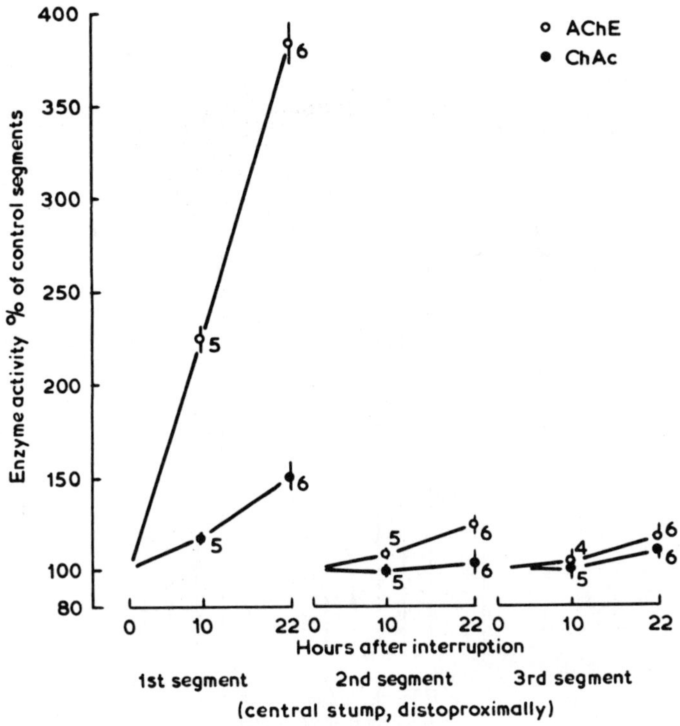

Fig. 3.4 The activities of AChE (open circles) and ChAc (filled circles) at the end of the central stump of rabbit peroneal nerve in the course of 22 h after the interruption of the nerve. The nerve was ligated at time 0; after 10 or 22 h, three 8 mm long segments were prepared from the end of the central nerve stump. The most distal segment (closest to the ligature) is shown on the left and described as the first segment. The most proximal segment is on the right. Abscissa: time in h; ordinate: enzymatic activity (mean ± S.E.M.) expressed as a percentage of activity in control nerve segments. The numerals beside individual points give the number of observations (after Tuček, 1975).

2–4 mm from the end of the nerve (Tuček, 1975; Fig. 3.5). This is another difference between the accumulation of ChAc and of AChE, since the latter enzyme accumulates in the most distal segment of the central nerve stump. The difference between the two enzymes may be explained on the basis of morphological observations indicating that an accumulation of intracellular organelles (mainly mitochondria, tubules and vesicles of endoplasmic reticulum) occurs at the ends of interrupted axons in such a way that the terminal parts of the axons are completely filled up with particulate material (Zelená *et al.*, 1968; Zelená, 1969; Kapeller and Mayor, 1969a). Since AChE is associated with the endoplasmic reticulum (Kása, 1968), it is not surprising that its activity increases in the area where the elements

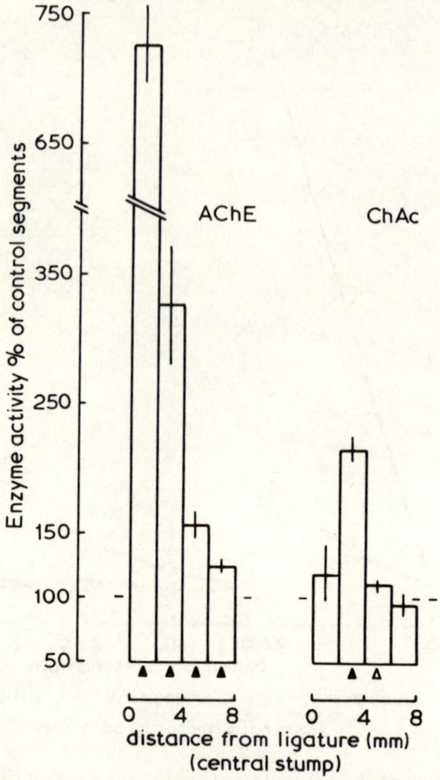

Fig. 3.5 Comparison of the distribution of AChE and ChAc at the end of the central stump of rabbit peroneal nerve, 22 h after the nerve had been ligated and transected distal to the ligature. Four 2 mm long segments were prepared from the most distal part of the nerve stump and the activities of AChE and ChAc were measured in the homogenates of these segments. The columns on the graph are arranged from the left to the right in the disto–proximal order; the left hand column of each block thus corresponds to the most distal segments (closest to the ligature). Abscissa: distance from the ligature; ordinate: enzyme activity, expressed as a percentage of the activity in control segments (mean ± S.E.M). The triangles indicate the statistical significance of the difference from values in the control segments; filled triangles, $p < 0.005$; open triangle, $p < 0.025$ (after Tuček, 1975).

of the endoplasmic reticulum accumulate. That the increase in the activity of ChAc occurs slightly more proximally supports the assumption (see Chapter 6.2) that the enzyme is contained in the axoplasm, which can accumulate only proximal to the accumulation of intra-axonal organelles.

The accumulation of ChAc proximal to the interruption can be prevented by injecting colchicine or vinblastine into a more proximal part of the nerve

(Dahlström *et al.*, 1975a; Wooten *et al.*, 1975; Dziegielewska *et al.*, 1976). These substances are known to cause the disintegration of microtubules and their effect on axonal transport is therefore usually interpreted as evidence for the role of microtubules in the mechanism of axonal transport. To a certain degree, such an interpretation is supported by observations that lumicolchicine, a derivative of colchicine with similar binding properties but without an effect on microtubules, does not affect the transport of ChAc (Dahlström *et al.*, 1975b). As with many other pharmacological agents, it is difficult to exclude the possibility that the actions of mitotic inhibitors on axonal transport are produced by some other, as yet uninvestigated mechanism of action which is different from their action on microtubules.

3.4.2 Proximo–distal transport of choline acetyltransferase in axons separated from neuronal perikarya

The view that the orthograde transport of ChAc continues in a nerve fibre separated from its cell body is supported by observations on isolated nerve segments *in vivo*, separated from the rest of the nerve by two ligatures (Fonnum *et al.*, 1973, 1976; Tuček, 1975; but see Partlow *et al.*, 1972, and Saunders *et al.*, 1973). As may be seen in Fig. 3.6, the activity of ChAc increased at the distal end of an isolated segment of rabbit peroneal nerve during the first 22 h after two ligatures had been placed round the nerve, 36 mm apart (Tuček, 1975). The activity at the proximal end of the segment was diminished but the total amount of enzyme in the segment did not change. This distribution of ChAc contrasts with that of AChE, the activity of which is increased at both ends of the isolated segment and decreased in the middle portion. The distribution of AChE in the isolated segment corresponds to what would be expected if the transport of AChE in the segment continues in both directions. On the other hand, the distribution of ChAc suggests that the enzyme is being moved in one direction only – to the distal end of the nerve segment. Fonnum *et al.* (1973, 1976) have, however, also observed an increase in the activity of ChAc at the proximal end of isolated nerve segments. This point will be discussed in Section 3.4.3.

A comparison between the accumulation of ChAc at the distal end of the central nerve stump, i.e. in the axons connected with the perikarya, and at the distal end of an isolated nerve segment, i.e. in the axons separated from the perikarya, indicates that the extent of the proximo–distal transport of ChAc is considerably reduced in the axons separated from the perikarya (Fig. 3.7). In two series of measurements, the amount of ChAc accumulating at the distal end of the central nerve stump during 22 h corresponded to the enzyme content of 3.96 mm or 2.63 mm of the control nerve. At the distal end of an isolated nerve segment, however, the content of ChAc was increased only by an amount corresponding to the content in 1.18 mm of the control nerve (Tuček, 1975). It is not yet possible to decide whether the diminished accumulation of ChAc was due to a decrease in the rate of transport, or to a decrease in the proportion of the transported enzyme (relative to the total enzyme content in the nerve), or if both factors played a role.

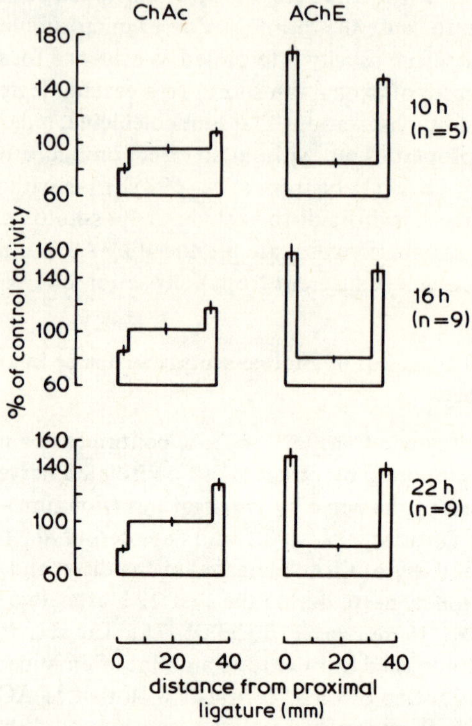

Fig. 3.6 The activities of ChAc and AChE in isolated segments of rabbit peroneal nerve. The segments were ligated at their proximal and distal ends and were left *in situ* 10, 16, or 22 h. The activities of the enzymes were then measured in the proximal part (about 4 mm long), middle part (about 28 mm long) and distal part (about 4 mm long) of the isolated segments. Abscissa: distance from the ligature on the proximal end of the segment; ordinate: enzymatic activity, expressed as percentage of activity in the corresponding segment from the contralateral control nerve. The bars express S.E.M. (after Tuček, 1975).

That the proximo–distal transport of ChAc continues in a transected nerve is also suggested by the observations described by Ekström and Emmelin (1971). In their experiments, the content of ChAc in the degenerating phrenic nerve was slightly increased when the enzyme was prevented from escaping towards the periphery by a ligature placed at the distal end of the nerve segment investigated. Partlow *et al.* (1972) and Saunders *et al.* (1973), however, did not find any translocation of ChAc within isolated nerve segments. The reason for their negative findings is not clear. In experiments on frog nerves *in vitro* (Partlow *et al.*, 1972), the conditions for revealing axonal transport of slowly transported enzymes were probably much less favourable than in experiments on warm blooded animals *in vivo.*

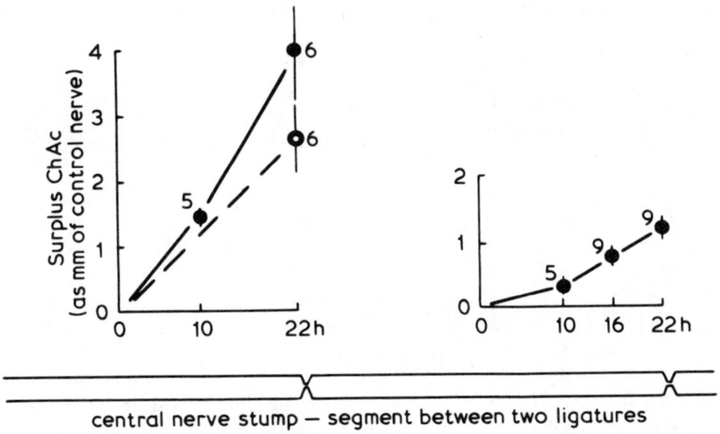

Fig. 3.7 The increase of the activity of ChAc at the end of the central nerve stump and at the distal end of an isolated segment of rabbit peroneal nerve during the 22 h following nerve interruption. The isolated segment was about 36 mm long. Abscissa: time after nerve interruption. Ordinate: the increase of enzyme activity, expressed as the length of the control nerve (mm) containing the same amount of enzyme as that accumulated proximal to the ligature. Data for the end of the central nerve stump were obtained in two different series of observations, which are expressed by filled or open circles. The bars indicate S.E.M. The numerals beside individual points give the number of observations (based on Tuček, 1975).

The negative results of Saunders *et al.* (1973) on the rat nerve might be connected with the use of very short isolated segments; in rabbits it is certainly difficult to observe the transport in very short segments (Tuček, unpublished).

Although the transport of ChAc in the peripheral nerve stump or isolated nerve segment continues, it does so for only a limited period of time. It certainly cannot continue after the formation of the so-called ovoids, i.e. after the loss of continuity of the axoplasmic column. When the activity of ChAc was measured in an 8 mm long segment of rabbit nerve immediately distal to a ligature (Tuček, 1974), it was found that 22 h after the ligation of the nerve the activity of ChAc had decreased by 19%; it did not change during the following 24 h, but in the course of the third day after ligation it fell steeply to 16% of the original value (Fig. 3.8). This observation is best interpreted as indicating that the proximo–distal transport continued during the first day, but was arrested during the second day, and on the third day, destruction of ChAc occurred. Some aspects of the transport of ChAc in the peripheral nerve stump are more fully discussed in Sections 3.4.3 and 3.4.4.

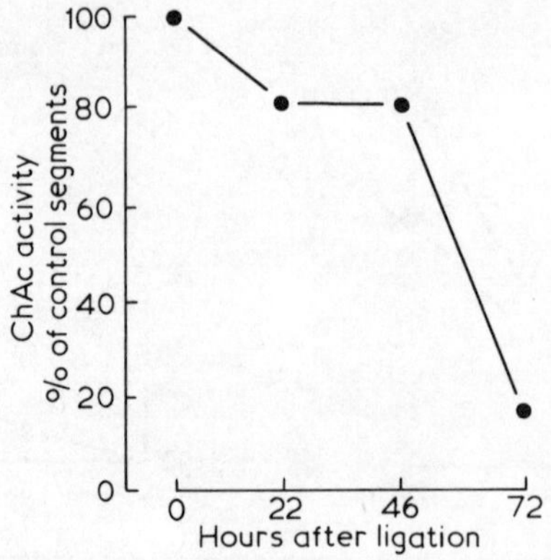

Fig. 3.8 ChAc activity at the proximal end of the peripheral nerve stump during the first 72 h after the nerve had been ligated and transected proximal to the ligature. The activity of ChAc was measured in 8 mm long segments immediately adjacent to the ligature and is expressed as percentage of the activity in control segments (based on Tuček, 1974).

3.4.3 Disto–proximal transport of choline acetyltransferase

The notion of retrograde transport of AChE is mainly based on the consistent observation that the activity of AChE is increased in the short segment of the nerve immediately distal to a ligature or to the site of nerve transection. In the case of ChAc, however, most investigators observed that the activity immediately distal to a ligature decreases during the first day after ligating the nerve (Partlow *et al.*, 1972; Kása *et al.*, 1973; Heilbronn and Pettersson, 1973; Tuček, 1974, 1975). In the experiments of Saunders *et al.* (1973) and Wooten and Coyle (1973), the activity of ChAc did not change distal to the ligature. Twenty hours after ligating the nerve, Frizell *et al.* (1970) did not find any change of ChAc activity in the nerve segment immediately below the ligature, but they observed a decrease in more distal segments. It was only in the studies of Fonnum *et al.* (1973, 1976) that an increase of ChAc activity was described in the nerve segment immediately distal to the site of interruption. A significant increase has been found only in the vagus nerve; the increase described for the hypoglossal nerve (4.4 ± 4.4% in a segment of 2.5 mm) is not convincing. It is difficult to decide whether the ChAc-containing parasympathetic preganglionic fibres in the vagus nerve are basically different from the ChAc-containing motor nerve fibres, used in all other investigations, or whether the observed increases of ChAc at the proximal ends of isolated segments of the vagus nerve might be due to the presence of cholinergic fibres running in the reverse (craniopetal) direction.

Experiments performed on rabbit peroneal nerve have revealed that the distributions of ChAc and AChE distal to a ligature are different (Tuček, 1974). In the first 2 mm of the peripheral nerve stump, the activity of ChAc diminishes, after 4 h,

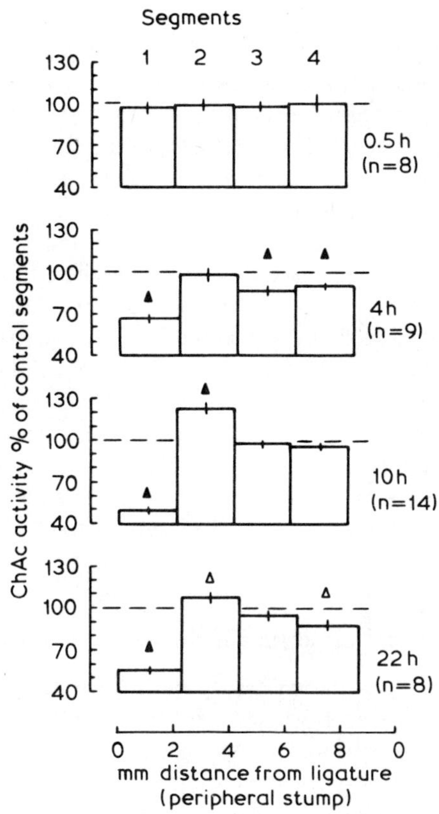

Fig. 3.9 Changes of ChAc activity in small segments from the proximal end of the peripheral stump of rabbit peroneal nerve. The nerve was ligated at time 0; after 0.5, 4, 10 or 22 h, the activity of ChAc was measured in four segments, approximately 2 mm long, from the proximal end of the peripheral nerve stump. Abscissa: distance (mm) from the ligature. Ordinate: ChAc activity, expressed as percentage of the activity in control segments (mean ± S.E.M.). The triangles indicate the statistical significance of the difference between the activity in each segment and its corresponding control; filled triangles, $p < 0.005$; open triangles, $p < 0.05$; n = number of animals (after Tuček, 1974d).

to 67% and, after 10 h, to 49% of the control value (Fig. 3.9). The activity of ChAc in the more distal 2 mm segment shows a slight, transient increase. The activity of AChE, on the other hand, measured in the same homogenates as ChAc, is very clearly increased in the first 2 mm of the peripheral nerve stump – by 94% after 4 h and by 164% after 10 h. It appears that the decrease of ChAc at the proximal end of the peripheral stump, similar to that at the proximal end of an isolated segment, (see Fig. 3.6) is caused not only by the continuing proximo–distal transport of the enzyme, but also by the accumulation of cellular organelles at the ends of the interrupted axons (Zelená *et al.*, 1968; Kapeller and Mayor, 1969b), which in its turn brings about passive translocation of the axoplasm and of the axoplasmic ChAc from the proximal ends of the axons to their more distal portions. The mild increase of ChAc activity 2–4 mm distal to the ligature then appears to be the consequence of this passive translocation of the axoplasm (Tuček, 1974, 1975).

Although the changes of ChAc activity at the proximal end of the peripheral nerve stump do not support the assumption of a retrograde streaming of ChAc, it is necessary to stress that they do not exclude it either. If the retrograde transfer system were operating at the same time as the more active orthograde system, it might be completely overshadowed so that there would be no accumulation, and perhaps even a decrease, of the enzyme at the proximal end of the peripheral nerve stump. The fact that AChE, cellular organelles and some enzymes associated with them, can accumulate at the central end of the peripheral nerve stump despite simultaneous orthograde transport, probably has a specific cause. For unknown reasons the intracellular organelles tend to become sequestered at the blind ends of the axons immediately below the ligature, and thus become eliminated from the bidirectional circulation in the neuron (Lubińska, 1964).

3.4.4 The size of the transportable portion of choline acetyltransferase in the axons

The existence of proximo–distal axonal transport of ChAc is beyond any doubt. A question which remains, however, is whether all ChAc present in the axons is subjected to proximo–distal transport, or whether the transport concerns only a certain proportion of it. In the case of the fast transport of AChE, the answer to this question has been obtained mainly from experiments on isolated nerve segments; these indicated, with a high degree of certainty, that the proximo–distal transport involves 5–10% of the total enzyme content in the nerve (see Section 3.3). It is not clear whether the remaining enzyme is stationary or is moving at a slow rate. In the case of ChAc, an attempt to use isolated nerve segments to find the size of the mobile fraction of the enzyme has been made by Fonnum *et al.* (1973, 1976). They found in studies on rabbit vagus nerve *in vivo* that the amount of ChAc accumulating at the distal end of isolated nerve segments is considerably smaller than that accumulating at the distal end of the central nerve stumps. They interpreted the low accumulation at the distal end of the isolated segments to mean that only a minor part of the total enzyme content in the axons is mobile, that this mobile enzyme moves rapidly and that the accumulation at the distal end of the segment stops as soon as all the mobile enzyme has reached the end of the segment. If this were so, the accumulation should occur rapidly and then stop. This is, indeed, what is found for AChE (Fig. 3.10), but in the case of ChAc, findings are discrepant. In the experiments of Fonnum *et al.* (1976) on rabbit vagus nerve, ChAc initially accumulated rapidly but after 3–5 h the accumulation slowed down although it did not stop. On the other hand, in experiments made by Tuček (1975) on the rabbit peroneal nerve, the activity of

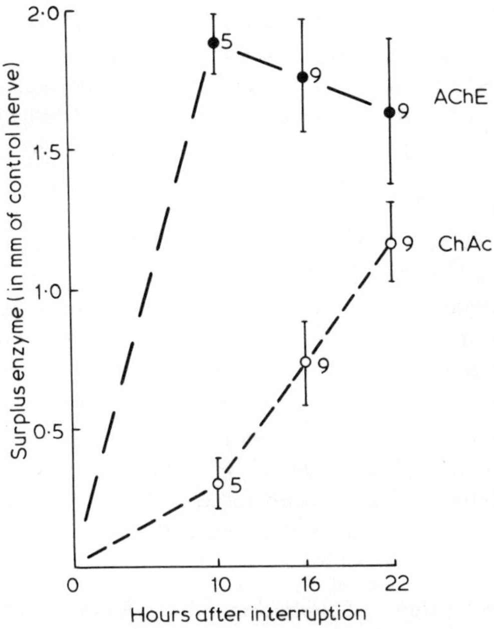

Fig. 3.10 Comparison of the increase of ChAc and AChE activity at the distal end of isolated segments of rabbit peroneal nerves *in situ* during the 22 h following a double interruption of the nerves. Filled circles correspond to AChE, open circles to ChAc. The increase in the activity above the original level is expressed as the length of the control nerve (mm) which contained the same amount of enzyme as that accumulated in the distal 4 mm of the isolated segment. Total length of the segment was about 36 mm. The bars indicate S.E.M. The number of observations is shown beside individual points (Tuček, 1975).

ChAc at the distal ends of the isolated segments increased continuously and linearly up to 22 h (Fig. 3.10). As already mentioned in Section 3.4.2, the rate of accumulation was much slower at the end of the isolated segment than at the end of the central nerve stump (Fig. 3.7). This indicates that the extent of the transport is considerably diminished after a loss of the continuity between neuronal bodies and their axons. It thus seems impossible to use isolated nerve segments (Fonnum *et al.*, 1973) or peripheral stumps of interrupted nerves (Dahlström *et al.*, 1975a; Dziegielewska *et al.*, 1976) in experiments to answer the question about the size of the mobile fraction of ChAc in normal nerves; these limitations probably also apply to the investigation of all substances moved by slow axonal transport.

At present, there is no unequivocal answer to the question about the true rate of transport of ChAc in the axons. If the transport involves all ChAc in the axons, then the rate at which it accumulates above ligatures on the nerve clearly indicates that

ChAc is moving slowly, at a rate of the order of 3–6 mm per day in mammalian nerves. If the mobile enzyme constitutes only a minor proportion of its total content in the nerve, then the rate of transport will be much faster than these values suggest. Experimental support for the view that the mobile portion represents only a small part of the ChAc in the axons is not convincing. For an investigator who inclines to the view that ChAc is transported by a slow mechanism, the problem remains as to whether this would be too slow to provide adequate transport of unstable proteins over long distances.

In terms of the slow transport of ChAc, it would be difficult to explain the observations described by Oesch and Thoenen (1973) that the activity of ChAc in the superior cervical sympathetic ganglia increased considerably as early as 24 h after an injection of reserpine. Since ChAc in the ganglia is present mainly in the terminals of preganglionic fibres and is supplied to them from neurons in the spinal cord, it would be impossible for the additional enzyme synthesized after the injection of reserpine to reach the ganglia within one day, if the enzyme were using the slow transport mechanism. The observations of Oesch and Thoenen (1973) have not, however, been confirmed in later investigations by Hendry (1976). In his experiments, reserpine was without effect on ChAc in the superior cervical ganglion.

3.4.5 Changes of the transport of choline acetyltransferase in old age and under pathological conditions

Age changes of ChAc transport have been investigated by Jablecki and Brimijoin (1975) in experiments on mice. The amount of enzyme accumulating above a ligature on the sciatic nerve was about the same between 2 and 6 weeks of age, but it later declined with age. At the age of 12 weeks it was less than 50%, and at the age of 36 weeks less than 30% of the amount accumulating at 6 weeks. It is thus evident that the amount of enzyme transported per unit time from the perikarya to the axons decreases with age – in spite of the fact that, in Jablecki's and Brimijoin's experiments, the activity of ChAc per mm length of the nerves increased up to the age of 36 weeks. From the accumulations above the ligatures, the authors calculated the average rate of ChAc transport, which would correspond to the true speed of ChAc transport if all the enzyme in the axons were mobile; they arrived at the conclusion that the average rate of transport decreases from 3.5 mm/day at 2 weeks to 0.2 mm/day at 36 weeks.

Among pathological conditions investigated in relation to the axonal transport of ChAc are ischaemia, diabetes and hereditary muscular dystrophy. Changes of ChAc activity and transport in peripheral nerves undergoing regeneration after transection are discussed in Chapter 7.7. The effect of ischaemia on ChAc and AChE transport has been investigated in experiments on isolated nerve segments *in vivo*, similar to those already described in Fig. 3.6. Under conditions of intact blood supply, the activity of ChAc increased at the distal end of the segments, and the activity of AChE at both ends, indicating that proximo–distal transport of ChAc, and proximo–distal and disto–proximal transport of AChE, were operating in the segments. When,

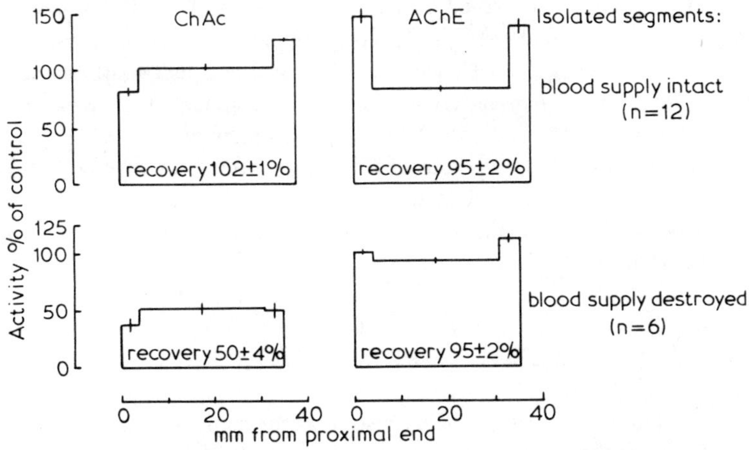

Fig. 3.11 The effect of ischaemia on the distribution of ChAc and AChE activity in isolated segments of rabbit peroneal nerves. Top: the segment was prepared with care to preserve the blood supply. Bottom: the segment was completely isolated from surrounding tissue and thus deprived of the blood supply. The segments were kept *in situ* 22 h and then taken out, divided into three parts approximately 4 mm, 28 mm, and 4 mm long, and homogenized. The activities of both enzymes were measured in the same homogenates. Abscissa: distance (mm) from the proximal end of isolated segments. Ordinate: enzyme activity, expressed as percentage of activity in the corresponding part of the intact contralateral control nerve. The bars show S.E.M. Data in individual blocks show the total enzyme activity found in the whole segment 22 h after it had been formed, expressed as a percentage of the activity found in the same length of the contralateral control nerve (after Tuček *et al.*, 1978b).

however, the segments were deprived of their blood supply, the translocation of ChAc and AChE to the appropriate ends of the segments was abolished or considerably reduced, indicating that axonal transport was arrested during ischaemia (Fig. 3.11; Tuček *et al.*,). In addition, the total activity of ChAc in the isolated segment diminished by 50% during 22 h of ischaemia, while in isolated control segments with preserved blood supply it remained at the level found in intact nerves. The effect of ischaemia on axonal transport of ChAc and AChE *in vivo* is in agreement with the effect of anoxia and metabolic inhibitors on axonal transport of radioactively labelled proteins in experiments *in vitro* (Ochs and Ranish, 1970; Ochs and Hollingsworth, 1971; Ochs, 1974). The intriguing question is, of course, whether those degrees of hypoxia which may occur in human patients with sclerotic changes of the arteries, anaemia or similar conditions, may also affect axonal transport of ChAc and other substances. Preliminary experiments in rats indicate that mild degrees of hypoxia are without effect (Řičný and Tuček, unpublished).

The effect of diabetes on axonal transport of ChAc and AChE has been investigated in rats in which diabetes had been produced by the administration of streptozotocine (Schmidt *et al.*, 1975). The rate of accumulation of ChAc and AChE above a ligature on the sciatic nerve was decreased by 40% and 20%, respectively; it returned to control values after the administration of insulin. In mice with hereditary muscular dystrophy, the calculated average rate of ChAc transport is lower than in normal animals. Although the activity of ChAc per mm nerve is increased, the amount of enzyme transported per unit time down the sciatic nerve is about 50% of normal (Jablecki and Brimijoin, 1974).

3.5 AXONAL TRANSPORT OF ACETYLCHOLINE

In adrenergic, cholinergic, and probably also in other neurons, the transmitters are mainly produced in the terminal portions of the axons; a minor part of the total transmitter synthesis occurs, however, in neuronal bodies and in the course of the axons. In vertebrates, ACh and noradrenaline are, therefore, regularly present in peripheral nerves containing motor and sympathetic fibres. It is not clear whether the transmitter compounds play some physiological role in the axons. Most probably, their presence there is a passive consequence of the presence of the enzymes and corresponding substrates necessary for their synthesis. Any transmitter produced in the axons is transported towards the nerve endings.

Axonal transport of noradrenaline has received much attention (reviews Dahlström and Häggendal, 1970; Dahlström, 1967b, 1971; Banks and Mayor, 1972; Dahlström and Heiwall, 1975). In sympathetic postganglionic axons, noradrenaline is contained in adrenergic storage granules and experiments on rat and cat show it to be transported proximo–distally within the granules at a speed estimated at 120–240 mm/day. Compared with the amount of noradrenaline which is produced in terminal parts of sympathetic nerve fibres, the amount of noradrenaline supplied via axonal transport is very low. Axonal transport is adrenergic storage granules to the nerve endings is physiologically important not for the supply of noradrenaline itself, but rather for the supply of structural constituents of the granules and the protein located in them.

Axonal transport of ACh has been investigated mainly in experiments on cut, crushed or ligated nerves. There is little doubt that the transport is responsible for most of the increase of ACh concentration observed at the end of the central stump of interrupted nerves (Evans and Saunders, 1967). In experiments on rat sciatic nerve, the rate of accumulation of ACh above the site of interruption of the nerve would correspond to a rate of proximo–distal transport equal to 24 mm/day if all ACh contained in the nerve were transported proximo–distally at the same rate (Dahlström *et al.*, 1974a). The true rate of transport is probably higher, but it does not involve all ACh in the axons; Dahlström *et al.* estimate that the mobile fraction of ACh in the nerve represents only 20% of the total ACh content, and that the rate of proximo–distal transport of mobile ACh is 120 mm/day. The estimate of the mobile fraction of ACh in the nerve is based on measurements of the decrease of ACh content in the peripheral nerve stump. It is difficult to make an exact estimate, since the decrease of ACh in the peripheral nerve stump immediately after nerve transection is rather variable (Häggendal *et al.*, 1971, 1973; Dahlström *et al.*, 1974a), and available data do not allow a clear distinction between the decrease caused by continuing proximo–distal transport and that caused by incipient Wallerian degeneration.

In sympathetic preganglionic nerve fibres, the accumulation of ACh above the site of interruption is much slower than in the sciatic nerve. At the same time, the proportion of mobile ACh is also smaller (5%), so that the rate of transport calculated for the preganglionic sympathetic fibres is 120 mm/day, just as for the sciatic nerve (Häggendal *et al.*, 1973). In the nerve segments separated from the cell bodies the transport of ACh continues: in the nerves interrupted at two sites simultaneously, the content of ACh increases proximal to both lesions (Häggendal *et al.*, 1971).

ACh probably has two forms in the peripheral nerves, and may be freely dissolved in the axoplasm or bound in the organelles, possibly in vesicles similar to synaptic vesicles. According to Prajmovski and Welsh (1948), rat nerves contain about 70% of ACh as free ACh; Welsch and Dettbarn (1970) find that in lobster nerves all the ACh is free; and according to Carlini and Green (1963) the ACh dissolved in the axoplasm represents about 2/3 of the total ACh content of rabbit nerves. In agreement with these findings and with further data on axonal transport, it seems very likely that the increase in the amount of ACh proximal to an interruption of a nerve is mainly caused by the accumulation of ACh-containing vesicles which are being transported proximo–distally by the fast axonal transport; at the same time, the ACh which is dissolved in the axoplasm is probably being moved by the slow transport mechanism (Dahlström *et al.*, 1974a). The assumption that the ACh accumulating above the site of nerve interruption is contained in some kind of intra-axonal organelles, is supported by observations that boiling at acid pH is necessary in order to extract it from the tissue (Heilbronn and Pettersson, 1973), and by the results of subcellular fractionations of the nerve segments immediately above the sites of the nerve crush (Dahlström *et al.*, 1974b).

The investigation of axonal transport of ACh on the basis of its accumulation proximal to the site of interruption of the nerve is complicated by the fact that mechanical damage to the nerve stimulates local synthesis of ACh and produces an increase in its content (Feldberg, 1943; Häggendal *et al.*, 1971); the mechanism of this phenomenon is not clear. This traumatic local synthesis is probably responsible for the small increase in the content of ACh observed in a short nerve segment immediately distal to the site at which the nerve had been crushed or ligated, and also for some of the much greater increase found proximal to the crush or ligature (Dahlström *et al.*, 1974a).

Axonal transport of ACh has also been demonstrated in intact nerves in experiments using the administration of radioactive precursors. After the injection of [^{3}H] choline into a giant cholinergic nerve cell of *Aplysia*, ACh is transported in its axon at two rates – 17 mm/day and 55 mm/day (Koike *et al.*, 1972); in the intact antennal nerve of *Leucophaea maderae*, ACh is transported at a speed of 120–130 mm/day (Schafer, 1973).

Axonal transport of ACh in rat sciatic nerve can be arrested by the administration of colchicine or vinblastine into the spinal cord or into the nerve (Dahlström *et al.*, 1974b; Dahlström and Heiwall, 1975; Heiwall *et al.*, 1976). When injected sub-epineurally, the alkaloids cause the accumulation of ACh in the nerve segment into which they have been injected. At the same time, they prevent the accumulation of ACh above a crush located more distally on the nerve. Just as in the case of the axonal transport of ChAc (see Section 3.4.1), the effects of colchicine and vinblastine on ACh transport may be associated with their action on the microtubules, but there is, again, the question of whether the alkaloids are also acting in some other way which is not yet understood.

The ACh which is supplied by axonal transport probably represents just a small portion of the total turnover of ACh in the nerve endings. This view is based on an analogy with adrenergic nerves and on a comparison between the transport and the turnover of ACh in preganglionic sympathetic fibres. In preganglionic fibres to the superior cervical ganglion of the rat, the amount of ACh accumulating within 12 h proximal to the site of their interruption represents no more than 2.5% of the total ACh store in the ganglion (Häggendal *et al.*, 1973). This seems to be very little, since it is known from experiments on cat sympathetic ganglia that the resting release alone can effect the exchange of all ACh in the ganglia within 8–16 h, and that the turnover of ACh in the ganglia is increased many times by nerve impulses (see Chapter 6.6; Birks and MacIntosh, 1961).

3.6 SUMMARY

In spite of enormous experimental effort, the phenomenon of axonal transport is poorly understood. The transport proceeds in two directions – proximo–distal (orthograde) and disto–proximal (retrograde). The proximo–distal transport seems to proceed in all axons with at least two different speeds:

(1) the so-called slow transport, 1–10 mm/day in mammalian nerves;
(2) the so-called fast transport, 200–400 mm/day in mammalian nerves.

Transport at intermediary speeds also occurs. Only a fast component has been demonstrated for disto–proximal transport. The slow transport involves mainly the soluble constituents of the axoplasm, whereas the fast transport involves mainly axonal organelles and membrane-bound enzymes. The fast transport is dependent on the supply of energy; the need for energy has not been clarified in the case of slow transport. The mechanism by which either kind of transport is effected is not known. Some hypotheses assume that the transport occurs at a continuum of velocities and that it is based on one common transport mechanism.

ChAc appears to be transported slowly in mammalian nerves, at a rate of 1–6 mm/day. Its transport probably involves all the enzyme in the axons and proceeds in the proximo–distal direction only; the transported enzyme is not associated with axonal organelles. There is, however, an alternative hypothesis which assumes that the transport concerns only a small part of ChAc in the axons, but that it proceeds at a high rate. Contradictions on this point are difficult to resolve, since there is no known way of determining the size of the mobile fraction of ChAc in the axons. Axonal transport of ChAc continues in the axons separated from nerve cell bodies, but its intensity is diminished. It is blocked by ischaemia.

ACh is also transported proximo–distally in cholinergic axons. The rate of its transport is estimated at 120 mm/day in mammalian nerves. The transport probably involves only the bound ACh in the axons, i.e. the ACh contained in some unidentified axonal organelles, about 20% of the total ACh content. The ACh supplied to the nerve endings via axonal transport represents a very minor part of the total amount of ACh which is necessary for synaptic transmission. Most ACh is synthesized in the nerve terminals, i.e. in the immediate vicinity of the synapses.

Axonal transport of AChE proceeds at a fast rate in both directions. The transported enzyme is associated with axonal organelles and represents a small part of the total AChE content in the axons. The transport of AChE in the axons is not dependent on the connection between the axons and the bodies of the nerve cells.

AUTHOR'S NOTE

L.P. Davies, W.P. Whittaker and H. Zimmermann (*Expl. Brain Res.* **30**, 493–510, 1977) have suggested that in *Torpedo marmorata* electromotor nerves, the proximo–distal transport of ChAc occurs at a velocity of 50–140 mm/day; the suggestion is based on the estimate that only about 15% of the axoplasmic enzyme is mobile.

4 Supply of acetyl groups for the synthesis of acetylcholine

4.1 INTRODUCTION

For some neurotransmitters, we have complete information about their precursors and even about the precursors of their precursors. For example there is no doubt about the chain of events leading to the synthesis of noradrenaline. It involves the consecutive transformation of four precursors, phenylalanine, tyrosine, dihydroxyphenylalanine and dopamine to noradrenaline, and the enzymes catalysing the individual steps of the transformation are well known. As far as is ACh concerned, however, only the parent substances have been established beyond doubt: acetyl–CoA and choline. There are no simple answers to the questions about the provenance of the acetyl groups of the acetyl–CoA and about the provenance of the choline. One of the big difficulties encountered in the research into the origin of acetyl groups in the acetyl–CoA used for ACh synthesis arises from the fact that ACh is synthesized exclusively in the cholinergic neurons, mainly in the cytoplasm (extramitochondrial space) of the terminal portions of their axons, whereas acetyl–CoA is produced in all cells of the nervous system, its synthesis being partly extramitochondrial but mainly intramitochondrial. In view of the complexity of brain structure and of possible changes in membrane permeability during isolation of subcellular fractions, it does not seem feasible at present to isolate that pool of acetyl–CoA which is localized specifically at the site of ACh synthesis, i.e. in the extramitochondrial space of presynaptic cholinergic nerve terminals, and to investigate it separately from other acetyl–CoA in the brain. For this and other reasons, there is surprisingly little certainty in our current understanding of the metabolism of acetyl groups in the brain as related to the biosynthesis of ACh. This chapter contains basic data on the role of acetyl–CoA in the main metabolic pathways, on the intracellular localization of enzymes forming acetyl–CoA in the brain, on experiments concerning the utilization of potential precursors of acetyl–CoA for the synthesis of ACh in the nervous tissue, and on the problem of transfer of acetyl–CoA from the mitochondrial matrix into the extramitochondrial space.

Many aspects of these problems have been discussed in earlier reviews by Hebb (1972), Tuček (1970, 1973b), Browning (1976) and Barker (1976a).

4.2 POSITION OF ACETYLCOENZYME A IN THE MAIN METABOLIC PATHWAYS AND ITS CONTENT IN THE BRAIN

Acetyl–CoA plays an important role in the metabolism of carbohydrates, fatty acids and some amino acids (Fig. 4.1). Its properties and metabolic functions have been thoroughly reviewed by Decker (1959).

During the catabolism of monosaccharides, acetyl–CoA is the connecting link between glycolysis and the Krebs cycle. It is produced by oxidative decarboxylation of pyruvate, catalysed by the pyruvate dehydrogenase complex (Reed *et al.*, 1972). The complex is formed by pyruvate dehydrogenase, dihydrolipoyl transacetylase, dihydrolipoyl dehydrogenase, pyruvate dehydrogenase kinase and pyruvate dehydrogenase phosphate phosphatase. Thiamine pyrophosphate, lipoic acid, coenzyme A, flavine adenine dinucleotide and nicotinamide adenine dinucleotide play the role of coenzyme in individual steps of oxidative decarboxylation of pyruvate. Acetyl–CoA formed from pyruvate reacts with oxaloacetate in a reaction catalysed by citrate synthase and yielding citric acid, which is further metabolized in the Krebs cycle.

Acetyl–CoA is also the connecting link between the oxidative cycle of the fatty acids and the Krebs cycle. Every cycle of the β-oxidation of fatty acids (see review by Greville and Tubbs, 1968) leads to the formation of a 3-ketoacyl–CoA, which then reacts with CoA in a reaction catalysed by 3-ketoacyl–CoA thiolase and yields acetyl–CoA and an acyl–CoA in which the acyl group is two carbons shorter than that in the original 3-ketoacyl–CoA. The acetyl–CoA thus formed also enters the Krebs cycle by condensation with oxaloacetate to citric acid in a reaction catalysed by citrate synthase.

During the catabolism of amino acids, acetyl–CoA is formed from substances which are also the intermediary products in the metabolism of carbohydrates and fatty acids, namely pyruvate, acetoacetate, 3-hydroxy-3-methylglutaryl–CoA and acetate. Pyruvate arises as an intermediary product during the catabolism of alanine, serine, threonine, glycine, cysteine and cystine; acetyl–CoA is formed from pyruvate by oxidative decarboxylation. Threonine yields acetyl–CoA also via acetate. Acetoacetate is formed during the catabolism of phenylalanine, tyrosine, tryptophan and lysine; it is then transformed to acetoacetyl–CoA which reacts with CoA in a reaction catalysed by acetoacetyl–CoA thiolase to form two molecules of acetyl–CoA. The catabolism of leucine yields 3-hydroxy-3-methylglutaryl–CoA, which is split to acetyl–CoA and acetoacetate in a reaction catalysed by 3-hydroxy-3-methylglutaryl–CoA lyase.

The utilization of acetyl groups of acetyl–CoA for oxidative metabolism in animal cells always occurs through the chain of reactions of the Krebs cycle.

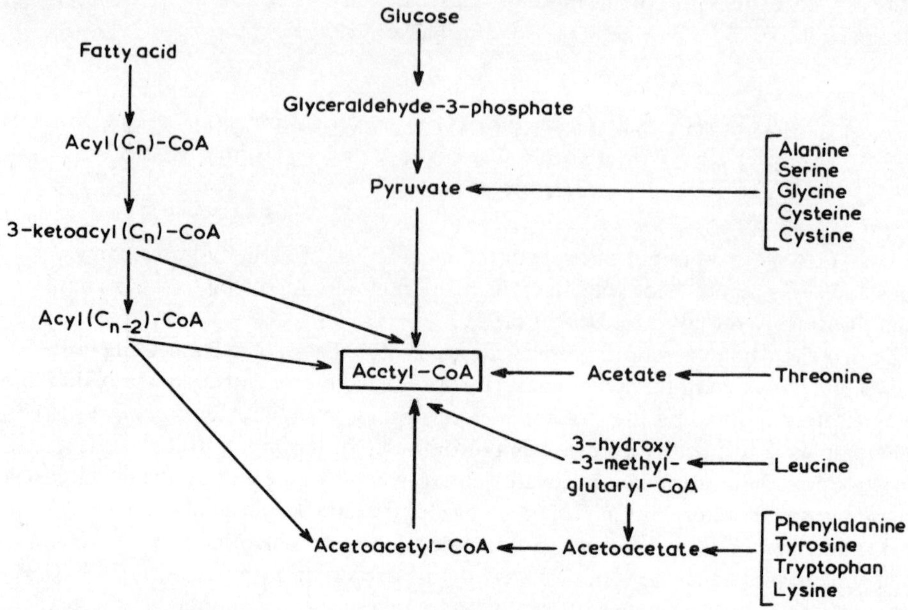

Fig. 4.1 The position of acetyl–CoA in the catabolism of fatty acids, glucose and amino acids.

Acetyl–CoA, however, is also used for many synthetic purposes, e.g. for the synthesis of fatty acids, steroids and acetylated compounds like acetylcarnitine, acetylaspartate, etc. Only the use of acetyl–CoA for the synthesis of ACh will be discussed in this chapter.

In view of the special features of cerebral metabolism it is important to consider the question of whether and how, acetyl–CoA may be formed from the carbon atoms of tricarboxylic and dicarboxylic acids – intermediates of the Krebs cycle. It is well known that the energy metabolism of the brain is based mainly (although not exclusively) on the utilization of glucose (reviews Bradford, 1968; McIlwain and Bachelard, 1971), but it is also known that after an injection of glucose or pyruvate with radioactively labelled carbon most radioactivity in the brain very soon appears in the large pool of brain amino acids, particularly of glutamic and aspartic acids (Busch, 1955; Gaitonde *et al.*, 1965). These amino acids can be used as a stock of fuel for the metabolism of the brain. In case of need they are oxidized in the Krebs cycle, into which they enter after the transformation of the glutamic acid to α-ketoglutaric acid and of aspartic acid to oxaloacetic acid. Acetyl–CoA can be formed from the oxaloacetic acid with oxaloacetic acid being first decarboxylated to pyruvic acid, which in turn is subjected to oxidative decarboxylation. The carbon atoms of the glutamic or α-ketoglutaric acid can be used for the production of acetyl groups of acetyl–CoA in two ways (Greville, 1969):

(a) In the orthograde direction of the Krebs cycle – by transformation of α-ketoglutarate to succinate, fumarate, malate and oxaloacetate, and then by the decarboxylation of oxaloacetate to pyruvate and by oxidation decarboxylation of pyruvate to acetyl–CoA; the metabolism of glutamate may also proceed via the so-called GABA shunt, i.e. by sequential transformations of glutamate to γ-aminobutyrate, succinic semialdehyde and succinate, with subsequent changes proceeding through oxaloacetate as indicated above.

(b) In the retrograde direction of the Krebs cycle – by transformation of α-ketoglutarate to isocitrate and citrate, followed by the cleavage of citrate to oxaloacetate and acetyl–CoA (D'Adamo and Haft, 1965; D'Adamo and D'Adamo, 1968). The cleavage of citrate to acetyl–CoA and oxaloacetate is catalysed by the enzyme ATP citrate lyase (see Section 4.3), which is different from citrate synthase, the enzyme responsible for the synthesis of citrate from acetyl–CoA and oxaloacetate in the initial reaction of the Krebs cycle.

The content of acetyl–CoA in the brain is very low, compared with the content of most other intermediates of basic metabolic pathways. As may be seen from data summarized in Table 4.1, it is in the range 2–14 nmol/g fresh weight.

Table 4.1 Acetyl–CoA content in the central nervous system

Organ	Concentration of acetyl–CoA (nmol/g)	References
Rat brain	3.91	Schuberth *et al.* (1965)
Brain of rat fed *ad libitum*	4.9	Schuberth *et al.* 1966b)
Brain of fed rat	8	Allred and Guy (1969)
Brain of rat fed *ad libitum*	6.2	Heinrich *et al.* (1973)
Brain of rat with avitaminosis B_1	3.6	
Brain of fed rat	3.0	Ruderman *et al.* (1974)
Brain of rat after 48 h starvation	4.8	
Brain of rat with streptozotocin diabetes	6.6	
Brain of rat with phloridzin diabetes	4.5	
Brain of rat fed *ad libitum*	9.4; 11.0; 14.2 (results from 3 experimental groups)	Reynolds and Blass (1975)
Brain of rat with avitaminosis B_1, fed *ad libitum*	8.9; 12.5; 16.7 (results from 3 experimental groups)	
Brain of mouse after 18 h starvation	2.86	Kato (1975)

Table 4.1 (*continued*) Acetyl–CoA content in the central nervous system

Organ	Concentration of acetyl–CoA (nmol/g)	References
Cerebelium of mouse after 18 h starvation	2.69	
Rat brain	5.1	Guynn (1976)
Rat brain; see original text for data on acetyl–CoA in 8 brain regions	5.5	Shea and Aprison (1977)

4.3 INTRACELLULAR LOCALIZATION OF ACETYLCOENZYME–A FORMING ENZYMES IN THE BRAIN

Considerations concerning the organization of the synthesis of ACh have to take into account data on the intracellular location for the synthesis of acetyl–CoA. This location is, of course, identical to the localization of the enzymes producing acetyl–CoA. The basic techniques used to discover the localization of enzymes in the cells are histochemistry and subcellular fractionation. It is mainly the latter method which has been successfully applied to the investigation of the enzymes forming acetyl–CoA in the brain and of ChAc. This chapter describes the method of subcellular fractionation, as usually applied to the brain, and summarizes available data on the subcellular localization of enzymes producing acetyl–CoA in the brain.

4.3.1 Subcellular fractionation of brain homogenates

Excellent reviews have been published explaining the theoretical basis of subcellular fractionation (Anderson, 1956) and summarizing the results of its use for the study of the localization of enzymes in cells outside the nervous system (De Duve *et al.*, 1962; Roodyn, 1965) and for the study of enzymes and transmitters within the nervous system (Whittaker, 1965; for recent comments on subcellular and cellular fractionation of the brain tissue see Morgan, 1976). Subcellular fractionation is based on the fact that, during the centrifugation of tissue homogenates in suitable media, the various particles of which the homogenate is composed sediment at different velocities. Two approaches are used for the separation of individual particle types:

(a) Differential centrifugation, i.e. repeated centrifugation of the homogenates at speeds which are increased in a stepwise sequence.

(b) Centrifugation in a density gradient. The separation of a mixture of particles is achieved by centrifugation, during which the particles are forced into a

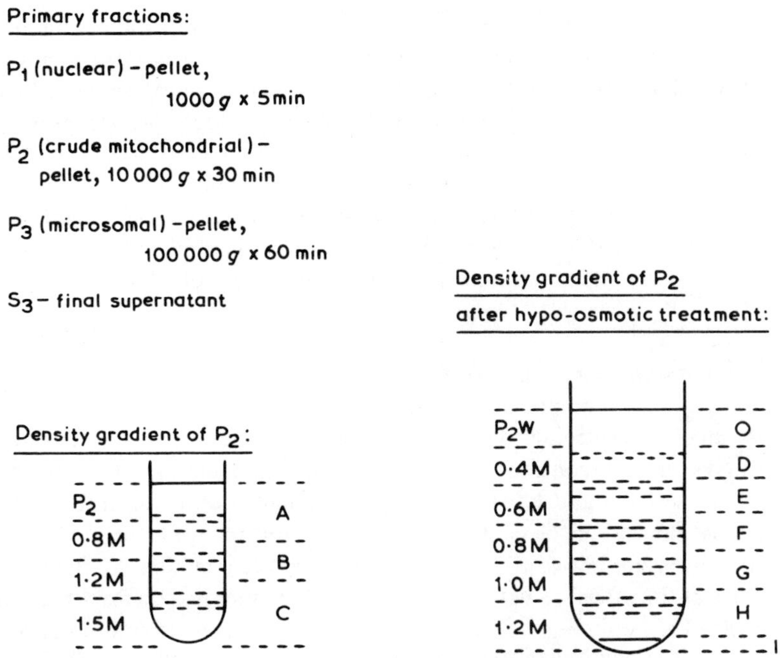

Fig. 4.2 Scheme of subcellular fractionation of brain homogenates by differential centrifugation (primary fractions) and density gradient centrifugation. See text for explanations.

medium the density of which increases from the top to the bottom of the centrifugation tube. The density increases either in comparatively sharp steps (discontinuous gradient) or gradually (continuous gradient). Depending on many factors, the sedimentation of various kinds of subcellular particles is arrested at various levels of the density gradients.

The technique of subcellular fractionation as performed in different laboratories differs in many features (e.g. in the choice of the homogenization medium, speed and duration of centrifugation, and composition and steepness of the density gradient). The fractionation scheme most widely used for studies of subcellular localization of enzymes in the brain has been that based on the investigations of Hebb and Whittaker (1958), Gray and Whittaker (1962) and Whittaker *et al.* (1964). It has been used in a great number of studies both from Whittaker's and from other laboratories (reviews Whittaker, 1965, 1969a). A short description of this type of fractionation follows (see also Fig. 4.2).

Differential centrifugation of brain homogenate

A homogenate prepared in 0.32M sucrose is centrifuged for 10 min at 800–1000 *g*. The pellet contains mainly cell nuclei and those cells which had escaped disintegration.

In order to reduce its contamination with other particles, it is resuspended once or twice in fresh aliquots of the original medium and recentrifuged at the same speed. The pellet is designated as faction P_1 or the nuclear fraction. The supernatant solutions from all centrifugations needed for the separation and washing of P_1 are combined (fraction S_1) and centrifuged for 30 min at 10 000 *g*. The pellet is designated as P_2 or the crude mitochondrial fraction. It contains mainly mitochondria, nerve endings and fragments of myelin. The supernatant solution (fraction S_2) is centrifuged 60 min at 100 000 *g*. The pellet is designated as P_3 or the microsomal fraction. Its main constituents are fragments of the endoplasmic reticulum and ribosomes. The supernatant solution (fraction S_3) contains soluble components of the cytoplasm.

Centrifugation on the density gradient

(a) Separation of basic components of the crude mitochondrial fraction. The pellet P_2 is resuspended in 0.32M sucrose and the suspension carefully pipetted as the uppermost layer on a discontinuous gradient, consisting (from the top to the bottom) of layers of 0.8M, 1.2M and 1.5M sucrose. The gradient is centrifuged for 120 min at 50 000 *g*. At the end of the centrifugation the fragments of myelin are concentrated mainly at the interface between 0.32M and 0.8M sucrose (fraction A), the isolated nerve endings at the interface between 0.8M and 1.2M sucrose (fraction B), and mitochondria at the interface between 1.2M and 1.5M sucrose (fraction C). It has been pointed out recently that fraction B may be contaminated by particles of glial origin (Henn *et al.*, 1976).

(b) Separation of basic constituents of the nerve endings after 'osmotic shock'. Isolated nerve endings (synaptosomes – see Whitaker, 1969a) are closed structures, whose surface has been resealed at the point at which they had been torn off the axons. They consist of the surface membrane of the presynaptic nerve ending (frequently with a portion of postsynaptic membrane attached to it as well), intraterminal axoplasm and intraterminal organelles, mainly the mitochondria and synaptic vesicles. When exposed to a hypotonic medium, the synaptosomes swell, their surface membrane is ruptured and their content is released. The osmotic sensitivity of the synaptosomes is exploited in the separation of their main components. Either fraction B from the density gradient or, more frequently, the crude mitochondrial fraction P_2 is exposed to hypotonic conditions. The pellet (deposited at the bottom of the tube by previous centrifugation) is suspended in water, the suspension is suitably stirred (e.g. by repeated sucking into and out of a pipette), and then it is put on the top (P_2W – see Fig. 4.2) of the discontinuous density gradient consisting (from the top to the bottom) of layers of 0.4M, 0.6M, 0.8M, 1.0M and 1.2M sucrose. The gradient is then centrifuged for 120 min at 50 000 *g*. Afterwards the gradient is divided into fractions O, D, E, F, G, H and I as shown in Fig. 4.2. Fraction O corresponds to the top layer of the gradient, originally formed by the hypotonically treated fraction, P_2W, and contains the soluble components of the cytoplasm of the nerve endings. Fraction D contains synaptic vesicles, while the main constituents of fractions E, F and G are emptied membranes ('ghosts') of the nerve endings. Fraction H contains mainly incompletely emptied nerve endings and fraction I the mitochondria.

4.3.2 Pyruvate dehydrogenase complex

The five enzymes of which the complex is composed have already been enumerated in Section 4.2. Pyruvate dehydrogenase, dihydrolipoyl transacetylase and dihydrolipoyl dehydrogenase together catalyse the reaction of oxidative decarboxylation of pyruvate which is summarized by the equation:

$$\text{pyruvate}^- + NAD^+ + CoA = \text{acetyl–CoA} + NADH + CO_2\,.$$

The recognition of the existence and functional role of pyruvate dehydrogenase kinase and pyruvate dehydrogenase phosphate phosphatase is a recent contribution to the understanding of the regulation of the complex (Linn *et al.*, 1969a, b). Pyruvate dehydrogenase kinase is responsible for the ATP-dependent phosphorylation of a serine moiety of pyruvate dehydrogenase. As a result of the phosphorylation, the pyruvate dehydrogenase complex is inactivated. Pyruvate dehydrogenase phosphate phosphatase reactivates it by removing the phosphate. Most data concerning the enzymatic regulation of the pyruvate dehydrogenase complex by pyruvate dehydrogenase kinase and pyruvate dehydrogenase phosphate phosphatase have been obtained on the heart, liver and adipose tissue. It has been demonstrated, however, that control by phosphorylation and dephosphorylation is also operating in the brain (Jope and Blass, 1975, 1976; Księżak, 1976). Investigations of this, and of other ways of regulating the pyruvate dehydrogenase complex have been reviewed by Denton *et al.* (1975).

Studies of the subcellular localization of the pyruvate dehydrogenase complex in organs other than the brain have shown that it is localized in the mitochondria (Sanadi, 1963). The same is also certainly true for the brain. A particulate fraction obtained from brain tissue homogenized in 0.9% KCl and centrifuged at 2000 *g* was found to perform the complete oxidation of pyruvate via the Krebs cycle (Green *et al.*, 1948). The ability of brain mitochondria to utilize pyruvate as a substrate for oxidative metabolism has been thoroughly analyzed by Balázs *et al.* (1964). In experiments with subcellular fractionation of rabbit brain homogenate, 96% of the total activity of the pyruvate dehydrogenase complex was found in the crude mitochondrial fraction (Fig. 4.3); when this fraction was further separated on a density gradient, most activity appeared in the mitochondrial subfraction C and a proportion in the nerve ending subfraction B, where it was probably localized in the intrasynaptosomal mitochondria (Tuček, 1967c).

During the 1960's, the question of the exact intramitochondrial localization of the pyruvate dehydrogenase complex and of most Krebs cycle enzymes and enzymes responsible for the oxidation and elongation of fatty acids, was the subject of a major controversy (see Tuček, 1970). At present, there is little, if any, doubt that

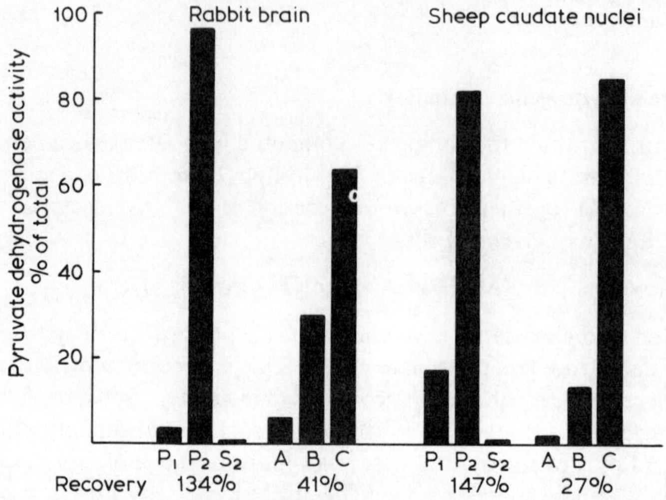

Fig. 4.3 The distribution of the pyruvate dehydrogenase complex in subcellular fractions of rabbit brain and sheep caudate nuclei. The fractions correspond to those on Fig. 4.2; S_2 is the supernatant after the sedimentation of the crude mitochondrial fraction P_2. Centrifugation on the density gradient was associated with considerable loss of activity of the pyruvate dehydrogenase complex; the greatest loss probably occurred in fraction C, containing purified mitochondria, which sediment to the bottom of the gradients (based on Tuček, 1967c).

the pyruvate dehydrogenase complex is located in the inner compartment of the mitochondria (Schnaitman and Greenwalt, 1968; Tubbs and Garland, 1968). It is probably not completely freely disolved in the mitochondrial matrix space (Denton *et al.*, 1975), but it is certainly separated from the cytosol by the very efficient and selective barrier represented by the inner mitochondrial membrane and by the much less restricitive outer mitochondrial membrane. Observations on the effect of treatment with ether on the activity of the pyruvate dehydrogenase complex in brain mitochondria (measured from the output of pyruvate-generated acetyl–CoA into the incubation medium) substantiate the localization of the complex in the matrix. Mild treatment with ether increased the production of acetyl–CoA 17 fold (Tuček, 1967c). Ether probably acted as a detergent (Tuček, 1967d) and increased the permeability of the inner mitochondrial membrane for acetyl–CoA.

4.3.3 Acetyl–CoA synthetase

The full name of this enzyme is acetate: CoA ligase (AMP), EC 6.2.1.1. It catalyses the reaction:

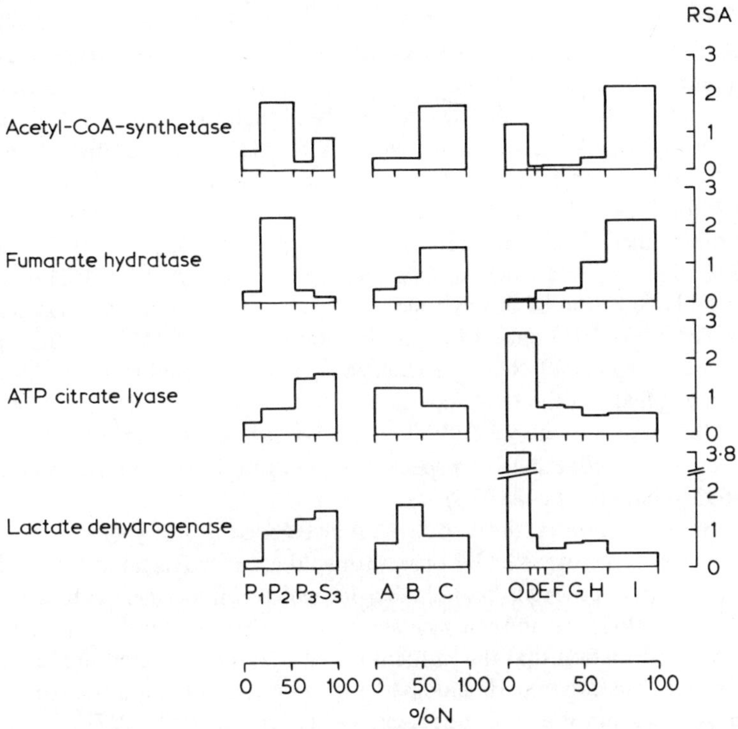

Fig. 4.4 Distribution of acetyl–CoA synthetase, fumarate hydratase, ATP citrate lyase and lactate dehydrogenase in subcellular fractions of sheep caudate nuclei. The fractions correspond to those in Fig. 4.2. The height of the columns indicates the relative specific activities (RSA) of the enzymes in the fractions. The relative specific activities are given by the ratio (per cent of enzyme recovered in the fraction)/(per cent of nitrogen recovered in the fraction). The width of the columns indicates the content of nitrogen in the fractions, expressed as a percentage of the content of nitrogen in the whole homogenate (or, in the case of fractions O–I, as a percentage of the content of nitrogen in the parent fraction P_2) (after Tuček, 1967b).

$$\text{Acetate} + \text{CoA} + \text{ATP} = \text{Acetyl–CoA} + \text{AMP} + \text{PP}_i$$

The literature on the enzyme has been reviewed by Sharkova (1968) and Groot, Scholte and Hülsmann (1976), among others. In the brain much of enzyme is located in the mitochondria, but some is found extramitochondrially. In Schuberth's (1965) experiments the activity of the enzyme which remained in the supernatant after the homogenate of the brain had been centrifuged at 100 000 *g* corresponded to approximately one half of the activity present in the mitochondrial fraction. Tuček (1967b) found that of the total activity recovered 58–67% was in the mitochondrial fraction and 17–25% was in the high speed supernatant (fraction S_3)

(Fig. 4.4). In the same experiments the high speed supernatant contained only 3–4% of the total recoverable activity of fumarate hydratase, an enzyme which is used as a mitochondrial marker in experiments with brain tissue. Presumably, this small amount of fumarate hydratase was present in the S_3 fraction as a result of damage to some mitochondria. The comparatively high proportion of the total activity of acetyl–CoA synthetase recovered in the S_3 fraction of brain homogenates suggests that this enzyme is located not only intramitochondrially, but also partly extramitochondrially. A bimodal localization of acetyl–CoA synthetase has also been found in other tissues (Aas and Bremer, 1968; Martin and Denton, 1970; Barth *et al.*, 1971, 1972; Snoswell and Koundakjian, 1972; Knowles *et al.*, 1974). The assumption of a bimodal localization of the enzyme is fully supported by the observations described by Tencati and Rosenberg (1973) and Reijnierse *et al.* (1975), although it does not agree with the work of Neidle *et al.* (1969), who recovered less than 6% of the total enzyme activity in the final supernatant (i.e. a smaller percentage than is found for some other typically mitochondrial enzymes). It has been suggested that the mitochondrial enzyme is contained in a specific population of brain mitochondria (Neidle *et al.*, 1969; Reijnierse *et al.*, 1975).

Inside the mitochondria, the acetyl–CoA synthetase is probably located in the matrix. This has been suggested by observations that, in the heart mitochondria, the activation of acetate proceeds behind a barrier which is impermeable to acetyl–CoA (Fritz and Yue, 1964), i.e. in the space enclosed by the inner mitochondrial membrane. More direct confirmation that the mitochondrial enzyme is located in the matrix has come from fractionation experiments performed on the mitochondria from the liver and the heart (Aas and Bremer, 1968; Aas, 1971; Scholte *et al.*, 1971), but data on the localization of the enzyme in brain mitochondria are not available. Investigation of this enzyme is difficult because of losses of its activity on density gradients (Tuček, 1967b; Neidle *et al.*, 1969; Tencati and Rosenberg, 1973) and inconsistent recoveries of its activity in other types of experiments (Aas and Bremer, 1968). By analogy with other tissues, however, it appears very likely that the enzyme is also located in the matrix in brain mitochondria.

4.3.4 ATP citrate lyase

The full name of this enzyme is ATP:citrate oxaloacetate lyase (CoA-acetylating and ATP-dephosphorylating), EC 4.1.3.8. Data on the enzyme have been reviewed by, among others, Spector (1972) and Srere (1972, 1975). It catalyses the reaction:

$$\text{Citrate} + \text{CoA} + \text{ATP} = \text{acetyl–CoA} + \text{oxaloacetate} + \text{ADP} + P_i.$$

Experiments on chicken liver (Srere, 1959), guinea pig brain and sheep caudate nuclei (Tuček, 1967b) and rat adipose tissue (Martin and Denton, 1970) indicate that the enzyme is located extramitochondrially. In subcellular fractionations of guinea pig brains more than 70% of enzyme activity is recovered in the final supernatant (S_3). Also in sheep caudate nuclei the highest proportion of the enzyme is in the high speed supernatant, but nearly 30% of the total activity is found in the microsomal fraction (Fig. 4.4). So far, it is not clear whether a proportion of the enzyme is indeed firmly attached to some of the ultrastructural elements sedimenting in the microsomal fraction, or if its presence in the microsomal fraction is caused by non-specific adsorption of the cytosolic enzyme.

4.3.5 3-ketothiolases

The term 3-ketothiolase (or β-ketothiolase) is used as a trivial name covering at least two enzymes, (1) acetyl–CoA acetyltransferase (= acetoacetyl–CoA thiolase, EC 2.3.1.9), and (2) acetyl–CoA acyltransferase (3-oxoacyl–CoA thiolase, EC 2.3.1.16). The reaction catalysed by these enzymes is described by the following equation:

$$RCOCH_2CO\text{–}CoA + CoA = RCO\text{–}CoA + CH_3CO\text{–}CoA.$$

Basic data on 3-ketothiolase have been reviewed by Gehring and Lynen (1972).

In several different rat tissues, Middleton (1973a,b) has found three types of 3-ketothiolase. These are cytoplasmic acetoacetyl–CoA thiolase, mitochondrial acetoacetyl–CoA thiolase (characteristically different from the cytoplasmic enzyme by its high sensitivity to stimulation by K^+), and mitochondrial 3-oxoacyl–CoA thiolase of general specificity. Only the first two enzymes had a measurable activity in the brain. By analogy with other tissues it is likely that in the brain, the mitochondrial acetoacetyl–CoA thiolase participates in the oxidation of fatty acids and ketone bodies, whereas the cytoplasmic enzyme provides acetyl–CoA for lipogenesis and the synthesis of cholesterol (Middleton, 1973b; Buckley and Williamson, 1973; Clinkenbeard *et al.*, 1973, 1975).

The intramitochondrial localization of 3-ketothiolases has been investigated mainly in experiments on liver mitochondria. The acetoacetyl–CoA thiolase has been found in their matrix (Clinkenbeard *et al.*, 1975). The 3-oxoacyl–CoA thiolase is localized in the inner mitochondrial compartment (Beattie, 1968; Tubbs and Garland, 1968), where the enzymes of the β-oxidation cycle possibly form a multienzyme complex (Garland and Yates, 1967), associated with the inner mitochondrial membrane (Landriscina *et al.*, 1970; Wit-Peeters *et al.*, 1971). Earlier findings from Green's laboratory, suggesting that the enzymes of the β-oxidation cycle are localized in the external mitochondrial membrane (Allmann *et al.*, 1966), were probably attributable to a fault in the procedure used for the separation of mitochondrial membranes: the phospholipase A, used to release the outer mitochondrial membranes, could simultaneously interfere with the integrity of the inner membranes (Brdiczka *et al.*, 1968).

Although evidence about the oxidation of fatty acids in brain mitochondria is much more limited than that concerning liver or muscle mitochondria, the available data for the brain are in good agreement with results obtained from other material. Brain mitochondria are able to oxidize fatty acids without the addition of CoA and

NAD to the incubation medium (Beattie and Basford, 1965, 1966). Carnitine stimulates the oxidation of palmitate by brain mitochondria, so long as the incubation medium is supplemented with exogenous CoA (Beattie and Basford, 1965). These observations indicate that the oxidation of fatty acids in the brain proceeds in a space which does not lose its CoA and NAD content during the isolation of the mitochondria and which is circumscribed by a barrier, impermeable to the esters of CoA, but permeable to the esters of carnitine. These are the properties of the inner compartment of the mitochondria, constituted by the mitochondrial matrix and inner mitochondrial membrane (Tubbs and Garland, 1968).

4.3.6 Carnitine acetyltransferase

The full name of the enzyme is acetyl–CoA: carnitine *O*-acetyltransferase, EC 2.3.1.7. It catalyses the reaction:

O-acetyl-(–)-carnitine + CoA = (–)-carnitine + acetyl–CoA.

Most findings point to a purely mitochondrial localization of the enzyme in the liver (Norum and Bremer, 1967; Brdiczka *et al.*, 1969; Snoswell and Koundakjian, 1972), muscle (Beenakkers and Henderson, 1967; Snoswell and Koundakjian, 1972), kidney (Snoswell and Koundakjian, 1972) and brain (McCaman *et al.*, 1966). In the heart, however, Marquis and Fritz (1965) found that a significant portion of the enzyme is in the soluble fraction of the homogenate. Evidence regarding the position of the enzyme inside the mitochondria is contradictory. Biochemical observations on the brain (McCaman *et al.*, 1966) and the liver (Norum and Bremer, 1967) and histochemical observations on the heart (Higgins and Barrnett, 1970) indicate that the enzyme is associated with mitochondrial membranes. In electron microscopic histochemical experiments on muscle mitochondria the final reaction product has been found on the outer surface of the inner membrane (Makita *et al.*, 1973).

Edwards *et al.* (1974) observed in experiments on several organs that carnitine acetyltransferase is bound to the mitochondria when they sedimented by centrifugation at low ionic strength in the presence of low concentrations of phosphate, but that it appears in the supernatant when mitochondria are isolated at high ionic strength in the presence of high concentrations of phosphate buffer. They concluded that the enzyme is bound to the mitochondrial membranes and is relatively easily released from them. It would seem necessary, however, to consider the possibility that the intracellular and intramitochondrial ionic strength in intact cells is sufficiently high to keep the enzyme in solution. In fact, Brdiczka *et al.* (1969) found that the enzyme is very easily solubilized in experiments with digitonin fractionation of liver mitochondria and came to the conclusion that most of the enzyme is present in a soluble form in the inner compartment of the mitochondria and at least 25% of the enzyme is dissolved in the outer compartment. The estimate of the amount of enzyme in the outer mitochondrial compartment was based on a comparison with glutamate dehydrogenase, an enzyme which the authors used as a marker for enzymes from the mitochondrial matrix. The estimate could be inaccurate if the low concentrations of digitonin used for the separation of outer mitochondrial membranes also caused some damage to the inner membranes and if leakage of carnitine acetyltransferase from the inner mitochondrial compartment occurred more easily than that of glutamate dehydrogenase.

Two types of experiment on intact mitochondria contradict the view that a significant part of carnitine acetyltransferase is located in the outer mitochondrial compartment. The activity of carnitine acetyltransferase found in intact liver mitochondria is very low; it increases many times after the mitochondria have been treated with triton (Barker *et al.*, 1968). Since the outer mitochondrial membrane is easily permeated by substances like carnitine, acetylcarnitine, CoA and acetyl–CoA (Garland and Yates, 1967; Tubbs and Garland, 1968), the experiments of Barker *et al.* (1968) suggest that the enzyme is located behind another barrier, presumably the inner mitochondrial membrane. A similar inference may be made from the experiments of Edwards *et al.* (1974) concerning the oxidation of acetyl–CoA and acetylcarnitine by bovine liver mitochondria. When the mitochondria are incubated in the presence of acetyl–CoA and carnitine, the acetyl groups are oxidized to a much lesser extent than during incubations in the presence of acetylcarnitine. If carnitine acetyltransferase were present in the intermembranous space, it ought to be able to ensure the transformation of acetyl–CoA to acetylcarnitine, which is able to penetrate the inner mitochondrial membrane and can be converted back to acetyl–CoA and oxidized in the matrix. The relative inaccessibility of mitochondrial carnitine acetyltransferase to exogenous acetyl–CoA and carnitine observed in mammalian liver mitochondria (Barker *et al.*, 1968; Edwards *et al.*, 1974) (but not in mitochondria from locust muscle – Beenakkers and Henderson, 1967) is a strong argument against the view that the mammalian enzyme is present in the outer compartment of the mitochondria. It is most likely that it is localized in the inner mitochondrial compartment but its position in this compartment and its relation to the inner mitochondrial membrane are not clear from the evidence available at present. Its possible role in the transport of acetyl–CoA is discussed in Section 4.5 (Fig. 4.10).

4.3.7 3-hydroxy-3-methylglutaryl–CoA lyase

The enzyme (HMG–CoA lyase, EC 4.1.3.4) catalyses the reaction:

$$\underset{\text{3-hydroxy-3-methylglutanyl–CoA}}{\mathrm{COOH{-}CH_2{-}\overset{\displaystyle OH}{\underset{\displaystyle CH_3}{\overset{|}{\underset{|}{C}}}}{-}CH_2{-}CO{-}CoA}} = \underset{\text{Acetoacetate}}{\mathrm{CH_3{-}CO{-}CH_2{-}COOH}} + \underset{\text{Acetyl–CoA}}{\mathrm{CH_3CO{-}CoA}}$$

Its function is important for two metabolic pathways: 1. formation of acetoacetate from acetoacetyl–CoA via HMG–CoA; 2. catabolism of leucine. In the first pathway, HMG–CoA is formed from acetoacetyl–CoA and acetyl–CoA in a reaction catalysed by 3-hydroxy-3-methylglutaryl–CoA synthase (HMG–CoA synthase, EC 4.1.3.5). HMG–CoA is then split to acetoacetate and acetyl–CoA by HMG–CoA lyase. This pathway does not lead to any net production of acetyl–CoA: as much acetyl–CoA is formed from HMG–CoA in its second step as is consumed for the synthesis of HMG–CoA in the first step. On the other hand, the activity of HMG–CoA lyase in the course of leucine catabolism leads to a net production of acetyl–CoA. HMG–CoA lyase has been found in several animal tissues, but it has been repeatedly reported to be absent from the brain (Bachhawat *et al.*, 1955; Knappe, 1957; McGary and Foster, 1969). Recently, however, Clinkenbeard *et al.* (1975) were also able to demonstrate the presence of HMG–CoA lyase in the brain. Its presence in the brain is consistent with data indicating the utilization of leucine in cerebral oxidative metabolism (Swaiman and Milstein, 1965; Chaplin *et al.*, 1976). The enzyme is purely mitochondrial in the liver and is located in the mitochondrial matrix (Clinkenbeard *et al.*, 1975); it may be conjectured that its localization in the brain is the same.

4.3.8 Other acetyl–CoA producing enzymes

Acetyl–CoA might also be produced in the course of reactions catalysed by citrate synthase (EC 4.1.3.7), acetyl–CoA carboxylase (EC 6.4.1.2), aspartate acetyltransferase (EC 2.3.1.17) and by several other enzymes; in living organisms, however, these reactions are connected with the utilization, not formation, of acetyl–CoA. Brain citrate synthase is located in the mitochondria as in other organs (Tuček, 1967b). Very little is known about brain acetyl–CoA carboxylase (Cheng, 1971a). Aspartate acetyltransferase is associated with particles which, on subcellular frationation of the brain, appear in the microsomal fraction (Goldstein, 1969). Enzymatic reactions involving CoA have been very completely reviewed by Jaenicke and Lynen (1960).

4.4 UTILIZATION OF PRECURSORS OF ACETYL GROUPS FOR THE SYNTHESIS OF ACETYLCHOLINE

Experiments concerning the utilization of various precursors of acetyl groups for the synthesis of ACh can be divided into three groups:

(1) experiments *in vitro* in which the synthesis of ACh is measured in the presence of various possible precursors without the use of isotopic labelling;
(2) experiments *in vitro* to study the incorporation into ACh of labelled atoms from radioisotopically labelled substrates present in the incubation medium;
(3) experiments *in vivo* to investigate the incorporation into ACh of labelled atoms after the administration of radioactively labelled substrates to living animals.

Experimental results obtained with these approaches will now be discussed. References to the literature concerning the utilization of various substrates for the synthesis of ACh are summarized in Table 4.2.

Table 4.2 References to observations on the utilization of various precursors of acetyl groups for the biosynthesis of acetylcholine

(A) *Precursors without isotopic label*

Precursor	Reference	Biological material
Acetate	Feldberg and Mann (1945)	Acetone powder or homogenate of rat brain
	Balfour and Hebb (1952)	Acetone-dried rabbit and guinea pig brain
	Severin and Lu (1962)	Nerve and muscle tissue of the cricket
	Buniatian *et al.* (1965)	Acetone-dried rat or guinea pig brain
	Tuček (1967a)	Isolated nerve endings from the brain of sheep, pig, dog, cat and rabbit
Citrate	Feldberg and Hebb (1947)	Acetone-dried rat and guinea pig brain
	Balfour and Hebb (1952)	Acetone-dried rabbit and guinea pig brain
	Severin and Lu (1962)	Nerve and muscle tissue of the cricket
	Tuček (1967a)	Isolated nerve endings from the brain of sheep, pig, dog, cat and rabbit
Pyruvate	Quastel *et al.* (1936)	Rat and guinea pig brain slices
	Mann *et al.* (1938, 1939)	Minced rat brain tissue; slices of rat and guinea pig brain
	Kahlson and MacIntosh (1939)	Cat sympathetic ganglion
	Johnson and Quastel (1953)	Minced rat brain
	Tuček (1967c)	Isolated nerve endings from rabbit and sheep brain
Lactate	Quastel *et al.* (1936)	Rat and guinea pig brain slices
	Mann *et al.* (1938)	Minced rat brain
	Kahlson and MacIntosh (1939)	Cat sympathetic ganglion
Glutamate	Quastel *et al.* (1936)	Rat and guinea pig brain slices
Acetoacetate	Stedman and Stedman (1937)	Minced bovine brain
Glucose	Quastel *et al.* (1936)	Rat and guinea pig brain slices
	Mann *et al.* (1938, 1939)	Minced rat brain, slices of rat and guinea pig brain
	Kahlson and MacIntosh (1939)	Cat sympathetic ganglion

Table 4.2 (*continued*) References to observations on the utilization of various precursors of acetyl groups for the biosynthesis of acetylcholine

(A) *Precursors without isotopic label*

Precursor	Reference	Biological material
Glucose	Welsh and Hyde (1944a)	Rat brain slices
	Harpur and Quastel (1949)	Acetone-dried bovine brain
	McLennan and Elliott (1950, 1951)	Rat brain slices
	Sattin (1966)	Rat brain slices
Fructose	Quastel *et al.* (1936)	Rat and guinea pig brain slices
	Harpur and Quastel (1949)	Acetone-dried bovine brain
Galactose	Quastel *et al.* (1936)	Rat and guinea pig brain slices
	Kahlson and MacIntosh (1939)	Cat sympathetic ganglion
Mannose	Kahlson and MacIntosh (1939)	Cat sympathetic ganglion
N-acetylated amino acids	Buniatian *et al.* (1965)	Acetone-dried mouse or rat brain
Acetylcarnitine	Thomitzek and Strack (1964)	Acetone-dried rat and guinea pig brain, crude mitochondrial fraction of guinea pig brain
Mesityl oxide	Alkonyi and Sándor (1969)	Acetone-dried rat and guinea pig brain
2-methyl-4-keto-penten-(1)-carboxylic(1) acid	Alkonyi and Sándor (1969)	Acetone-dried rat and guinea pig brain

(B) *Isotopically labelled precursors in vitro*

Precursor	References	Biological material
Acetate	Browning and Schulman (1968)	Rat brain slices (negative result)
	Nakamura *et al.* (1970)	Rat and guinea pig brain slices
	Cheng and Nakamura (1970)	Lobster nerve
	Sollenberg and Sörbo (1970)	Rat brain slices

Table 4.2 (*continued*) References to observations on the utilization of various precursors of acetyl groups for the biosynthesis of acetylcholine

(B) *Isotopically labelled precursors in vitro*

Precursor	Reference	Biological material
Acetate	Israël and Tuček (1974)	Slices of electric organ of *Torpedo*
	Morel (1975, 1976)	Slices of electric organ of *Torpedo*
	Dreyfus (1975)	Rat skeletal muscle
	Zimmermann and Whittaker (1977)	Perfused electric organ of *Torpedo*
	Zimmermann and Denston (1977b)	Perfused electric organ of *Torpedo*
	Dunant *et al.* (1977)	Slices of electric organ of *Torpedo*
Citrate	Cheng and Nakamura (1970)	Lobster nerve
	Nakamura *et al.* (1970)	Rat and guinea pig brain slices
	Lefresne (1974)	Isolated nerve endings from rat brain (negative result)
Pyruvate	Browning and Schulman (1968)	Rat brain slices
	Cheney *et al.* (1969)	Rat brain homogenate
	Nakamura *et al.* (1970)	Rat and guinea pig brain slices
	Cheng and Nakamura (1970)	Lobster nerve
	Cheng (1972)	Lobster nerve
	Lefresne *et al.* (1973)	Rat brain slices
	Lefresne (1974)	Rat brain slices and isolated nerve endings
	Israël and Tuček (1974)	Slices of electric organ of *Torpedo*
	Dreyfus (1975)	Rat skeletal muscle
	Lefresne *et al.* (1975)	Rat striatal synaptosomes
	Gibson *et al.* (1975)	Rat brain mince
	Thomas *et al.* (1976)	Rat brain mince
	Molenaar and Polak (1976)	Rat brain slices
	Morel (1976)	Slices of electric organ of *Torpedo*
Glutamate	Nakamura *et al.* (1970)	Rat and guinea pig brain slices

Table 4.2 (*continued*) References to observations on the utilization of various precursors of acetyl groups for the biosynthesis of acetylcholine

(B) *Isotopically labelled precursors* in vitro

Precursor	Reference	Biological material
Acetoacetate	Itoh and Quastel (1970)	Rat brain slices
Glucose	Browning and Schulman (1968)	Rat brain slices
	Sharkawi and Schulman (1969a,b)	Rat brain slices and homogenate
	Sollenberg and Sörbo (1970)	Rat brain slices
	Itoh and Quastel (1970)	Rat brain slices
	Lefresne *et al.* (1973)	Rat brain slices
	Lefresne (1974)	Rat brain slices and isolated nerve endings
	Lefresne *et al.* (1975)	Rat striatal synaptosomes
	Thomas *et al.* (1976)	Rat brain mince
Bicarbonate	Nakamura *et al.* (1970)	Rat brain slices

(C) *Isotopically labelled precursors* in vivo

Precursor	Reference	Biological material
Acetate	Fitzgerald and Cooper (1967)	Rabbit corneal epithelium
	Tuček and Cheng (1970, 1974)	Rat brain
Citrate	Fitzgerald and Cooper (1967)	Rabbit corneal epithelium
	Tuček and Cheng (1970, 1974)	Rat brain
Pyruvate	Fitzgerald and Cooper (1967)	Rabbit corneal epithelium
	Cheney *et al.* (1969)	Rat brain (s.c. administration of precursor)
	Tuček and Cheng (1970, 1974)	Rat brain
Lactate	Tuček and Cheng (1970, 1974)	Rat brain
Glutamate	Kumar (1971)	Rat brain
	Tuček and Cheng (1970, 1974)	Rat brain (negative result)

Table 4.2 (*continued*) References to observations on the utilization of various precursors of acetyl groups for the biosynthesis of acetylcholine

(C) *Isotopically labelled precursors in vivo*

Precursor	Reference	Biological material
Acetoacetate	Tuček and Cheng (1970, 1974)	Rat brain
3-hydroxybutyrate	Tuček and Cheng (1970, 1974)	Rat brain
Glucose	Fitzgerald and Cooper (1967)	Rabbit corneal epithelium
	Tuček and Cheng (1970, 1974)	Rat brain
Leucine	Tuček and Cheng (1970, 1974)	Rat brain

4.4.1 Precursors without isotopic labelling

When brain tissue, some of its subcellular fractions, or brain extracts are incubated in a suitable medium, the content of ACh in the tissue and in the incubation medium increases. For the synthesis of ACh to occur *in vitro,* the preparations of brain tissue have to be incubated in the presence of substances which can serve as precursors of acetyl groups. It has been found in the course of many years of research that the brain tissue is able to use, for the synthesis of ACh, a number of precursors – acetate, citrate, glucose, fructose, lactate, pyruvate, acetoacetate, acetylcarnitine, glutamate, *N*-acetylated amino acids, methyl-keto-pentencarboxylic acid and mesityl oxide (see first part of Table 4.2). Experiments without labelled precursors usually do not permit quantitative comparisons between different substrates from the point of view of their importance for the synthesis of ACh *in vivo*. Although they demonstrate that the nervous tissue is capable of synthesizing ACh in the presence of certain substances, they do not prove that the acetyl groups of the newly synthesized ACh originate from these substances. Studies using nervous tissue which is severely damaged (e.g. experiments with extracts or homogenates of brain tissue) may easily produce misleading results both with unlabelled and with labelled substrates; it may happen that, after the destruction of the spatial and structural organization of the cells, the metabolites used for the synthesis of ACh include some which would not get into the cytoplasm of cholinergic nerve endings in intact tissue.

4.4.2 Isotopically labelled precursors *in vitro*

The use of radioactively labelled precursors for the investigation of the origin of acetyl groups of ACh in the brain is comparatively recent. Browning and Schulman (1968) observed in experiments with slices of brain tissue that labelled atoms from [1-^{14}C] glucose, [6-^{14}C] glucose and [2-^{14}C] pyruvate are incorporated into ACh. On the other hand, no incorporation of labelled carbon from [2-^{14}C] acetate was observed; this negative finding has to be accepted with reserve since acetate was present in the incubation medium as the only oxidizable substrate. The non-utilization of acetate could therefore have been caused by the lack of ATP which is necessary for its activation. Poor utilization of acetate for the synthesis of ACh in the brain slices has been confirmed, however, in experiments in which labelled acetate was present in the medium together with unlabelled glucose (Nakamura and Cheng, 1969; Nakamura *et al.,* 1970; Sollenberg and Sörbo, 1970). On the other hand, acetate is actively used for the synthesis of ACh in rat skeletal muscle (i.e., in intramuscular branches and endings of the motor nerve) (Dreyfus, 1975).

The utilization of glucose and pyruvate for the synthesis of ACh in mammalian brain has been confirmed in many studies (see Table 4.2). Itoh and Quastel (1970) compared the utilization of [2-^{14}C] glucose and [3-^{14}C] acetoacetate in brain slices. In rats aged 1–3 days both substrates were used for synthesis of ACh approximately equally; in adult rats the utilization of glucose was nearly three times higher. Both substrates were present in the medium in a 5 mM concentration. Compared with conditions *in vivo*, this concentration must have favoured the utilization of acetoacetate because its physiological concentration in the brain is much lower, 41 μM (Hawkins *et al.*, 1971), and its utilization in the brain increases proportionally to its concentration (Hawkins *et al.*, 1971; Ruderman *et al.*, 1974). [2-^{14}C] pyruvate and [6-^{14}C] glucose are used for the synthesis of ACh to an equal degree (Lefresne *et al.*, 1973). All ACh synthesized during an incubation with glucose or pyruvate originates from these added precursors. This implies that under conditions of incubation *in vitro*, brain tissue does not use, for the synthesis of acetyl groups of ACh, any endogenous precursors of acetyl groups (in contrast to the utilization of endogenous sources of choline – see chapter 5).

Controversial findings have been reported regarding the role of citrate as a precursor of acetyl–CoA for the synthesis of brain ACh. The possibility that citrate supplies the acetyl groups for ACh is very important in view of the fact that citrate is generally regarded as the carrier of acetyl groups across the inner mitochondrial membrane (see Section 4.5 and Greville, 1969). Nakamura *et al.* (1970) have observed that, during incubation of brain or striatal slices in the presence of non-radioactive glucose and [2-^{14}C] pyruvate or [1,5-^{14}C] citrate, the incorporation of radioactivity from citrate into ACh is 2–3 orders of magnitude lower than that from pyruvate. Lefresne (1974) found that no label was incorporated from citrate into ACh in experiments with rat synaptosomes. Sollenberg and Sörbo (1970), however, arrived in an indirect way at the conclusion that all the carbon atoms from glucose which, in their experiments with brain slices, appeared in the acetyl group of ACh, must have passed through the citrate stage (i.e. that the two-carbon groups reached ACh by the pathway: glucose → pyruvate → acetyl–CoA → citrate → acetyl–CoA → ACh). These authors compared the ratio between the amount of ^{3}H and ^{14}C incorporated into ACh when [6-^{3}H] glucose and [6-^{14}C] glucose, mixed together, were used as the precursors for the synthesis. The ratio ^{3}H/^{14}C in ACh was 1/3 lower than the ^{3}H/^{14}C ratio in glucose in the incubation medium. This change corresponds to the comparative loss of ^{3}H (relative to ^{14}C) atoms which must occur when the [2-^{3}H] acetyl–CoA (as compared to [2-^{14}C] acetyl–CoA) undergoes the initial reaction of the Krebs cycle with oxaloacetate to form citrate (Bartley *et al.*, 1965).

It is not easy to explain the contradiction between Sollenberg and Sörbo's conclusion about the role of citrate as an ACh precursor and the negligible utilization of citrate when it is present in the incubation medium during experiments with brain slices (Nakamura *et al.*, 1970) and with synaptosomes (Lefresne, 1974). There are weak points both in the evidence suggesting that citrate is not important as an ACh precursor and in the evidence that it is important. Whether the labelled citrate enters the cells and is utilized in their metabolism has not been checked in experiments on brain slices or synaptosomes; the non-incorporation of label from citrate into ACh would seem of importance only if, at the same time, the label is incorporated into other compounds, e.g. CO_2. In this respect, more complete evidence for the non-utilization of citrate for ACh synthesis has been obtained in experiments *in vivo* (Tuček and Cheng, 1974; see Section 4.4.3). On the other hand, the relative loss of

^3H as compared to ^{14}C in Sollenberg and Sörbo's (1970) experiments with ACh synthesis from double-labelled glucose may be only partly due to the involvement of the citrate synthase catalysed reaction and can be explained without postulating that ACh originates from citrate. A big loss of ^3H atoms from the original position 6 in glucose necessarily occurs in the reactions of the Krebs cycle. If [2-^3H] acetyl–CoA and [2-^{14}C] acetyl–CoA (both compounds arising from [6-^3H] glucose and [6-^{14}C] glucose) enter the Krebs cycle by condensation with oxaloacetate and pass through one whole turn of the cycle back to oxaloacetate, and if this oxaloacetate is then transformed by consecutive decarboxylations to pyruvate and to acetyl–CoA, all the original ^{14}C atoms, but only 1/6 of the original ^3H atoms are found in the acetyl–CoA thus formed (see Mahler and Kordes, 1966; Cheng, 1971b). The loss of ^3H atoms can also be caused by the exchange of hydrogen between the acetyl group of acetyl–CoA and water; such an exchange can be catalysed by citrate synthase (Eggerer, 1965; Srere, 1967) and ATP citrate lyase (Das and Srere, 1972), without being connected with either the synthesis or the cleavage of citrate.

The observations discussed so far have concerned the origin of acetyl groups of ACh in the nervous tissue of mammals. Experiments on the synthesis of ACh in the nervous tissue of lower animals indicate that they may utilize the precursors of acetyl groups differently from mammalian brain. An example of a tissue with an extremely rich cholinergic innervation is the electric organ of some fish. In the electric organ of *Torpedo marmorata* incubated *in vitro*, acetate is very actively used for the synthesis of ACh, whereas pyruvate is used about five times less actively and glucose is used very little (Fig. 4.5; Israël and Tuček, 1974). Possibly, acetate is a more important metabolite in fish than in mammals. When trout are kept in conditions of anoxia, short chain fatty acids accumulate in their muscles, in place of the lactic acid found in mammals (Blažka, 1958). The low utilization of glucose may be connected with the low concentration of hexokinase in some organs of the fish (Black *et al.*, 1961). Similarly in experiments on lobster nerves acetate was found to be the best precursor of the acetyl groups of ACh; pyruvate, citrate, glucose and other substrates are used considerably less (Cheng and Nakamura, 1970).

4.4.3 Isotopically labelled precursors *in vivo*

The interpretation of results obtained in the experiments *in vitro* (Table 4.2) is beset by a number of problems. Two are particularly important:

(a) The permeability of membranes can be easily changed during the preparation of brain slices and their incubation in a not entirely physiological medium. Of special importance is the possibility of changes in the permeability of the inner mitochondrial membrane to acetyl–CoA (see Section 4.5).
(b) The concentrations of substrates used in experiments *in vitro* differ considerably from the concentrations at which these substrates are present under conditions *in vivo*.

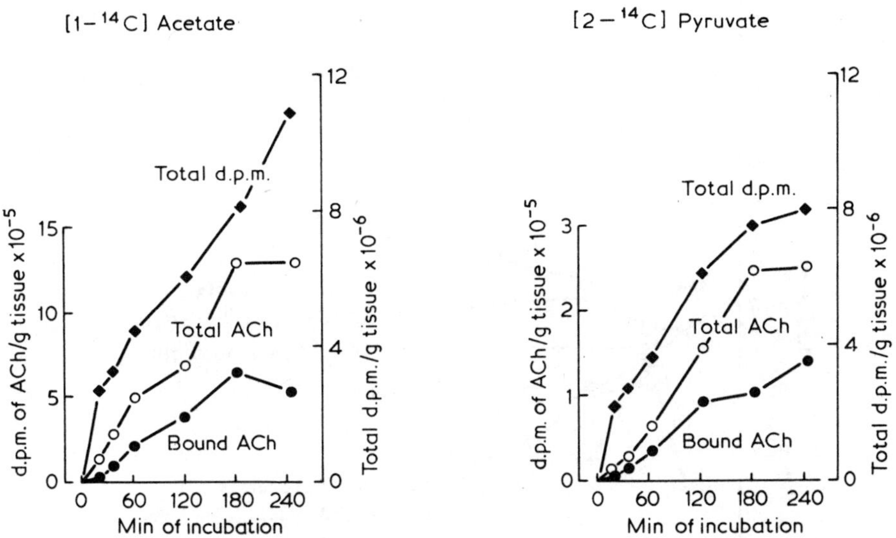

Fig. 4.5 The synthesis of [^{14}C] ACh in slices of the electric organ of *Torpedo marmorata* incubated in the presence of [1-^{14}C] acetate or [2-^{14}C] pyruvate. Abscissa: duration of incubation in min. Ordinate: total radioactivity in the tissue (filled squares, scale on the right), radioactivity in total ACh (open circles, scale on the left), and radioactivity in the bound ACh (filled circles, scale on the left); note that the scale on the left is different for acetate and pyruvate (after Israël and Tuček, 1974).

The design and interpretation of experiments *in vivo*, however, are also subject to many difficulties. These include among others:

(a) The route of administration of labelled precursors to the brain. After the administration to the whole body (intravenous, intraperitoneal or subcutaneous), the precursor may first be metabolized in the liver or in other organs and the labelled atoms may be supplied to the brain only afterwards.
(b) The blood–brain barrier. This can prevent the penetration of some exogenous precursors into the brain from the blood, although the same precursors arise in the brain endogenously during its metabolism.
(c) Differences in the penetration of precursors. Even after the administration of the precursors into the cerebrospinal fluid it is necessary to take into account the possibility that the precursors may enter some cells (neurons or glia) more easily than others, and also that their penetration into some parts of the cell (e.g. the nerve endings) may be easier or more difficult than into other parts of the same cell.
(d) Dilution of injected labelled precursors in the endogenous pool of the same (unlabelled) substances. This dilution entirely changes the specific radioactivity of the precursors. The degree of dilution depends not only on the concentration of the

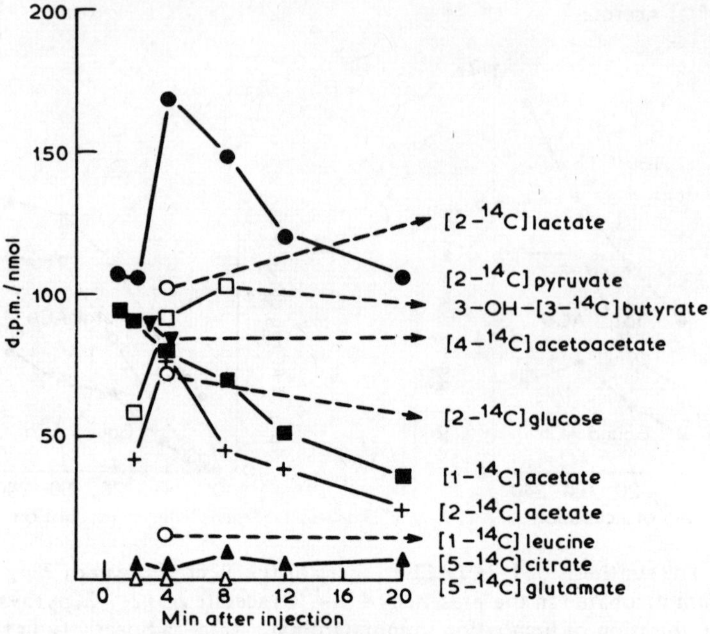

Fig. 4.6 Specific radioactivities of the acetyl group of ACh in rat brain, normalized for the same total radioactivity in the brain, 1–20 min after intracisternal injections of various precursors. The injected radioactivity was 6.25 μCi per rat for each substrate (after Tuček and Cheng, 1974).

endogenous precursor in the brain, but also on the rate of its metabolic turnover; the picture is even more complicated in view of the fact that the rate of metabolic 'flow' may be different in various cells and also in various parts of the same cell.

Experiments *in vivo* related to the question of the origin of the acetyl group of ACh have been described by Fitzgerald and Cooper (1967), Cheney *et al.* (1969), Kumar (1971), and Tuček and Cheng (1970, 1974). Fitzgerald and Cooper (1967) injected the labelled substrates into the anterior chamber of the rabbit eye and measured the radioactivity of ACh in the corneal epithelium. Labelled atoms from acetate were incorporated into ACh much more actively than those from glucose, pyruvate or citrate. Cheney *et al.* (1969) observed that, after a subcutaneous injection of [3-^{14}C] pyruvate to rats, the radioactivity appeared in brain ACh. Kumar (1971) observed that the same happened after intracisternal injection of uniformly labelled glutamate.

A number of possible precursors of acetyl groups of acetyl–CoA were compared from the point of view of their incorporation into ACh, lipids, proteins, glutamate, glutamine and citrate in experiments on rats by Tuček and Cheng (1970, 1974). In animals killed at intervals from 1–20 min after intracisternal injections of labelled

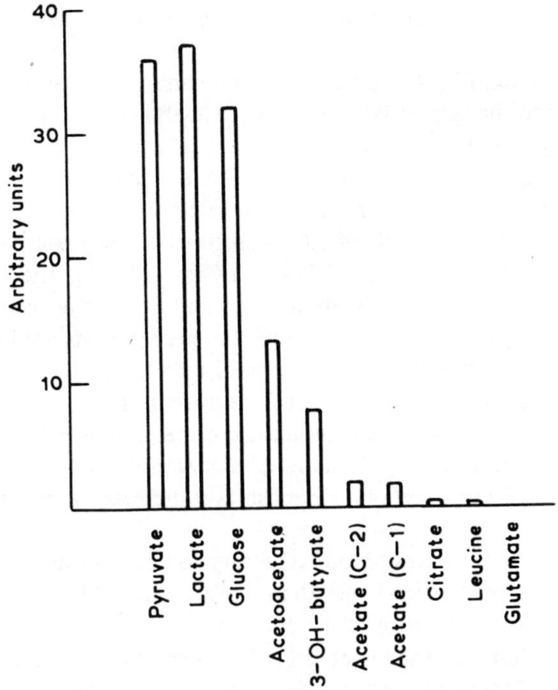

Fig. 4.7 The contribution of various precursors to the synthesis of acetyl groups of ACh in the brain of rats. The diagram is based on measurements of specific radioactivity of the acetyl groups of ACh in the brain 4 min after intracisternal injections of ^{14}C-labelled precursors (see Fig. 4.6). The likely contribution of different precursors to the synthesis of ACh has been calculated from the specific radioactivities of ACh actually measured, taking into account the unequal dilution of the injected precursors by the endogenous pools of the same substances in the brain and other modifying circumstances. It is expressed in arbitrary units. See text for explanation of why the contributions of acetoacetate, 3-hydroxybutyrate and acetate, as calculated here, probably overestimate the role which these substances play in the biosynthesis of ACh. See original work for details (after Tuček and Cheng, 1974).

precursors, the highest radioactivity of brain ACh was found after injections of [2-^{14}C] pyruvate (Fig. 4.6). It reached the peak value 4 min after the injection. The radioactivities of ACh measured in the brain extracts were recalculated to take into account the inequality of the injected amounts of the precursors and of their endogenous pools, the fact that the molecules of some precursors yielded one, and others two, molecules of acetyl–CoA, the fact that the labelled atoms from some positions virtually cannot pass into acetyl–CoA, and some other complicating factors (see Tuček and Cheng, 1974, for details). The calculation produced a set of comparative values reflecting the extent to which the precursors used participated in the synthesis of ACh in the rat brain. The comparison of various precursors is summarized in Fig. 4.7.

As may be seen from Fig. 4.7, pyruvate, lactate and glucose were the substrates contributing most to the synthesis of ACh. Since acetyl–CoA is produced from lactate and from glucose via pyruvate, it appears that pyruvate is the most important source of acetyl–CoA for the synthesis of ACh. According to Fig. 4.7, acetoacetate and 3-hydroxybutyrate can also contribute significantly to the synthesis of ACh. Their contribution to the synthesis of ACh was, however, probably overestimated in the experimental conditions used by Tuček and Cheng (1974). The concentration of both substrates in the brain is extremely low (41 and 84 nmol/g according to Hawkins *et al.*, 1971). Therefore, even though the preparations used were of the highest specific activity available, the injection of labelled acetoacetate and 3-hydroxybutyrate must have caused a significant local increase in their concentrations in the brain. Since the utilization of these compounds in the brain is proportional to their concentration (Hawkins *et al.*, 1971; Ruderman *et al.*, 1974), the injection of exogenous acetoacetate and 3-hydroxybutyrate must have increased their utilization beyond normal values.

The utilization of acetate was found to be very low and, in the light of more recent data, it was probably even lower than is indicated in Fig. 4.7. Tuček and Cheng (1974) based their estimate of the contribution of acetate to the synthesis of ACh on the assumption that the injected [1-^{14}C] acetate had been diluted in an endogenous pool of 110 nmol acetate/g tissue; this figure, which is the concentration of acetate found in rat heart, was used since no data were then available for the brain. According to data published by Guynn and Veech (1975), however, the concentration of acetate in rat brain is only 20–30 nmol/g, so that the dilution of injected acetate was approximately four times less than supposed by Tuček and Cheng (1974); therefore, the estimate of the contribution of acetate to the synthesis of ACh should likewise be approximately four times lower than that given in Fig. 4.7. As may be seen from Fig. 4.7, citrate and leucine contributed very little to the synthesis of ACh and virtually no glutamate was used.

In view of the likely role of citrate as the transporter of acetyl groups from the intramitochondrial to the extramitochondrial space for the synthesis of fatty acids (Lowenstein, 1968; Greville, 1969) and of the contradiction between, on one side, the low incorporation of radioactivity from citrate into ACh both *in vitro* (Nakamura *et al.*, 1970; Lefresne, 1974) and *in vivo* (Tuček and Cheng, 1974) and, on the other, the results of Sollenberg and Sörbo (1970), discussed in Section 4.4.2, special attention has been paid to several aspects of the utilization of citrate in Tuček and Cheng's (1974) experiments. It was found that the radioactive citrate was metabolized very quickly after intracisternal injections; as early as 2 min after the intracisternal injections of [1,5-^{14}C] citrate, less than 7% of the total radioactivity in the brain was recovered in the form of citrate; 93% of injected citrate had already been transformed to other compounds. It is likely that citrate penetrates the nerve endings to about the

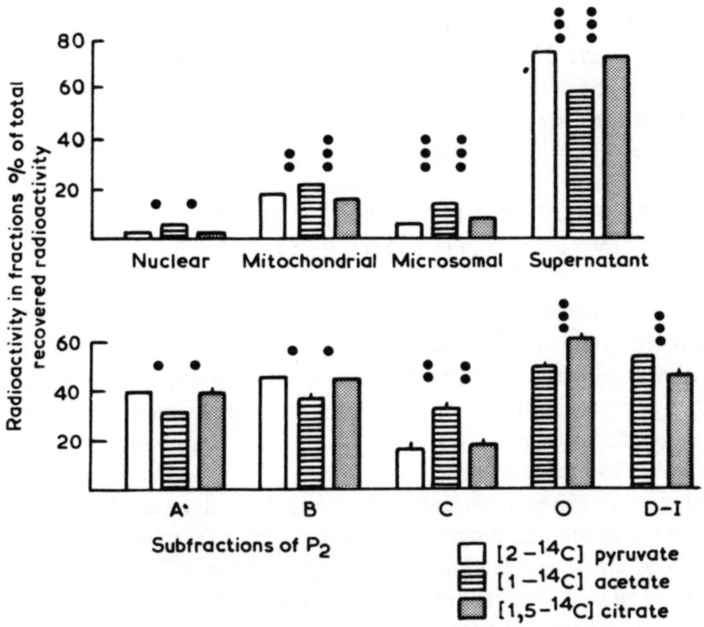

Fig. 4.8 The distribution of radioactivity in subcellular fractions of rat brain 4 min after intracisternal injection of [2-^{14}C] pyruvate, [1,^{14}C] acetate and [1,5-^{14}C] citrate. The upper histogram shows the primary fractions – nuclear (P_1), crude mitochondrial (P_2), microsomal (P_3) and final supernatant (S_3). The lower histogram shows subfractions of P_2, obtained by centrifugation on a density gradient; for description of fractions see Fig. 4.2. The hypo-osmotically treated fraction P_2 was separated into fraction O and into another fraction, designated as D–I and representing the sum of fractions D, E, F, G, H and I; pyruvate was not used in experiments with hypo-osmotic treatment of P_2. The height of the columns indicates what percentage of total radioactivity, recovered in all fractions of the homogenate or in all subfractions of P_2, was present in the corresponding fraction or subfraction. The bars express S.E.M. In most cases the S.E.M. was too low to be shown on the scale used. The statistical significance of the difference between neighbouring columns (i.e. between pyruvate and acetate or between acetate and citrate) is expressed by black circles: ●, $p < 0.05$; ●●, $p < 0.01$; ●●●, $p < 0.005$ (after Tuček and Cheng, 1974).

same degree as pyruvate, since the distribution of radioactivity in brain subcellular fractions after the injections of [1,5-^{14}C] citrate and [2-^{14}C] pyruvate was virtually identical (Fig. 4.8). The low utilization of citrate could not have been due to an inhibitor action of citrate on the metabolic turnover of ACh (caused, for example, by chelation of Ca^{2+} ions), because non-radioactive citrate injected together with radioactive pyruvate or acetate did not alter the incorporation of radioactivity from these precursors into ACh. Taken together, these observations contradict the view that citrate acts as the transporter of acetyl groups from the inner mitochondrial compartment for the synthesis of ACh and that it is the immediate precursor of the acetyl–CoA used for the synthesis of ACh.

4.5 TRANSFER OF ACETYL GROUPS ACROSS THE INNER MITOCHONDRIAL MEMBRANE

Experiments with radioactively labelled precursors indicate that the acetyl groups of ACh in rat brain originate from glucose and pyruvate. In order to be used for the synthesis of ACh in the cytoplasm of the nerve endings, the acetyl–CoA which is formed from pyruvate in the inner mitochondrial compartment has to pass through the inner and outer mitochondrial membranes. The outer membrane is probably easily permeable to most small molecules including coenzyme A and its esters. The inner membrane, however, is virtually impermeable to most small molecules; some substances can pass the membrane through the mediation of specialized carriers (see Chappell, 1968; Tubbs and Garland, 1968; Klingenberg, 1970). The very low permeability of the inner mitochondrial membrane to CoA and acetyl–CoA is indicated by the following observations:

(1) CoA penetrates into only 70–75% of intramitochondrial water (Yates and Garland, 1966), and acetyl–CoA into only 60–70% (Garland and Yates, 1967);
(2) during preparation, standing and incubation, mitochondria retain a portion of their CoA, most probably that portion which is located in the inner mitochondrial compartment (Garland *et al.*, 1965; Beattie and Basford, 1965, 1966; Lowenstein, 1964, 1968);
(3) mitochondria oxidize free acetate (which passes through the inner mitochondrial membrane) much faster than acetyl–CoA (Fritz and Yue, 1964). The assumption that the inner mitochondrial membrane is permeable to acetyl–CoA is also supported by analogy with other molecules of similar size, e.g. NADH, which is not oxidized by the respiratory chain of the mitochondria when added to a suspension (Lehninger, 1964).

The problem of the transport of acetyl groups of acetyl–CoA from the mitochondria into the cytoplasm has been much discussed in connection with the problem of the supply of acetyl–CoA for extramitochondrial synthesis of fatty acids. Several mechanisms have been proposed by which the acetyl groups of intramitochondrial acetyl–CoA could be transferred to the extramitochondrial space (see, for example, Srere, 1965; Kornacker and Lowenstein, 1965; Greville, 1969; Fig. 4.9):

(a) Via citrate. Acetyl–CoA inside the mitochondria is condensed with oxaloacetate to form citrate. Citrate then passes with the help of a carrier into the cytosol where it is split, with the participation of CoA, by ATP citrate lyase to oxaloacetate

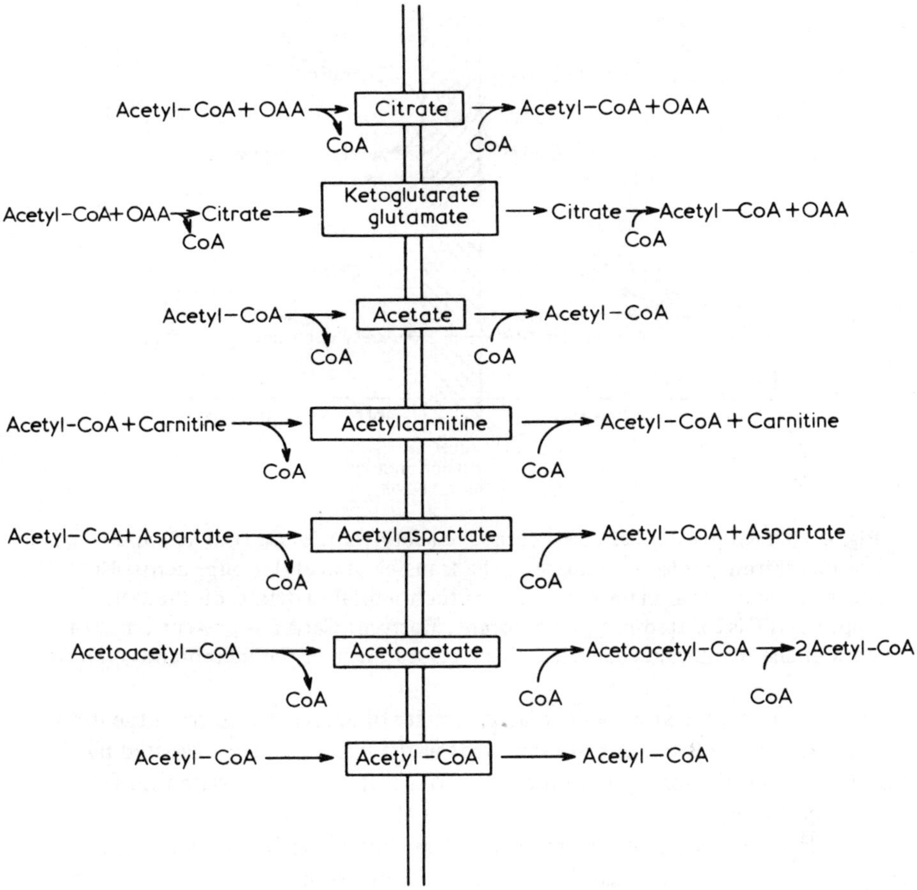

Fig. 4.9 Schematic representation of several possibilities for the transport of intramitochondrial acetyl groups for extramitochondrial acetyl–CoA. The two vertical lines represent the inner mitochondrial membrane.

and acetyl–CoA. Citrate is regarded as being mainly responsible for the supply of intramitochondrial acetyl groups for the extramitochondrial synthesis of fatty acids (Lowenstein, 1968; Greville, 1969; see, however, objections raised by Rous, 1971).

(b) Via α-ketoglutarate or glutamate. Intramitochondrial citrate is transformed to these substances, which then leave the mitochondria (probably with the help of a carrier) and are transformed back to citrate extramitochondrially. Citrate is split by ATP citrate lyase in the presence of CoA to acetyl–CoA and oxaloacetate. The existence of this pathway in the nervous tissue has been demonstrated by D'Adamo and D'Adamo (1968).

(c) Via acetylcarnitine, which is formed from acetyl–CoA in the inner mitochondrial

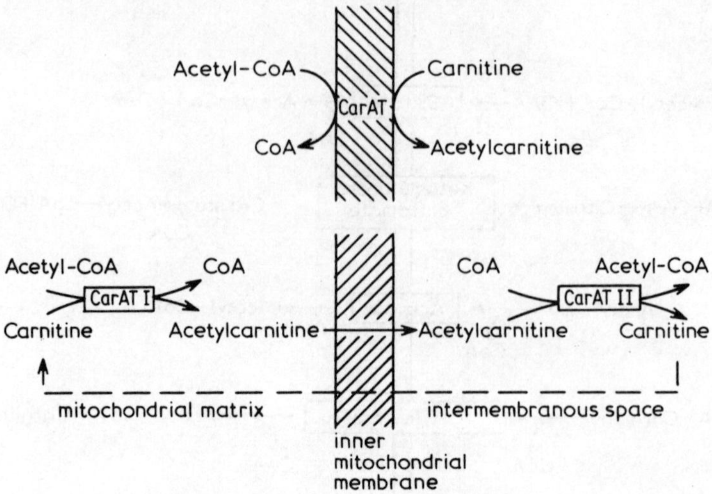

Fig. 4.10 Two possibilities how carnitine acetyltransferase (CarAT) and acetylcarnitine could participate in the transfer of acetyl groups across the inner mitochondrial membrane. The mitochondrial matrix is on the left. Top: CarAT is located in the membrane. Bottom: CarAT is present on both sides of the membrane; acetylcarnitine passes through the membrane.

compartment. Acetylcarnitine-mediated transfer of acetyl groups from the mitochondria during the synthesis of fatty acids in the liver has been suggested by the observation that the incorporation of ^{14}C from acetate and pyruvate into fatty acids is increased by the administration of carnitine (Bressler and Katz, 1965). The mechanism of the assumed transfer is not clear. Either the whole molecule of acetylcarnitine passes through the inner mitochondrial membrane, or the acetyl group of acetylcarnitine which is present in the mitochondrial matrix, is transferred to coenzyme A which is present in the intermembranous space. The first possibility requires the presence of carnitine acetyltransferase both in the inner compartment of the mitochondrion and also somewhere outside the inner compartment. The alternative mechanism assumes that the enzyme is located inside the internal mitochondrial membrane is such a way that it is able to react with the substrates on both sides of the membrane (Fig. 4.10).

(d) Via acetate, which is produced in the mitochondria by the hydrolysis of acetyl–CoA, diffuses through the mitochondrial membranes and is utilized for the synthesis of new acetyl–CoA extramitochondrially.

(e) Via acetoacetate. This mechanism has been proposed by Rous (1976). She suggests that acetoacetyl–CoA, which is formed intramitochondrially, is deacylated by mitochondrial acetoacetyl–CoA deacylase and that the acetoacetate thus produced leaves the mitochondria. In the cytosol, it is converted to acetoacetyl–CoA

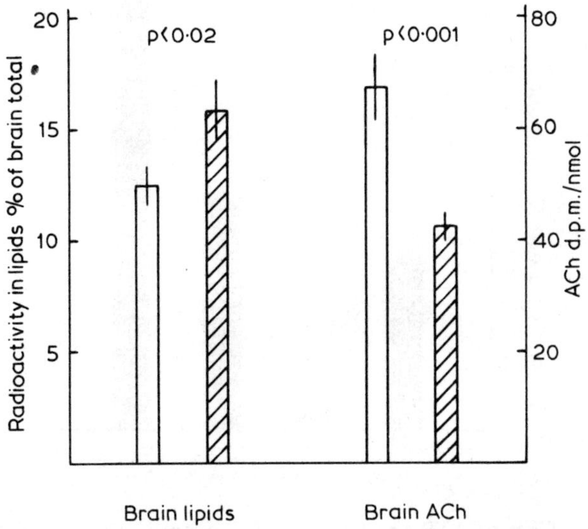

Fig. 4.11 The influence of carnitine on the incorporation of ^{14}C from [1-^{14}C] acetate into brain lipids (left) and into brain ACh (right). White columns: rats were injected intracisternally with [1-^{14}C] acetate, with no other treatment. Hatched columns: 34 min before the intracisternal injection of [1-^{14}C] acetate, rats received an intraperitoneal injection of 40 μmoles D, L-carnitine. In both cases the animals were killed 4 min after the injection of [1-^{14}C] acetate. The scale on the left: radioactivity in lipids, expressed as percentage of total radioactivity in the brain. The scale on right: normalized specific radioactivity of brain ACh (d.p.m. per nmole). The statistical significance of the differences between the groups without and with carnitine is shown at the top of the graph. See Tuček and Cheng (1974) for details.

in a reaction catalysed by acetoacetyl–CoA synthetase, and acetyl–CoA is then formed from this acetoacetyl–CoA by the action of acetoacetyl–CoA thiolase. It seems likely that the cells of the brain are capable of producing extramitochondrial acetyl–CoA from acetoacetate in the blood, by the coupled action of cytosolic acetoacetyl–CoA synthetase and cytosolic acetoacetyl–CoA thiolase (Buckley and Williamson, 1973; Patel and Owen, 1976).

(f) Via acetylated amino acids, particularly *N*-acetylaspartate (D'Adamo *et al.*, 1968; Rous, 1973).

(g) By direct transport or diffusion of acetyl–CoA from the mitochondria, possibly occurring *in vivo*, despite negative evidence obtained in experiments *in vitro* and mentioned earlier in this section.

It would be expected that a compound serving as the physiological carrier of

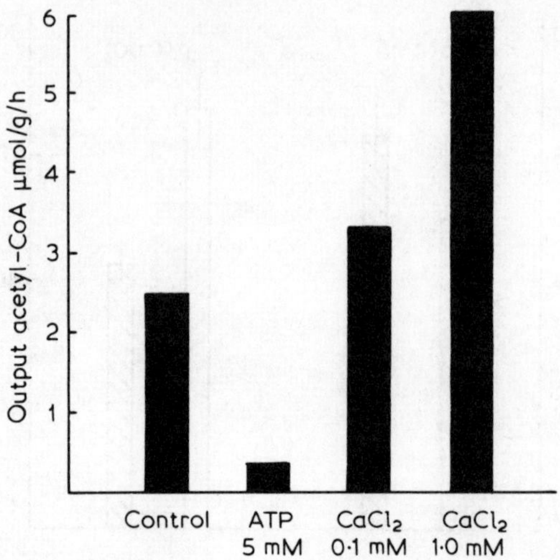

Fig. 4.12 The effect of ATP and $CaCl_2$ on the output of acetyl–CoA from rabbit brain mitochondria (P_2 fraction) into the incubation medium. Acetyl–CoA was formed in the mitochondria from pyruvate. After the permeability of the mitochondrial membranes had been increased by treating them with ether, $CaCl_2$ lost its effect on the amount of acetyl–CoA released into the incubation medium and the effect of ATP was considerably diminished. ADP has the same effect as ATP. Therefore it is likely that in these experiments Ca^{2+} and ATP acted mainly on mitochondrial membranes, not on the pyruvate dehydrogenase complex. (Based on Tuček, 1967c).

acetyl groups for ACh synthesis will be very efficiently used for ACh synthesis after being injected to the brain. Surprisingly, most compounds considered as acetyl carriers in Fig. 4.9 proved, on injection, to be poorly used for ACh synthesis. Judging by the comparatively low incorporation of labelled atoms from citrate, glutamate, acetate, acetoacetate, and acetylaspartate (Tuček and Cheng, 1974 and unpublished results) into brain ACh, none of these compounds seems to play the role of acetyl carrier for ACh synthesis. Some indirect evidence indicates that acetylcarnitine is also unlikely to play this role. The administration of carnitine to rats increases the incorporation of ^{14}C from acetate into lipids, but decreases its incorporation into ACh (Fig. 4.11, Tuček and Cheng, 1974). When rat striatal synaptosomes synthesize labelled ACh from [2-^{14}C] pyruvate, the radioactivity of ACh produced from this substrate is not reduced by the addition of a high concentration of unlabelled acetylcarnitine into the medium; if [^{14}C] acetylcarnitine were the carrier of pyruvate acetyl groups from [^{14}C] pyruvate for the synthesis of [^{14}C] ACh, the addition of unlabelled acetylcarnitine into the incubation medium should lower the resulting specific radioactivity of [^{14}C] ACh (Lefresne, 1974).

Although it is generally regarded as unlikely that acetyl–CoA leaves the mitochondria as such, i.e. that there is direct exchange of acetyl–CoA and CoA between the mitochondria and the extramitochondrial space, such a possibility should not be entirely dismissed, particularly in view of the failure to demonstrate other means of acetyl groups transfer. Tuček (1967c) measured the output (leakage ?) of acetyl–CoA from the mitochondria in a system in which acetyl–CoA had been produced in the mitochondria from pyruvate; the incubation medium contained partially purified ChAc and choline, so that the acetyl–CoA leaving the mitochondria was transformed to ACh. The amount of ACh formed in the medium was measured after the end of the incubation. Under basal conditions, mitochondria released 2.5 μmol acetyl–CoA/g tissue/h. This constituted only a small portion of the total amount of acetyl–CoA produced in them; after the mitochondria had been treated with ether, the release of acetyl–CoA rose to 40–50 μmol/g tissue/h. The output of acetyl–CoA from intact mitochondria could be increased by adding Ca^{2+} ions to the incubation medium and decreased by adding ATP or ADP (Fig. 4.12). Ca^{2+} ions are known to cause swelling of the mitochondria, whereas ATP and ADP cause their contraction. Cycles of swelling and contraction proceed in the mitochondria *in vivo* (Lehninger, 1964). Possibly, significant amounts of acetyl–CoA might leave the mitochondria during the periods of swelling. Although the amount of acetyl–CoA leaving the mitochondria under basal conditions in Tuček's (1967c) experiments is low in comparison with its total production in the mitochondria, it is not negligible: it represents more acetyl–CoA than can be formed in guinea pig brain or in sheep caudate nuclei by their ATP citrate lyase and the same amount as or more than, can be formed by their acetyl–CoA synthetase (Tuček, 1967b).

Polak *et al.* (1977b) reported recently that the release of acetyl groups from brain mitochondria incubated with pyruvate is increased in the presence of a cytoplasmic extract. They suggested that a proportion of acetyl groups leave the mitochondria in the form of an unidentified intermediate, different from acetyl–CoA, acetylcarnitine, acetate, or citrate, and that the intermediate is transformed to acetyl–CoA by a cytoplasmic enzyme. The possibility that the cytoplasmic extract acts by altering the permeability of the inner mitochondrial membrane for acetyl–CoA or by affecting the activity of the pyruvate dehydrogenase complex ought to be considered.

4.6 COMMENT ON THE SPECIES, ORGAN AND AGE DIFFERENCES IN THE UTILIZATION OF ACETYL GROUPS OF VARIOUS ORIGIN

Data on the utilization of various sources of acetyl groups for the synthesis of ACh in mammals are largely based on the single experimental object, i.e. on the rat brain. These data, obtained in experiments *in vivo* and *in vitro*, point to an important role of pyruvate as the source of acetyl–CoA for the synthesis of ACh. It would be premature, however, to generalize from the findings on the rat brain to other animal species or classes; it would even seem premature to generalize from them to parts of the nervous system other than the brain. It has been pointed out in Section 4.4.2 that, in comparison with the rat, the *Torpedo* fish and the lobster use much more acetate for the synthesis of ACh. Big differences in the utilization of various sources of acetyl groups for the synthesis of lipids have been found between the ruminant and monogastric mammals (for references see Tuček, 1967a; Škarda and Bílek, 1973). In this case, the differences are connected with the important role which the volatile fatty acids play in the metabolism of ruminants. Although experiments comparing the utilization of acetate and citrate in isolated nerve endings from several animal species (Tuček, 1966d, 1967a) did not reveal important differences in the utilization of acetate for the synthesis of ACh, species differences in other aspects of neuronal metabolism cannot be ruled out *a priori.* It is impossible to decide without further experimental study whether the high utilization of acetate for the synthesis of ACh in rabbit cornea (Fitzgerald and Cooper, 1967) has to be interpreted as a result of 'organ' specificity (i.e. as a special feature of the metabolism of the nerve endings in the cornea), or of species specificity. The finding of the high utilization of acetate for the synthesis of ACh in rat diaphragm (Dreyfus, 1975), in contrast to its low use for the synthesis of ACh in rat brain, indicates that the 'organ' differences can be large.

In the brain of newborn animals, the activity of pyruvate dehydrogenase is low (Wilbur and Patel, 1974), whereas the activity of acetoacetyl–CoA thiolase is high (Page *et al.*, 1971; DeVivo *et al.*, 1976). The utilization of ketone bodies (acetoacetic acid and 3-hydroxybutyric acid) by the brain is higher during early postnatal ontogeny than at later stages of development (Drahota *et al.*, 1965; Itoh and Quastel, 1970; Hawkins *et al.*, 1971; DeVivo *et al.*, 1975). In the light of these observations, it will not be surprising to find that the relative importance of various precursors of the acetyl group of ACh also varies with age. The observation of the high utilization of acetoacetate for the synthesis of ACh in the brain slices from 1–3 day old rats (Itoh and Quastel, 1970) supports such assumption. The need for further study of problems mentioned in this chapter seems evident.

4.7 SUMMARY

The immediate precursor of the acetyl groups of ACh in living cells is acetyl–CoA. The enzymes forming acetyl–CoA in the brain are localized in the mitochondria (pyruvate dehydrogenase complex, 3-oxoacyl–CoA thiolase, carnitine acetyltransferase), in the cytoplasm (ATP citrate lyase), or in both the mitochondria and cytoplasm (acetoacetyl–CoA thiolase, acetyl–CoA synthetase). Quantitatively the most important sources of acetyl–CoA in the cells are the oxidative decarboxylation of pyruvate and the β-oxidation of fatty acids; in both cases, acetyl–CoA is formed in the inner mitochondrial compartment.

Experiments with various preparations of the brain tissue *in vitro* revealed that the brain tissue can synthesize ACh when it is incubated in the presence of many compounds which serve as remote precursors of acetyl–CoA. In the light of experiments with radioactively labelled precursors *in vivo* and *in vitro*, pyruvate is the most likely source of acetyl groups for the acetyl–CoA used for ACh synthesis in rat brain; data for the brain tissue of other mammals are not available. Acetate is important as the precursor of acetyl groups for the synthesis of ACh in the electric organ of *Torpedo* and in lobster nerves.

It is not clear how the acetyl groups of the acetyl–CoA which is formed in the mitochondrial matrix from pyruvate pass into the extramitochondrial space, where the synthesis of ACh occurs. The inner mitochondrial membrane is generally considered to be impermeable to acetyl–CoA. A number of substances (citrate, α-ketoglutarate, glutamate, acetylcanitine, acetate, acetoacetate, acetylated amino acids) have been proposed to act as carriers of acetyl groups from the mitochondria for metabolic reactions proceeding extramitochondrially. Experimental observations do not confirm the participation of the supposed acetyl carriers in ACh synthesis in the brain. The possibility that acetyl–CoA leaves the mitochondria as such and is used directly for the extramitochondrial synthesis of ACh cannot be entirely dismissed with the evidence available at present time.

AUTHOR'S NOTE

A.C. Kato, P. Lefresne, Y. Berwald-Netter, J.C. Beaujouan, J. Glowinsky and F. Gros (*Biochem. biophys. Res. Commun.* **78**, 350–356, 1977) have described the use of glucose and acetate for the synthesis of ACh in a cholinergic neuroblastoma clone. P. Lefresne, M. Hamon, J.C. Beaujouan and J. Glowinsky (*Biochimie* **59**, 197–215, 1977) have provided further analysis of the utilization of pyruvate for ACh synthesis in rat striatal synaptosomes. J.P. Blass and G.E. Gibson (in *Cholinergic Mechanisms* and *Psychopharmacology,* D.J. Jenden, ed. Plenum Press, New York, in press) have given a summary of data on the relations between the metabolism of carbohydrates and ACh.

5 Supply of choline for the synthesis of acetylcholine

5.1 INTRODUCTION

Although choline is a simple compound and is essential for the life of cells, it appears that the cells of nervous tissue are unable to synthesize it. They are able, however, to release free choline from its esters. In addition, their surface membranes are equipped with carriers for the uptake of choline from the extracellular fluid. Choline is supplied to the brain via the blood stream both as free choline and in the form of phospholipids. This Chapter gives a short account of the biosynthesis of choline in animal organisms, its content in the blood plasma, cerebrospinal fluid and the brain, its transfer across neuronal membranes, its transport from the liver to the brain and its utilization in the synthesis of ACh *in vitro* and *in vivo*. Some of these problems have recently been reviewed by Sparf (1973), Ansell and Spanner (1975), Barker (1976a) and Freeman and Jenden (1976).

5.2 BIOSYNTHESIS OF CHOLINE

Choline is the trivial name for (2-hydroxyethyl) trimethylammonium hydroxide, its chemical formula being $HO^{-} \cdot (CH_3)_3N^{+} \cdot CH_2 \cdot CH_2OH$. So far, only one pathway leading to its synthesis has been discovered in animal organisms (Fig. 5.1; Bremer and Greenberg, 1960, 1961; Bremer *et al.*, 1960; Bjǿrnstad and Bremer, 1966; review by Voskresenskii and Maksimovich, 1967). In this pathway, choline is formed not as free compound, but as the choline moiety of phosphatidylcholine. The pathway may be described as starting from phosphatidylserine, which is decarboxylated to phosphatidylethanolamine. Phosphatidylethanolamine is then consecutive methylated to phosphatidylmonomethylethanolamine, phosphatidyldimethylethanolamine, and phosphatidylcholine (lecithin). Adenosylmethionine is the source of methyl groups used for the methylations (Gibson *et al.*, 1961). The formation of phosphatidylcholine, as just described, occurs mainly in the liver (Bjǿrnstad and Bremer, 1966). The

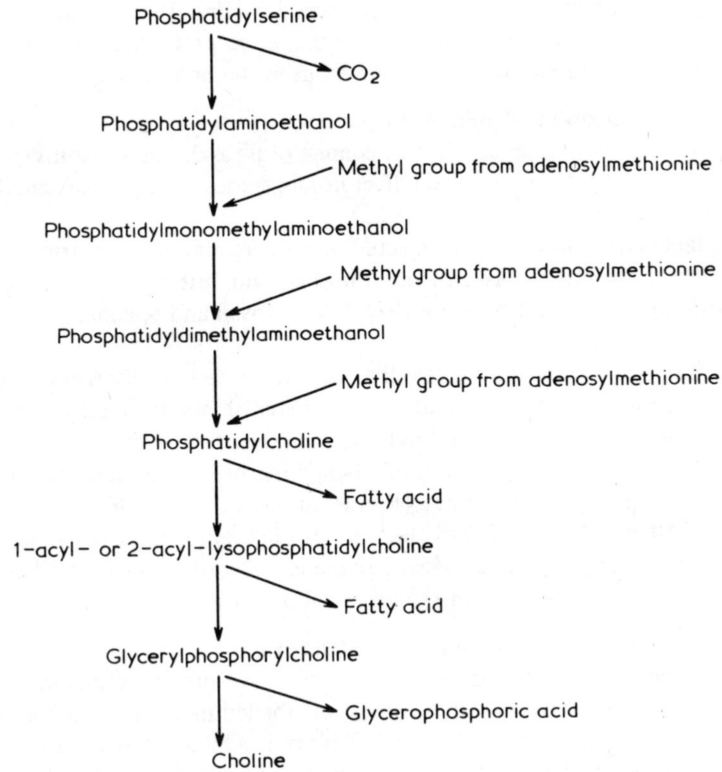

Fig. 5.1 Summary of the biosynthesis of choline.

degradation of phosphatidylcholine, finally leading to the formation of free choline, usually starts with the splitting off of glycerol-bound acyl groups (Thompson, 1973), which is catalysed by phospolipases A_1 and A_2. In this way, lysophosphatidylcholine and then glycerylphosphorylcholine are formed. The latter compounds is then hydrolysed to glycerophosphate and choline in a reaction catalysed by glyceryl-phosphorylcholine diesterase (L-3-glycerylphosphorylcholine glycerophosphoydrolase, EC 3.1.4.2).

There is no doubt that free choline may be formed in the brain from phosphatidyl-choline by the pathway just described. The presence of glycerylphosphorylcholine diesterase in the brain has been shown by Dawson (1956); it is distributed rather uniformly in various brain regions and appears to be preferentially associated with presynaptic membranes (Mann, 1976). The release of choline from glycerylphos-phorylcholine appears to be of primary importance, although the brain also contains phospholipase D (Saito and Kanfer, 1973) and lysophospholipase D (Wykle and Schremmer, 1974), which catalyse the direct release of choline from phosphatidyl-choline and lysophosphatidylcholine respectively; phospholipase D may possibly be responsible for the base exchange reactions of phospholipids in the brain (see Kanfer, 1972, for references).

While there is no doubt that the brain can release choline from choline-containing compounds, a number of observations indicate that *de novo* synthesis of choline, in either the free or lipid-bound form, does not occur in the brain tissue:

(a) Brain homogenates incubated in the presence of adenosylmethionine do not methylate phosphatidylmonomethylethanolamine or phosphatidyldimethylethanolamine under conditions in which liver homogenates effect intense methylation (Chojnacki *et al.*, 1964; Marshall *et al.*, 1965).

(b) When labelled ethanolamine is injected into the lateral brain ventricle, labelled phosphatidylethanolamine is formed from it in the brain, but no subsequent formation of labelled phosphatidylcholine is detectable (Ansell and Spanner, 1967, 1968a).

(c) Brain microsomes (i.e. the subcellular fraction formed mainly from particles of endoplasmic reticulum) do not catalyse the transfer of labelled methyl groups from adenosylmethionine to phospholipids; in this respect, they differ from liver microsomes, which execute the transfer of labelled methyl groups and the formation of choline-labelled phosphatidylcholine (Bremer and Greenberg, 1961).

(d) In the presence of labelled choline, slices of the brain form labelled ACh; no labelled ACh is produced, however, when choline is replaced by labelled ethanolamine, serine or methionine (Browning and Schulman, 1968).

Despite these observations, certain inconsistencies in the time course of labelling and in the relations between the specific radioactivities of presumed precursors and products, observed after intravenous injections of labelled methionine, ethanolamine or phosphate, led Kewitz *et al.* (1974, 1975; Kewitz and Pleul, 1976) to suggest that new choline is formed in the brain by methylation of free ethanolamine. This suggestion is based on indirect evidence only and most, if not all, of the observed inconsistencies in the relations between specific radioactivities of precursors and products can be explained by taking into account the following important features of choline metabolism in the brain:

(a) the inhomogeneity of the brain phosphatidylcholine pool, with a large proportion of brain phosphatidylcholine turning over very slowly and a small proportion turning over at an intermediate or rapid rate;

(b) the uncertainty about the levels of free choline in the brain and in the blood plasma as ascertained in various investigations (see Section 5.3.3 and Table 5.3);

(c) the possibility that free choline in the brain originates from phosphatidylcholine or lysophoasphatidylcholine of the blood plasma.

Haubrich *et al.* (1975c) found that the concentration of ACh in the brain increased after the administration of dimethylethanolamine. This observation would favour the view that choline is produced directly from dimethylethanolamine in the brain, but it was not confirmed in subsequent work by Zahniser *et al.* (1977).

5.3 THE CONTENT OF CHOLINE IN THE BLOOD PLASMA, CEREBROSPINAL FLUID AND BRAIN

5.3.1 Choline content in the blood plasma

As may be seen from data listed in Table 5.1 on the concentration of choline in the blood plasma, most investigators have reported the plasma concentrations of unesterified choline in various animal species to be in the range 5–25 μM. The results of Spanner *et al.* (1976) are an exception; they found that the choline concentrations in rat and human blood plasma are less than 1 μM. Repeated measurements performed in the same individuals indicate that the concentration of choline in the blood plasma is comparatively stable (Bligh, 1952; Appleton *et al.*, 1953) and no evidence of a circadian rhythm in plasma choline concentrations has been found (Haubrich *et al.*, 1976). The injection or infusion of choline brings about an increase of choline concentration in the blood plasma, followed by a rapid return to the initial state (Bligh, 1953; Appleton *et al.*, 1953; Gardiner and Paton, 1972; Kuntscherová, 1972; Choi *et al.*, 1975); this point is illustrated by Fig. 6.12. Surplus choline supplied by the infusions is taken up mainly by the liver and kidneys (Bligh, 1953; Haubrich *et al.*, 1975a; Gardiner and Paton, 1972) and by other abdominal visceral organs and lungs (Gardiner and Paton, 1972). As will be discussed in Section 5.5, the concentration of choline in the blood plasma leaving the brain is higher than in the blood plasma entering it. In rats kept on a choline-deficient diet the concentration of blood plasma choline falls to about one half of control values (Wang and Haubrich, 1975; Haubrich *et al.*, 1976).

Recent reports indicate that the results of measurements of blood plasma choline are strongly influenced by the way in which the blood samples are treated before assay. Wang and Haubrich (1975) demonstrated that the concentration of choline was unchanged when samples of plasma were kept for 3 h on ice, but that it more than doubled when samples were kept for 3 h at 22.5°C. Spanner *et al.* (1976) reported a similar finding for both rat and human plasma, but not for rabbit plasma in which the concentration of free choline was stable also at room temperature. In addition, they stressed the necessity of centrifuging the blood samples at 4°C in order to prevent the post mortem rise in unesterified plasma choline. It is not clear to what extent the very low concentrations of blood plasma choline reported by these authors (0.25 μM for rats and 0.72 and 0.90 μM for 2 observations on man) reflect the more careful prevention of hydrolysis of choline esters or whether other factors may be responsible.

5.3.2 Choline content in the cerebrospinal fluid

A comparison of choline concentrations in the blood plasma (Table 5.1) with those in cerebrospinal fluid (0.4–5.1 μM, see Table 5.2) indicates that there is less unesterified choline in the cerebrospinal fluid. The difference is seen best in studies

Table 5.1 Concentration of choline in the blood plasma*

Species	Concentration of choline (μM)		References
Cat	6		Bligh (1952)
	7.3		Wang and Haubrich (1975)
Dog	9		Bligh (1952)
	10.5		Schuberth and Sundwall (1971)
	5.5		Wang and Haubrich (1975)
Guinea pig	15.4		Wang and Haubrich (1975)
Mouse	15		Schuberth and Sundwall (1971)
	12.6		Wang and Haubrich (1975)
Rabbit	24		Bligh (1952)
	10.1		Schuberth and Jenden (1975)
	5.2		Spanner *et al.* (1976)
Rat	7		Kuntscherová (1971)
	12.3	(whole blood)	Dross and Kewitz (1972)
	10–15		Sparf (1973)
	16.7		Saelens *et al.* (1973)
	14.4		Wang and Haubrich (1975)
	10		Freeman *et al.* (1975a)
	11		Choi *et al.* (1975)
	13		Racagni *et al.* (1975)
	8.2		Haubrich *et al.* (1976)
	8	(diet without choline)	Cohen and Wurtman (1976)
	15.3	(diet with 20 mg choline per day)	
	32.6	(diet with 129 mg choline per day)	
	0.25		Spanner *et al.* (1976)
Rhesus monkey	15.1		Wang and Haubrich (1975)
Man	8–18		Bligh (1952)
	22–63		Appleton *et al.* (1953)
	10.9		Aquilonius *et al.* (1970)
	10.9		Schuberth and Sundwall (1971)
	15.9		Wang and Haubrich (1975)
	12.7		Aquilonius *et al.* (1975)
	0.81		Spanner *et al.* (1976)

* Results included in the table have been obtained from arterial blood plasma, or from venous blood plasma other than that flowing from the brain.

Table 5.2 Concentration of choline in the cerebrospinal fluid

Species	Concentration of choline (μM)		Reference
Cat	0.4–3.6		Gardiner and Domer (1968)
Dog	1.1		Bowers (1967b)
	4.6	(ventricular CSF)	Aquilonius *et al.* (1970)
	2.3	(cisternal CSF)	
	4.6	(ventricular CSF)	Schuberth and Sundwall (1971)
	1.9	(cisternal CSF)	
Rabbit	5.1		Schuberth and Jenden (1975)
Man	1.1		Bowers (1967b)
	1.8		Jönsson *et al.* (1969)
	2.2		Aquilonius *et al.* (1970)
	2.2		Schuberth and Sundwall (1971)
	2.4		Aquilonius *et al.* (1971)
	3.35		Welch *et al.* (1976)
	2.2		Growdon *et al.* (1977)

in which the cerebrospinal fluid and the plasma have been investigated simultaneously. Aquilonius *et al.* (1970) found 2.2 μM choline in human cerebrospinal fluid and 10.9 μM in the plasma; in rabbit corresponding values were, respectively, 5.1 and 10.1 μM (Schuberth and Jenden, 1975). It seems important to confirm that the reported differences between the cerebrospinal fluid and the blood plasma persist when the assays are performed under strictest conditions suggested for prevention of the hydrolysis of choline esters (Wang and Haubrich, 1975; Spanner *et al.*, 1976; Mann and Hebb, 1977).

An interesting point is that choline is not distributed uniformly throughout the cerebrospinal fluid. The existence of a ventriculo–lumbar gradient in its concentration, the lumbar concentration being lower, is likely in view of the differences between the ventricular and cisternal concentrations (Aquilonius *et al.*, 1970; Schuberth and Sundwall, 1971) and between the concentrations in samples taken soon and later after lumbar puncture (Welch *et al.*, 1976).

Choline in the cerebrospinal fluid probably originates from unesterified choline in the extracellular fluid of the brain. This, in its turn, comes from two sources:

(1) from unesterified choline of the blood plasma;
(2) from choline esters hydrolysed in the cells of the brain. After infusions of labelled choline, or its administration in the diet, the pools of choline in the blood plasma and in the cerebrospinal fluid become labelled, but the specific radioactivity in the cerebrospinal fluid never reaches that in the plasma (Schuberth and Jenden, 1975). This is best explained on assumption that, on its passage through the

extracellular space of the brain, the labelled choline from the blood plasma is continuously diluted by unlabelled (or less labelled) choline released from the brain cells and originating from choline esters, mainly from phospholipids. Although labelled choline from the blood reaches the cerebrospinal fluid very rapidly, its concentration in the cerebrospinal fluid is not directly dependent on its concentration in the blood plasma. It changes only slightly during short term intraarterial infusions of choline in cats (Gardiner and Domer, 1968), but it does increase after long term oral administration of choline to man (Growdon *et al.*, 1977). Choline is probably removed from the cerebrospinal fluid via the choroid plexus like other quarternary ammonium compounds (Tochino and Schanker, 1965).

5.3.3 Choline content in the brain

The data on the concentration of unesterified choline in the brain, summarized in Table 5.3, reveal that, during the last decade, the values reported from different laboratories underwent a marked reduction. This is particularly conspicuous in the case of data on choline concentrations in rat brain: from values well above 100 nmol/g the concentrations have decreased to below 40 nmol/g in most recent reports and to below 10 nmol/g in the study by Mann and Hebb (1977). This trend to lower values stemmed from the realization that a post mortem increase in free choline occurs in the brain (Schuberth *et al.*, 1970a,b; Dross and Kewitz, 1972; Aprison *et al.*, 1974; Hanin and Schuberth, 1974; Stavinoha and Weintraub, 1974b; Choi *et al.*, 1975; Freeman *et al.*, 1975b; see Section 5.4 for discussion) and that the rapid inactivation of brain enzymes and the prevention of non-enzymatic formation of free choline are therefore of the utmost importance in establishing the concentrations existing in the brain *in vivo*.

Dross and Kewitz (1972) tried to circumvent the problem of post mortem changes by measuring their rate and extrapolating the choline concentration present at the moment of death from concentrations found in the brain at different times after death. They arrived at a value of 27.5 nmol/g. Stavinoha and Weintraub (1974b) demonstrated the importance of rapid inactivation of brain enzymes by comparing the content of choline in rat brains homogenized 5 min after the animal had been killed by microwave with that in rat brains irradiated and homogenized 5 min after the animal had been killed by cervical dislocation. When denaturation of the brain enzymes by microwave was delayed for 5 min, the concentration of choline increased from 26.3 to 148.3 nmol/g.

Although many investigators have found the technique of microwave irradiation useful for rapid inactivation of brain enzymes before the assay of choline concentration, the lowest concentration of free choline in the brain, and probably the most complete prevention of post mortem choline formation, has been obtained using the method of freeze-blowing the brain (Mann and Hebb, 1977). The concentration of free choline has been found to be 8.7 nmol/g in the cerebrum and 14.9 nmol/g in the cerebellum. The importance features of the technique used by Mann and Hebb

Table 5.3 Content of choline in the central nervous system

Species	Region	Choline content (nmol/g)	Reference
Mouse	Brain	115	Schuberth *et al.* (1969)
	Brain	131.5	Saelens *et al.* (1970)
	Brain	68.1	Schuberth and Sundwall (1971)
	Brain	68.8	Collier *et al.* (1972)
	Brain	65.1	Consolo *et al.* (1972)
	Brain	57.4	Jenden *et al.* (1972)
	Brain	38.2	Ladinsky *et al.* (1972b)
	Cerebellum	36.4	
	Brain	43	Sparf (1973)
	Brain	43.4	Jenden *et al.* (1974)
	Brain	33	Cheney *et al.* (1975b)
	Brain	30	Cheney *et al.* (1975c)
	Brain	29.2	Gibson and Blass (1976)
	Brain	28	Haubrich and Wang (1976)
	Brain	51.6	Jenden *et al.* (1976)
	Cortex	30.5	Nordberg and Sundwall (1976)
	Cerebellum	18.6	
	Medulla	46.7	
	Midbrain	41.3	
	Striatum	41.4	
	Hippocampus	27.4	
Guinea pig	Brain	141	Haubrich *et al.* (1974)
Rat	Brain	170	Ansell and Spanner (1968b, 1971)
	Brain	274	Hanin *et al.* (1970)
	Brain	67.7	Reid *et al.* (1971)
	Brain	107	Browning (1972)
	Brain	71.2	Ladinsky *et al.* (1972a)
	Brain	42; 27.5 *	Dross and Kewitz (1972)
	Brain	77.7	Sethy *et al.* (1973)
	Cortex	35.1	
	Striatum	127	
	Hypothalamus	111.3	
	Midbrain	67.8	
	Brainstem	66.6	
	Hippocampus	54.9	
	Cerebellum	38.1	
	Brain	58.8	Sethy and VanWoert (1973)
	Cortex	73	Saelens *et al.* (1973)
	Midbrain	74	
	Brainstem	83	

* The value of 27.5 nmol/g has been obtained by subtracting the post mortem increase of free choline from the measured value of 42 nmol/g.

Table 5.3 (*continued*) Content of choline in the central nervous system

Species	Region	Choline content (nmol/g)	Reference
Rat	Brain	39	Sparf (1973)
	Cerebrum	25	Shea and Aprison (1973)
	Brain	21	Eade *et al.* (1973)
	Brain	50	Hanin and Schuberth (1974)
	Cortex	22.1	Stavinoha *et al.* (1974)
	Striatum	43	
	Medulla–pons	34.7	
	Hippocampus	36	
	Cerebellum	17.6	
	Brain	25.6	Stavinoha and Weintraub (1974a)
	Brain	26.3	Stavinoha and Weintraub (1974b)
	Striatum	43	Stavinoha *et al.* (1974)
	Striatum	79.4	Consolo *et al.* (1975)
	Brain	28.3	Schmidt and Speth (1975)
	Cortex	28	Racagni *et al.* (1975)
	Striatum	32	
	Brain	46.4	Choi *et al.* (1975)
	Brain	22.7	Freeman *et al.* (1975b)
	Brain	75.4	Smith *et al.* (1975)
	Brain	26.8	Cohen and Wurtman (1975)
	Telencephalon	85.2	Smith *et al.* (1975)
	Diencephalon–mesencephalon	69.6	
	Pons–medulla	85.4	
	Cerebellum	72	
	Cortex	22.1	Modak *et al.* (1975)
	Striatum	43	
	Hippocampus	36	
	Medulla	34.7	
	Cortex	17	Haubrich *et al.* (1975b)
	Striatum	29	
	Brain	28	Cheney *et al.* (1975b)
	Striatum	35	Haubrich *et al.* (1975c)
	Brain	38	Haubrich *et al.* (1976)
	Striatum	39–43	Racagni *et al.* (1976)
	Striatum	43	Costa *et al.* (1976)
	Hippocampus	45	Zsilla *et al.* (1976)
	Cortex	26	
	Striatum	39	
	Brainstem	36	

Table 5.3 (*continued*) Content of choline in the central nervous system

Species	Region	Choline content (nmol/g)	Reference
Rat	Cerebrum	24	Cohen and Wurtman (1976)
	Cerebrum	8.7	Mann and Hebb (1977)
	Cerebellum	14.9	

(1977) are, in addition to rapid freezing, the extraction of choline at –70°C, the avoidance of an acid extraction medium, and the removal (by ionic exchange) of substances from which free choline might be formed.

The concentration of free choline in the brain may be increased by intravenous infusions of choline (Racagni *et al.*, 1975) or by administering very large amounts of choline in the diet (Cohen and Wurtman, 1976). In animals raised on choline-deficient diets the content of choline is lowered in many organs and in the blood plasma, but it does not differ from controls in the brain (Haubrich *et al.*, 1976).

Compared with the low concentration of free choline, cerebral concentrations of compounds containing esterified choline appear enormous: 1 g of brain tissue contains 380 nmol phosphorylcholine, 50 nmol cytidine diphosphate choline, 400 nmol glycerylphosphorylcholine, 14 700 nmol phosphatidylcholine, 620 nmol choline plasmalogen, 3650 nmol sphingomyelin, and 16 nmol ACh (Ansell and Spanner, 1968b, 1970, 1975).

5.4 FACILITATED UPTAKE OF CHOLINE BY THE BRAIN TISSUE

Despite its positive charge, choline passes very rapidly from the blood to the brain. After intravenous injections of [^{3}H] choline to mice the content of [^{3}H] choline in the whole brain was highest in animals sacrificed only 0.5 min after injection (Aquilonius *et al.*, 1973) while the radioactivity in the fraction of the nerve endings was highest in animals sacrificed 90 s after the injection (Schuberth *et al.*, 1970b). The rapid passage of choline into the brain has been observed in many other studies (Schuberth *et al.*, 1969; Haubrich *et al.*, 1972, 1975a,b; Jenden *et al.*, 1974; Nordberg and Sundwall, 1976).

The entry of choline into the brain depends on the activity of a choline-specific transport system in the blood–brain barrier (Partridge and Oldendorf, 1977) and on the activity of choline-specific carriers in the membranes of neural and glial cells. The existence of saturable carrier system for choline at the level of the blood–brain barrier has been suggested by the results of experiments in which mice were injected with increasing doses of radioactively labelled choline and the uptake of

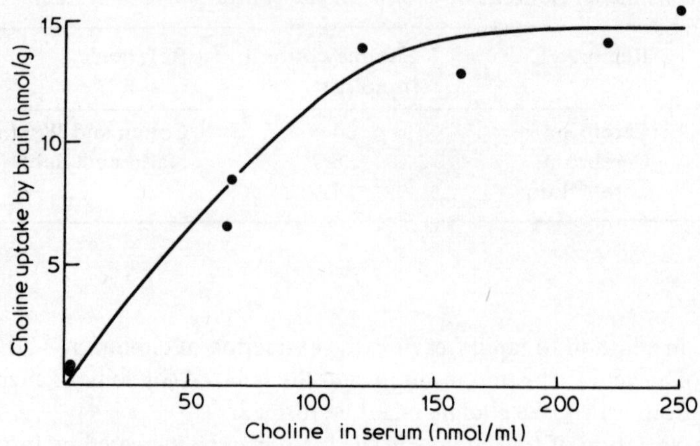

Fig. 5.2 The relation between the concentration of radioactive choline in the blood serum and its uptake by the brain in experiments on mice *in vivo*. Abscissa: concentration of [^{3}H] choline in the serum (nmoles per ml). Ordinate: amount of choline taken up by the brain (nmoles per g brain weight). Measurements were performed 1 min after i.v. injection of varying amounts of [^{3}H] choline. Each point corresponds to 1 animal. The shape of the curve indicates that the mechanism for choline uptake by the brain is saturated at high concentrations of choline in the blood (after Diamond, 1971).

label by the brain was measured (Fig. 5.2; Diamond, 1971). The uptake increased with increasing concentrations of labelled choline in the blood, but when the concentration of labelled choline in the blood serum exceeded about 120 μM, the amount of label recovered in the brain did not increase further. An interesting feature of Diamond's (1971) experiments was that phenobarbital reduced the uptake of choline by the brain by about 50%.

The presence of a carrier for choline in the membranes of nerve cells was initially demonstrated by Hodgkin and Martin (1965) in the giant axons of *Loligo*, and the first observations indicating the presence of a choline carrier in brain tissue were described by Schuberth *et al.* (1966a) and Quastel (1966). Schuberth *et al.* (1966a) noted that on incubation in a medium with radioactively labelled choline the content of radioactivity in brain slices increased, so that after incubation for 90 min the concentration of labelled atoms in the slices was three times higher than in the medium. Most (77%) of the label in the tissue remained in the form of choline. The uptake of choline had two components. One of them was saturated by higher concentrations of choline in the medium and required the presence of glucose and oxygen and was inhibited by dinitrophenol; the other component, which most probably corresponded to the diffusion of choline, was not saturated even at very high concentration of choline in the medium. Subsequently, saturable uptake of choline, obeying Michaelis–Menten kinetics and clearly based on the function of a carrier system, was demonstrated in isolated nerve endings (Potter, 1968; Marchbanks, 1968b; Diamond and Kennedy, 1969; Haga, 1971), in subcellular fractions containing mitochondria (Marchbanks, 1968b; Diamond and Milfay, 1972), in microsomes and synaptic vesicles (Diamond and Milfay, 1972), and in cultures of neural and glial cells (Massarelli *et al.*, 1974a; Lanks *et al.*, 1974). A carrier system for choline has also been discovered in the membranes of many cells outside the nervous system (see Diamond and Milfay, 1972, for references).

An important step forward was the discovery that there are at least two carrier systems for choline in the membranes of brain cells, differing in their affinity for the transported substances. This was first proposed by Haga (1971) and confirmed by Yamamura and Snyder (1972, 1973), Haga and Noda (1973), Whittaker *et al.* (1972), Dowdall and Simon (1973), Kuhar *et al.* (1973) and by many others. The affinity of the carrier for the transported substances may be expressed, with some qualification, by the value of K_m. This is analogous to the Michaelis constant used in enzymology and corresponds to the concentration of the substance at which its transport proceeds at a velocity equal to 1/2 of the maximal velocity attainable. Yamamura and Snyder (1973) found in homogenates of rat striatum a high affinity carrier with a K_m for choline equal to 1.4 μM and a low affinity carrier with a K_m equal to 93 μM. Corresponding values in homogenates of brain cortex were 3.1 μM and 33 μM, while in homogenates of the cerebellum, which has a very small cholinergic component, only the low affinity carrier with a K_m equal to 41 μM was found (Fig. 5.3). Similarly, Haga and Noda (1973) concluded from experiments on crude mitochondrial fractions that there are two choline carriers in rat brain – one with a K_m of 4–8 μM and another with a K_m of about 40 μM. The synaptosomes from the optic lobes of *Loligo pealii* and *Loligo forbesi* are both equipped with a high affinity carrier with a K_m of about 2 μM, whereas the low affinity carriers have K_m of 37 μM and 117 μM respectively (Dowdall and Simon, 1973).

Kinetic data similar to those illustrated in Fig. 5.3 and indicating the simultaneous presence of a high and low affinity carrier for choline have been obtained in experiments on many parts of the nervous system or on innervated tissues, e.g. cat retina (Neal and Gilroy, 1975), guinea pig intestinal muscle (Pert and Snyder, 1974), rat sympathetic ganglia (Bowery and Neal, 1975), mouse minced brain cortex (Carroll and Goldberg, 1975), chick iris (Suszkiw and Pilar, 1976), segmental ganglion of the leech (Adamič, 1975), nervous tissue of *Aplysia* (Schwartz *et al.*, 1975), suboesophageal ganglia of the snail (Osborne, 1976), and cultured neuroblastoma cells (Massarelli *et al.*, 1974c).

The high and low affinity carriers for choline differ not only in their K_m but also in their localization, properties and functional significance. The high affinity carrier appears to be localized in the axons and their endings. In *Aplysia*, the high affinity uptake in the cell bodies of cholinergic neurons is very low, whereas it is high in the neuropil and nerves (Eisenstadt *et al.*, 1975). It is absent from the denervated ciliary ganglia (i.e. from the bodies of cholinergic neurons; Suszkiw *et al.*, 1976; Suszkiw and Pilar, 1976), but it is present in the axonal terminals of ciliary ganglion cells

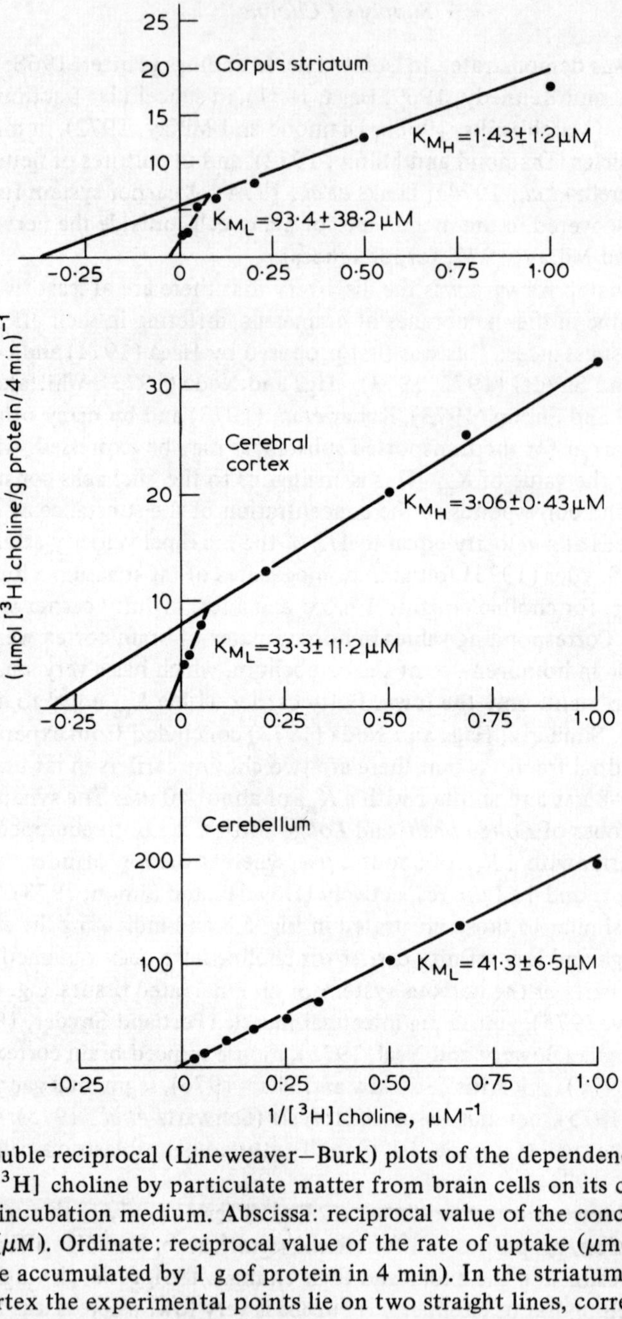

Fig. 5.3 Double reciprocal (Lineweaver–Burk) plots of the dependence of the uptake of [^{3}H] choline by particulate matter from brain cells on its concentration in the incubation medium. Abscissa: reciprocal value of the concentration of choline (μM). Ordinate: reciprocal value of the rate of uptake (μmoles of [^{3}H] choline accumulated by 1 g of protein in 4 min). In the striatum and cerebral cortex the experimental points lie on two straight lines, corresponding to the high affinity and low affinity uptake systems for choline. Only the low affinity system is present in the cerebellum. K_m values corresponding to individual straight lines are shown on the graph. The subscripts L and H indicate low and high affinity uptake respectively (after Yamamura and Snyder, 1973).

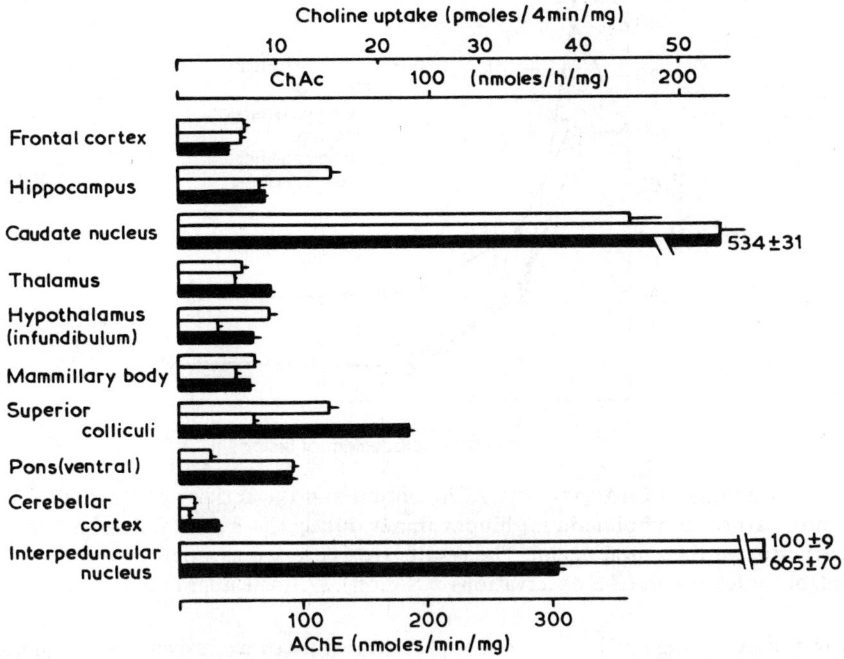

Fig. 5.4 Comparison of the high affinity uptake of choline (white columns), ChAc activity (dotted columns) and AChE activity (black columns) in crude synaptosomal preparations from various parts of rat brain. The uptake of choline is expressed in pmoles choline/4 min/mg protein, the activity of ChAc in nmoles ACh/h/mg protein, the activity of AChE in nmoles acetylthiocholine/min/mg protein. The crude synaptosomal preparation corresponded to a sucrose homogenate, from which the big particles had been removed by 10 min centrifugation at 1000 *g*. Choline uptake was measured at a concentration of 430 nM (after Sorimachi and Kataoka, 1974b).

(Suszkiw and Pilar, 1976). Both types of uptake can be found in the nerve ending fraction isolated from rat brain homogenates on density gradients, but only the low affinity uptake is present in the purified mitochondrial fraction (Yamamura and Snyder, 1973). The high affinity carrier differs from the low affinity carrier by its greater dependence on the presence of sodium (Yamamura and Snyder, 1973; Haga and Noda, 1973; Eisenstadt *et al.*, 1975; Suszkiw and Pilar, 1976), by its greater sensitivity to metabolic inhibitors – cyanide and dinitrophenol; (Yamamura and Snyder, 1973; Dowdall and Simon, 1973), to ouabain (Yamamura and Snyder, 1972, 1973; Dowdall and Simon, 1973; Eisenstadt *et al.*, 1975) and to hemicholinium-3 (Haga and Noda, 1973; Dowdall and Simon, 1973).

From the point of view of the physiology of cholinergic synapses, the most interesting aspect of findings concerning the carrier for choline in the brain is the

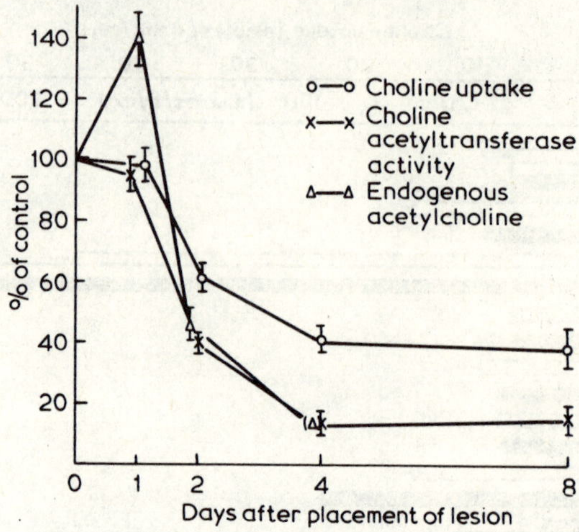

Fig. 5.5 Changes of ChAc activity, ACh content and the activity of the high affinity carrier for choline in rat hippocampus during the 8 days following the destruction of the septal nuclei. The results are expressed as a percentage of control values (mean of 5 observations ± S.E.M.). (After Kuhar *et al.*, 1973).

possibility that the high affinity carrier is present mainly or exclusively in cholinergic neurons and that its function is, therefore, closely connected with the synthesis of ACh. The following experimental observations support this idea:

(a) When various parts of the brain are compared, a very good correlation can be found between the activity of ChAc and the activity of the high affinity choline carrier (Fig. 5.4; Sorimachi and Kataoka, 1974b). Yamamura and Snyder (1973) found the high affinity carrier in synaptosomes from the striatum and cerebral cortex, but not in those from the cerebellum, which contains few cholinergic components; Carroll and Buterbaugh (1975a) did find the high affinity choline uptake system in cerebellar synaptosomes, but its maximal capacity was lower than in brain areas containing more cholinergic neurons.

(b) Most of the choline transported by the high affinity system is acetylated to ACh, but in the case of choline transported by the low affinity system the acetylation involves only a small part of the transported substance (Haga, 1971; Haga and Noda, 1973; Yamamura and Snyder, 1972, 1973; Simon *et al.*, 1976).

(c) Lesions made in the medial septal area, causing the degeneration of cholinergic fibres and endings in the hippocampus, considerably lower the high affinity uptake of choline in the hippocampus; the lowering of uptake proceeds in parallel with the lowering of the activity of ChAc and of ACh content (Fig. 5.5; Kuhar *et al.*, 1973). A similar simultaneous decrease of ChAc, ACh and the high affinity choline carrier was observed in the interpeduncular nucleus after lesions made in the medial habenular area (Kuhar *et al.*, 1975).

(d) The postnatal increase of the high affinity uptake of choline in the striatum and hippocampus coincides remarkably with the increase of ChAc activity in these areas (Sorimachi *et al.*, 1974; Sorimachi and Kataoka, 1975).

(e) In experiments on hippocampal slices, an increased concentration of K^+ ions caused the release of ACh from neurons which gained choline via the high affinity uptake (Mulder *et al.*, 1974). Preincubation of brain slices (Polak *et al.*, 1977a) or of synaptosomes (Murrin and Kuhar, 1976; but cf. Barker, 1976b) in the presence of a high concentration of K^+ ions increased the subsequent high affinity uptake only if Ca^{2+} ions (necessary for ACh release) were present in the medium during preincubation.

(f) When the diaphragm was incubated with 2 μM choline, the uptake of choline in the region containing nerve terminals did not differ from the uptake in 'aneural' areas of the muscle; if, however, the incubation was performed with much less choline (12 nM), the uptake was considerably higher in the nerve ending region as compared with that in the 'aneural' area (Chang and Lee, 1970).

(g) The high affinity uptake was no longer detectable in minces of intestinal longitudinal muscle after the myenetric plexus had been removed (Pert and Snyder, 1974).

(h) Comparison of different animal species reveals a positive correlation between the content of ACh in the nervous system and the rate of high affinity uptake of choline (Whittaker and Dowdall, 1975; Dowdall *et al.*, 1976).

The view that the high affinity carrier for choline is a specific component of the membranes of cholinergic nerve endings accords well with data indicating that ACh is synthesized preferentially from the choline which is supplied by the high affinity carrier (see Section 5.6 and chapter 6.9). On the other hand, several observations on cell cultures are at variance with the assumption that the high affinity choline uptake is specific for cholinergic neurons. The high affinity uptake has also been observed in glial cells (Richelson and Thompson, 1973; Massarelli *et al.*, 1974b), in glioblastoma cells (Massarelli *et al.*, 1974b), and in non-cholinergic neuroblastoma cells (Richelson and Thompson, 1973; Massarelli *et al.*, 1974c, 1976; Lanks *et al.*, 1974). The high affinity transport in cell cultures appears to be different, however, from the uptake system described in preparations from the mature nervous system. It is less dependent on the presence of sodium ions and less sensitive to the inhibitory action of hemicholinium-3 (Lanks *et al.*, 1974) and also its kinetics are different (Massarelli and Mandel, 1976). Despite these differences, the observations on non-cholinergic neuroblastoma cells and on glia in culture suggest the need for caution in accepting the view that the high affinity uptake of choline in the living brain is specific for cholinergic neurons. Relevant to this point is the observation by Bowery and Neal (1975) that the high affinity uptake in sympathetic ganglia still persists after preganglionic nerve section when the cholinergic terminals should have degenerated.

The low affinity uptake of choline most probably represents an example of facilitated diffusion, i.e. of carrier-mediated transfer proceeding along the electrochemical gradient independently of an energy supply. In the case of the high affinity

Table 5.4 Effects of inhibition of oxidative metabolism by cyanide ions, 2,4-dinitrophenol (DNP) or by the omission of glucose on the high affinity uptake of choline

Animal	Preparation	Concentration of choline (μM)	Concentration of CN^- (mM)
Rat	Nuclei-free	0.5	1
	homogenate of the	0.5	
	striatum	0.5	
Rat	Synaptosomes from	3.7	4
	the brain	3.7	
Rat	Crude synaptosomal–	1	1
	mitochondrial fraction	1	
	from the hippocampus	1	
Guinea pig	Mince of innervated	0.2	0.25
	longitudinal	0.2	
	intestinal muscle		
Chick	Mixed neuronal–glial	0.5	
	cell culture from		
	embryonic brain		
Loligo	Synaptosomes from	1	2
	the head ganglion	1	
Aplysia	Circumoesophageal	20	1.3
	ganglia	20	
Helix pomatia	Suboesophageal	0.5	0.5
	ganglia	0.5	
		0.5	

uptake it is still not possible to decide with certainty whether it is based on active transport (i.e. transfer against the electrochemical gradient and dependent on a supply of energy) or on facilitated diffusion. None of the studies on the uptake of choline by brain tissue has analysed the problem of equilibrium distribution of choline along the electrochemical gradient. In view of the presence of a positive charge on choline and a negative charge on the inner side of cell membranes one would expect that the concentration of choline in the tissue would be higher than in the medium even if the substance is distributed entirely passively.

In studies following the distribution of radioactively labelled atoms originally present in choline, the tissue/medium ratio of radioactivity will be elevated also, because much of the tissue label will be present in choline metabolites. It may be appropriate to recall here that Yamamura and Snyder (1973) showed that as much as 88% of [^{3}H]choline transported into the subcellular particles of the brain via the high affinity system was converted to [^{3}H]ACh. The ratio of the concentration of

Table 5.4 (*continued*) Effects of inhibition of oxidative metabolism by cyanide ions, 2,4-dinitrophenol (DNP) or by the omission of glucose on the high affinity uptake of choline

Concentration of DNP (μM)	Concentration of glucose (mM)	Uptake of choline (% of control)	Reference
	11	27	Yamamura and Snyder (1973)
0.2	11	40	
	0	100	
	10	98	Haga and Noda (1973)
0.2	10	96	
	11	56	Simon and Kuhar (1976)
0.1	11	85	
	0	67	
	11	107	Pert and Snyder (1974)
1	11	64	
1	?	61	Massarelli *et al.* (1974a)
	10	10	Dowdall and Simon (1973)
0.1	10	65	
	6	102	Eisenstadt *et al.* (1975)
0.2	6	88	
	5	73	Osborne (1976)
0.5	5	70	
	0	100	

label in the tissue to that in the medium has indeed been found to be higher than 1.0 in various experiments in which tissues have been incubated in the presence of radioactively labelled choline: in brain slices (Schuberth *et al.*, 1966a; Quastel, 1966), subcellular particles of nervous tissue (Marchbanks, 1968b; Dowdall and Simon, 1973; Carroll and Buterbaugh, 1975b; but cf. Potter, 1968), in the retina (Neal and Gilroy, 1975), and in snail ganglion (Osborne, 1976). Cooke and Robinson (1971) found in experiments with brain slices that the tissue/medium ratio of unmetabolized [^{3}H]choline was only 1.1. In experiments with cultured neuroblastoma cells exposed to [^{3}H]choline, the concentration of labelled compounds within the cells exceeded the radioactivity in the medium by a factor of 20 (Lanks *et al.*, 1974). It can, however, be calculated from data provided in this study, that the concentration of unmetabolized choline in the cells was lower than in the medium, with most of intracellular label being present in phosphorylcholine. This example demonstrates particularly clearly how misleading it may be to identify a high tissue/medium ratio of radioactive label with the presence of an active uphill transport process.

As far as the effect of metabolic inhibition on the uptake of choline is concerned, there is a general concensus that metabolic inhibitors have little effect on choline uptake studied under conditions favouring the low affinity system, i.e. in the presence of high concentrations of choline (Marchbanks, 1968b; Diamond and Kennedy, 1969; Yamamura and Snyder, 1973; Dowdall and Simon, 1973; Suszkiw *et al.*, 1976). Data regarding the effect of metabolic inhibitors on the high affinity uptake of choline, summarized in Table 5.4, are controversial. Although metabolic inhibitors strongly reduced the uptake in some experiments (Yamamura and Snyder, 1973; Dowdall and Simon, 1973), they had little or no action in others (Haga and Noda, 1973; Pert and Snyder, 1974; Simon and Kuhar, 1976; Osborne, 1976; Massarelli *et al.*, 1974a; Eisenstadt *et al.*, 1975). The dependence of the high affinity uptake of choline on an energy supply, as suggested by some of the observations in Table 5.4, might indicate that this is a case of energy-dependent active transport. It is possible, however, that the supply of energy is necessary, not for the uptake of choline as such, but for other processes influencing the distribution of choline between the medium and the tissue. Such processes include the maintenance of the membrane potential and the formation of energy-rich intermediary compounds which are required for the metabolic turnover of choline in the cells (e.g. the formation of acetyl–CoA for the synthesis of ACh, or of ATP for the synthesis of phosphorylcholine). In view of these problems and of discrepancies in available data, the results of experiments with metabolic inhibitors cannot provide the answer to the question whether the facilitated uptake of choline occurs by facilitated diffusion or by active transport.

An important feature of the facilitated transport of choline in the nervous tissue is its sensitivity to many physiologically and pharmacologically active compounds. One of the important compounds affecting the uptake of choline is ACh. Its inhibitory action on choline uptake was first observed by Potter (1968) and later confirmed by many other investigators. The effect of ACh is comparatively strong. Yamamura and Snyder (1973) reported that in homogenates of rat striatum the high affinity uptake was decreased by 75% in the presence of 10 μM ACh, while Simon *et al.* (1975) found a decrease of 50% in the presence of 12 μM ACh. Among the many drugs having an inhibitory effect on choline uptake are chlorpromazine, atropine, bretylium, guanethidine, eserine and neostigmine (Diamond and Kennedy, 1969; Yamamura and Snyder, 1973; Guyenet *et al.*, 1973a; Pert and Snyder, 1974; Osborne, 1976). Other inhibitors include choline analogues (Simon *et al.*, 1975; Holden *et al.*, 1975; Barker and Mittag, 1975) and neurotoxic snake venoms acting presynaptically (Dowdall *et al.*, personal communication). In contrast to ACh and the other inhibitory substances, noradrenaline (Carroll and Buterbaugh, 1975b), prednisone and dexamethasone (Veldsema-Currie *et al.*, 1976) have been found to stimulate the uptake of choline.

Ionic requirements of the high affinity uptake in cerebral synaptosomes have been most systematically investigated by Simon and Kuhar (1976). They found, as already mentioned, that the uptake was characteristically dependent on the presence of Na^+

ions, but it was not altered by the omission of magnesium or calcium from the incubation media. This latter observation suggesting that calcium is unimportant disagrees with the finding of Pert and Snyder (1974) on minces of innervated intestinal muscle. In their experiments, the omission of calcium decreased the uptake of choline by more than 50%. The high affinity uptake in brain synaptosomes was reduced in the absence of chloride anions. It was maximal with potassium concentration between 0.35 and 4.8 mM, but it was reduced at both lower and higher potassium concentrations. The reduction was about 50% in the presence of 35 mM K^+ (Simon and Kuhar, 1976) and more than 90% in the presence of 62 mM K^+ (Murrin and Kuhar, 1976). The reduction of choline uptake *during* potassium-induced depolarization is in marked contrast to the increase of uptake observed *after* the end of depolarization; this will be discussed below. It seems likely that much of the observed reduction of uptake during depolarization is based on the reduction of the electrochemical gradient driving the positively charged choline ions into the interior of the cells.

Friesen and Khatter (1971) observed that the content of choline in sympathetic ganglia was increased after a period of electrical stimulation of preganglionic nerve fibres.

Profound changes in the rate of high affinity choline uptake have been discovered in synaptosomes prepared from animals immediately after they had been exposed to conditions producing changes in synaptic activity or transmitter release in the brain (Simon and Kuhar, 1975; Atweh *et al.*, 1975; Simon *et al.*, 1976). In animals sacrificed 30 min after the administration of pentobarbital or chloral hydrate, the sodium-dependent uptake of choline in hippocampal synaptosomes was reduced to less than 1/2 of control values. On the contrary, after the administration of pentylenetetrazole (producing convulsions), atropine or scopolamine (both increasing the release of ACh) the uptake was increased (Atweh *et al.*, 1975; Simon *et al.*, 1976). Direct addition of the drugs to the suspension of synaptosomes was without effect. The inhibitory action of pentobarbital on the uptake by hippocampal synaptosomes could be reversed by direct electrical stimulation of the cholinergic septal–hippocampal tract. All these observations suggest that there is a direct relationship between the activity of nerve terminals, or the release of ACh, and the sodium-dependent uptake of choline.

A similar conclusion follows from experiments with synaptosomes or cortical slices exposed to depolarizing agents *in vitro*. The high affinity uptake was considerably increased in synaptosomes (Barker, 1976b; Murrin and Kuhar, 1976) and in cortical slices (Polak *et al.*, 1977a,b) which had been incubated in the presence of high concentrations of K^+ immediately before the measurement of the uptake of choline. Preincubation with veratridine had a similar effect (Murrin and Kuhar, 1976). The depolarization by high K^+ or by veratridine produced an increase in the subsequent high affinity uptake of choline only when Ca^{2+} ions were present during depolarization (Murrin and Kuhar, 1976; Polak *et al.*, 1977a,b; but cf. Barker, 1976b). Since potassium causes depolarization both in the presence and in the absence of Ca^{2+} ions, these observations suggest that the post-depolarization increase in the high affinity uptake of choline is not initiated by the depolarization as such, but by the release of ACh and the consequent change of ACh concentration in the nerve terminals or by some other action of potassium.

Whittaker and Dowdall (1975) preincubated squid synaptosomes in the presence of various concentrations of ACh. After the synaptosomes had been washed, the high affinity uptake of choline was inhibited to differing degrees depending on the concentration of ACh with which the synaptosomes had been equilibrated. Jenden *et al.* (1976) measured the content of ACh and the high affinity uptake of choline in the synaptosomes prepared from the brain of mice subjected to elctroshock or treated with drugs increasing (pentobarbital, oxotremorine) or decreasing (atropine, pentylenetetrazole) the content of ACh in the brain. They observed an inverse relationship between the concentration of ACh in the synaptosomes and the rate of uptake of choline. The most likely explanation for these observations and those described above seems to be that there is a negative feedback between the concentration of ACh in the nerve endings and the high affinity uptake of choline. As has been stated earlier in this chapter, ACh has a negative effect on choline uptake when it is present in the incubation medium, i.e. on the outside of nerve terminal membrane. The observations indicating that the uptake of choline depends on the concentration of ACh in the nerve terminals suggest that the high affinity carrier also can be influenced by the ACh which is on the inside of the nerve terminal membrane. Dowdall (1975) presented an interesting idea how the intraterminal ACh might act (Fig. 5.6).

There is, however, the possibility that the effects of stimulation or depolarization of the nerve endings on the high affinity uptake of choline are related to some action of the nerve impulses or of depolarization other than the release of ACh. Such a possibility is suggested by the results of experiments on the uptake and release of choline analogues by sympathetic ganglia (Collier and Ilson, 1977). When ganglia are perfused with [^{3}H] homocholine (2-hydroxypropyltrimethylammonium) or with [^{14}C] triethylcholine (2-hydroxyethyltriethylammonium), both drugs accumulate in the ganglion and the accumulation is increased by preganglionic stimulation. The increased accumulation is preganglionic and is most probably based on the activity of the high affinity carrier for choline, since it is blocked by hemicholinium-3 and by choline. Stimulation causes an increase in the accumulation of choline analogues only if Ca^{2+} ions are present in the perfusion fluid during the stimulation. The effect of stimulation is not dependent on the release of ACh; however, since stimulation also increases the uptake of choline in the presence of high concentrations of Mg^{2+} ions, that is, under conditions when the release of ACh is blocked. Thus it appears that stimulation increases the uptake of choline analogues by a Ca^{2+}-dependent mechanism, but that this mechanism is not identical with transmitter release. Barker (1976b) has, however, shown in experiments with brain synaptosomes, that increasing the concentration of Mg^{2+} ions prevented the increased high affinity uptake of choline produced by high concentration of K^+.

An important point which still requires further investigation for a full understanding of the mechanism of the high affinity uptake of choline is the relation

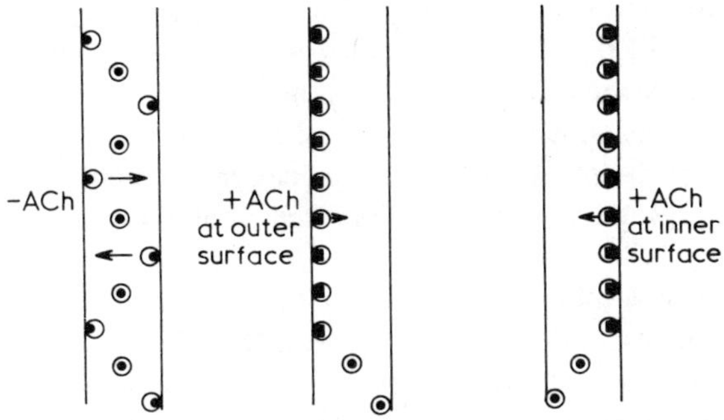

Fig. 5.6 Hypothetical model for the inhibition of choline uptake by ACh.
Left: Uptake of choline in the absence of ACh. The interaction between choline and a hydrophilic pocket in a hypothetical carrier molecule results in the formation of a carrier–choline complex that has a hydrophilic core (full small circle) surrounded by a hydrophobic shell and is thus able to move freely in the membrane.
Centre: ACh present at the outer surface of the membrane competes with choline and forms a complex with the carrier in which the hydrophilic core (full rectangle) is not completely surrounded by a hydrophobic shell – thus reducing the mobility of the carrier molecule in the membrane.
Right: The same as the centre figure, but with ACh present at the inner surface of the membrane. (After Dowdall, 1975).

between uptake and acetylation. The fact that most of the choline which is taken up by the high affinity carrier is immediately transformed to ACh makes it extremely difficult to study the properties of the transport system alone. The relation between the transport of choline and its acetylation appears to be flexible. Under certain conditions, such as the lack of glucose or the inhibition of ChAc, the synthesis of ACh is inhibited, but the uptake is not changed (Jope, 1977). It should be possible to dissociate uptake and acetylation completely if we could find an analogue of choline which will be transported by the high affinity carrier, but which will not be acetylated. Initial steps in this direction have been made in experiments with homocholine and tetraethylcholine. Their uptake in sympathetic ganglia appears to be independent of their acetylation (Ilson *et al.*, 1977; Collier and Ilson, 1977).

5.5 THE SUPPLY OF CHOLINE TO THE BRAIN AND ITS OUTPUT FROM THE BRAIN

Since the brain is unable (or has only an extremely limited ability) to synthesize choline (see Section 5.2), it is evident that choline must be supplied to the brain from choline producing organs, mainly the liver (Bjørnstad and Bremer, 1966) via the blood stream. In view of the presence of a constant concentration of free choline in the blood plasma and of the existence of carriers for choline in the membranes of brain cells, it appears likely that the brain utilizes the unesterified choline of the blood plasma. Experimental findings indicate, however, that the free choline of the blood plasma represents only a part of the total amount of choline which is supplied to the brain. Apparently, much choline is provided in a bound form, probably mainly in lipoproteins and lysophosphatidylcholine, free choline then being released in the brain.

So long as we assume that no significant *de novo* synthesis of free or bound choline occurs in the brain, the most telling evidence that much of the choline is supplied to the brain in a bound form comes from measurements of arterio-venous differences in the concentrations of free choline in the blood flowing through the brain. Dross and Kewitz (1972) found that in the rat the concentration of free choline in the arterial blood is 12.3 μM, in the blood from the femoral vein it is 12.7 μM, and in the blood from the jugular vein 19.4 μM. The observed arterio-venous difference indicates that there is a net output of free choline from the brain of 7.2 nmol/g brain/min. Higher levels of choline in venous relative to arterial blood plasma of the cerebral circulation have been found in man by Aquilonius *et al.* (1975) and in rats by Freeman *et al.* (1975), Choi *et al.* (1975), and by Spanner *et al.* (1976), who did not find elevated venous levels in rabbits. Erythrocytes in the jugular vein also contain more free choline than do those in the arterial blood (Spanner *et al.*, 1976). We thus face the interesting situation that an organ believed to be unable to synthesize new choline in any form acts as a producer of its unesterified variety.

If the free choline released from the brain originates from bound choline present in the arterial blood, one would expect that a negative arterio–venous difference of free choline will be paralleled by a positive arterio–venous difference of bound choline. Unfortunately, the arterio–venous difference of bound choline required to compensate for the output of free choline is so small, in comparison with the total content of bound choline in the blood, that it will be difficult to demonstrate. The problem is that the concentration of lipid-bound choline in the blood plasma of rats is of the order of 1140 nmol/ml (Spanner *et al.*, 1976), so that it does not have to change by more than 1% in order to account for the reported arterio–venous differences of free choline across the brain.

Direct experimental evidence is available, however, that the brain can indeed utilize bound choline supplied to it in the form of lysophosphatidylcholine. Illingworth and Portman (1972) injected squirrel monkeys intravenously with lysophosphatidylcholine labelled in the acyl group [^{14}C] and in the choline moiety [^{3}H]. The lysophosphatidylcholine was partly acylated to phosphatidylcholine and partly hydrolysed, with label appearing in, among other substances, free choline and ACh in the brain. The radioactive label recoverable from brain was about 1% of that injected. The uptake of lysophosphatidylcholine from the blood by peripheral organs has been shown earlier by Stein and Stein (1966). Contrary to experiments with lysophosphatidylcholine, virtually no radioactivity entered the brain in experiments in which liposomes containing choline-labelled phosphatidylcholine were injected intracardially in rats (Mann, 1976). At the same time, however, intracardial injections of choline-labelled plasma lipoproteins were followed by the rapid appearance of the label in the brain; a small portion of label could be recovered in free choline and ACh (Mann, 1976).

The results of experiments in which animals were injected with labelled precursors of choline support the view that choline, normally synthesized in the liver, is transported to the brain in a bound form. In rats injected with labelled ethanolamine or dimethylethanolamine, phosphatidylcholine with a labelled choline moiety was formed in the liver. Phosphatidylcholine, similarly labelled, was also found in the blood plasma and in the brain, but the free choline in the liver, blood and brain was not measurably labelled. It appears that the labelled choline group of brain phosphatidylcholine reached the brain as an integral part of plasma phosphatidylcholine or lysophosphatidylcholine and not as free choline (Ansell and Spanner, 1971; Spanner *et al.*, 1976).

A similar conclusion has been drawn from experiments, on organs other than the brain, in which an attempt was made to dilute the radioactivity of extrahepatic lipid-bound choline by injections of unlabelled choline (Bjørnstad and Bremer, 1966). In these experiments, phosphatidylcholine labelled in the choline moiety was formed in the liver after the administration of methyl-labelled methionine. If the labelled choline moiety was transported from the liver to other organs as free choline, it should be possible to reduce the specific radioactivity of phosphatidylcholine in these organs by injection of large amounts of unlabelled choline. No such reduction could be achieved, however, again suggesting that labelled choline was transported from the liver in a bound form.

When [^{14}C]choline is injected intravenously into rats, the pool of free choline in the brain becomes radioactive. The peak of specific radioactivity of free choline in the brain reaches its maximum in less than 1 min and then decreases in parallel with the specific radioactivity of free choline in the blood serum (Fig. 5.7 – Dross and Kewitz, 1972). Even when it is at its maximum, however, the specific radioactivity of free choline in the brain does not exceed 10% of the specific radioactivity of free choline in the blood serum. This observation indicates that labelled choline passes easily across the hemato–encephalic barrier, but that it is then diluted by unlabelled choline continuously released from choline containing compounds in the brain. As a result, the specific radioactivity of free choline in the brain always remains lower than in the blood (Dross and Kewitz, 1972). Similarly, the specific labelling of free choline in the cerebrospinal fluid remains considerably lower than that in the blood plasma when [^{3}H]choline is administered in the died or by infusion (Schuberth and Jenden, 1975).

Observations on the time course of labelling of free choline in the brain, cerebrospinal fluid and blood plasma, after intravenous or oral administrations of labelled choline, have provided the basis for estimates of how much the free choline formed in the brain from esterified choline and from the plasma contribute to the turnover of the free choline pool in the brain. Different estimates have been obtained for

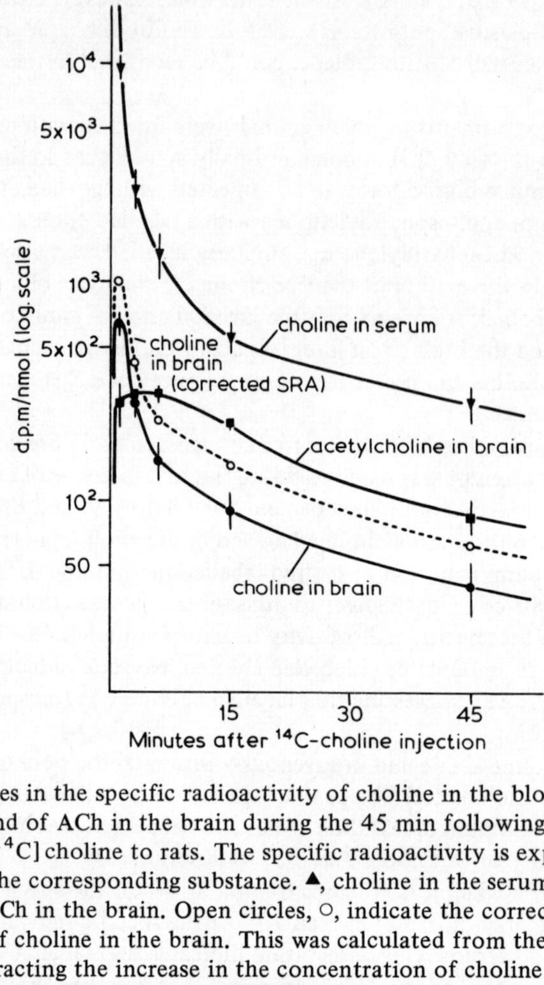

Fig. 5.7 Changes in the specific radioactivity of choline in the blood serum and in the brain, and of ACh in the brain during the 45 min following an i.v. injection of 20 μCi of [^{14}C] choline to rats. The specific radioactivity is expressed in d.p.m. per nmole of the corresponding substance. ▲, choline in the serum; ●, choline in the brain; ■, ACh in the brain. Open circles, ○, indicate the corrected specific radioactivity of choline in the brain. This was calculated from the experimental values by subtracting the increase in the concentration of choline in the brain which occurs during the time between killing the animal and the arrest of brain metabolism (after Dross and Kewitz, 1972).

different mammalian species. In rabbits, the difference between the labelling of choline in the blood plasma and in the cerebrospinal fluid after the administration of [^{3}H] choline indicates that free choline from the plasma is responsible for about 50% of the supply to the free choline pool in the brain (Schuberth and Jenden, 1975). In mice, the contribution of free choline from the plasma is about 80% (Schuberth and Jenden, 1975, based on data from Hanin and Schuberth, 1974), whereas in rats it is only about 12% (Schuberth and Jenden, 1975, based on data from Dross and Kewitz, 1972) or, according to Choi *et al.* (1975), 7%.

The formation of free choline from endogeneous stores of bound choline in the brain is revealed by the post mortem increases in choline concentration in the brain (Schuberth *et al.*, 1970a,b; Dross and Kewitz, 1972; Hanin and Schuberth, 1974; Stavinoha and Weintraub, 1974b; Choi *et al.*, 1975; Freeman *et al.*, 1975b; Dross, 1975; Freeman and Jenden, 1976; Jenden *et al.*, 1976). During the first minutes after death, the content of unesterified choline increases in the brain of rats at a rate of 20.5 nmol/g brain tissue/min. The increase does not seem to be caused by the immediate breakdown of the brain tissue, but rather by the continued formation of free choline from its precursors (mainly probably from glycerylphosphorylcholine) at a time when its utilization (mainly for the synthesis of lipids) and removal by the venous blood have been arrested (Dross and Kewitz, 1972). The formation of free choline in the brain can also be observed during the incubation of brain slices *in vitro*; the concentration of choline increases both in the tissue and in the incubation medium (Bhatnagar and MacIntosh, 1967; Browning, 1971; Collier *et al.*, 1972; Lefresne *et al.*, 1973).

5.6 THE SOURCE OF CHOLINE FOR THE SYNTHESIS OF ACETYLCHOLINE

There is no doubt that free choline from the blood plasma can be used, to some extent at least, for the synthesis of ACh in cerebral cholinergic neurons. After the administration of labelled choline intravenously (Schuberth *et al.*, 1969, 1970b; Dross and Kewitz, 1972; Haubrich *et al.*, 1972, 1975a,b; Aquilonius *et al.*, 1973; Sparf, 1973; Saelens *et al.*, 1973; Jenden *et al.*, 1974; Nordberg and Sundwall, 1975, 1976; Schuberth and Jenden, 1975; Choi *et al.*, 1975; Atweh and Kuhar, 1976), subcutaneously (Kuntscherová *et al.*, 1974), intraventricularly (Barker *et al.*, 1972), intracortically (Charkin and Shideman, 1968; Chakrin *et al.*, 1968; Chakrin and Whittaker, 1969) or with the diet (Hanin and Schuberth, 1974; Schuberth and Jenden, 1975) the labelled atoms very soon appear in the brain ACh. The incorporation into ACh occurs so rapidly, particularly after intravenous administration, that is it virtually certain that choline enters the nerve cells directly, without being previously metabolized, and that it is used for the synthesis of ACh immediately after it enters the cells.

In experiments *in vitro* it is, however, not necessary to add choline to the extracellular fluid (i.e. the incubation medium), which shows that the brain tissue is fully able to ensure the synthesis of ACh from endogenous sources. For example, the initial rate of synthesis of ACh in slices of corpus striatum (measured during 10 min of incubation) was shown by Lefresne *et al.* (1973) to be unaltered when the concentration of choline in the medium varied from 0 to 2000 μM. The addition of choline to the medium increased by only 18% the amount of ACh accumulating in striatal slices during an incubation lasting 3 h (Lefresne *et al.*, 1973). It is easier to explain this small increase as a result of a shift in the equilibrium between reaction substrates and products (see chapter 6.9) than as a consequence of overcoming lack of choline in the tissue.

The content of ACh and choline in brain slices is reduced after incubation in a medium without Na^+; when the tissue is subsequently incubated in the presence of Na^+ and labelled choline, it produces labelled ACh, but the specific radioactivity of the newly formed ACh is less than half the specific radioactivity of the choline in the medium. Moreover, the initial concentration of ACh can be restored by the addition of Na^+ alone; the addition of choline to the medium is not necessary (Collier *et al.*, 1972). These findings indicate that endogenous choline is being used for the synthesis of ACh. This conclusion is further supported by experiments with the formation of the so-called surplus ACh (see chapter 6.4) in sympathetic ganglia perfused with a solution containing labelled choline and a ChE inhibitor. The specific radioactivity of the surplus ACh corresponds to only 35% of the specific radioactivity of choline in the perfusion fluid (Collier and Katz, 1971).

It is evident that, for the synthesis of ACh, cholinergic neurons can use both free choline, supplied by the blood, and endogeneous choline, released in the cells of the nervous tissue from larger molecules. There are, however, strong reasons for supposing that the synthesis of ACh is based on the preferential use of the free choline which the presynaptic nerve endings obtain from the extracellular fluid. Experiments with the addition of [^{2}H] choline to the diet show that within less than 24 h the ratio between labelled and unlabelled ACh in the brain equals the ratio between labelled and unlabelled choline in the blood plasma. The pool of choline in the brain from which ACh is synthesized therefore appears to be in a dynamic equilibrium with the pool of choline in the blood plasma (Hanin and Schuberth, 1974). Guyenet *et al.* (1975) observed preferential use of choline from the extracellular fluid for the synthesis of ACh by rat striatal synaptosomes incubated in a medium with radioactive choline. The specific radioactivity of ACh in the synaptosomes corresponded to the specific radioactivity of choline in the medium and was substantially higher than the specific radioactivity of choline in the synaptosomes.

The following experimental observations together with some others suggest that the high affinity carrier for choline in the membranes of cholinergic nerve terminals plays an important if not entirely specific role in ensuring the supply of choline for the synthesis of ACh:

(a) Hemicholinium-3 is a competitive inhibitor of the high affinity uptake of choline. In the presence of increasing concentrations of hemicholinium-3, the synthesis of ACh in the synaptosomes decreases linearly with the increasing inhibition of the uptake (Guyenet *et al.*, 1973a,b).

(b) Very low concentrations of the detergent Triton X-100 reduce the high affinity uptake of choline by the synaptosomes. In the concentration range of 0.001–0.006% Triton X-100, the synthesis of ACh in the synaptosomes decreases in proportion to the decrease of high affinity uptake of choline (Lefresne *et al.*, 1975). When the synthesis of ACh is lowered by Triton X-100, the inhibitory effect of hemicholinium-3 on the synthesis of ACh is also decreased; this supports the view that the reduction of the synthesis of ACh, achieved by Triton X-100, is caused by a partial blockade of the high affinity uptake of choline (Lefresne *et al.*, 1975).

(c) The synthesis of ACh is considerably lowered in an incubation medium without Na^+ ions (Guyenet *et al.*, 1975). The negative effect of low Na^+ on the synthesis of ACh can be prevented by the addition of 1 mM choline to the incubation medium (Guyenet *et al.*, 1975). The lowered synthesis of ACh under conditions of low Na^+ is apparently caused by the decrease of the high affinity choline uptake, which is known to be Na^+ dependent (Haga and Noda, 1973; Yamamura and Snyder, 1973).

(d) In cortical slices, hemicholinium-3 only slightly reduces the high affinity uptake of choline, measured after incubation in low K^+ medium, but it prevents the increase of the uptake, occurring after incubation in a high K^+ medium and associated with the increased synthesis of ACh (Polak *et al.*, 1977b).

(e) The high affinity uptake is stimulated by procedures causing the release of ACh and is inhibited by agents reducing the turnover of ACh. Relevant findings *in vivo* and *in vitro* have been discussed in Section 5.4.

Guyenet *et al.* (1975) and Lefresne *et al.* (1975) proposed on the basis of their experimental observations that there is a close functional link between the high affinity choline carrier and the molecule of ChAc, and that the high affinity carrier of choline plays an important role in the regulation of ACh synthesis. The view that ACh is synthesized mainly from the choline supplied by the high affinity carrier does not contradict the observations indicating that the nervous tissue has large endogenous stores of choline, from which it can ensure the synthesis of ACh. It is possible that choline is produced from endogeneous stores (e.g. from glycerylphosphorylcholine) in glial cells and passes from them into the extracellular fluid to be taken up by the high affinity carrier into the cholinergic nerve endings. In contrast, the synthesis of ACh occurring in the nerve cell bodies may be based on the supply of choline by the low affinity carrier (Suszkiw *et al.*, 1976) and on the utilization of choline released in the neurons from phospholipids.

The view that the synthesis of ACh in cholinergic nerve endings depends on the utilization of free choline from the extracellular fluid and on the activity of the high affinity choline carriers is in good agreement with experimental results indicating the re-utilization of the choline which is formed in synaptic gaps from synaptically released ACh. When preganglionic sympathetic fibres are stimulated by two series of impulses, the ability of the ganglion to release ACh into the perfusion fluid during the second stimulation period is considerably diminished if eserine is present in the perfusion fluid during the first stimulation period (Perry, 1953). The presence of eserine causes the inhibition of ChE during the first stimulation period; the released ACh cannot therefore be hydrolysed and its choline cannot be taken up by the presynaptic endings and re-used for the synthesis of new ACh. This evidently causes an abnormally rapid exhaustion of the store of ACh available for release. The store of ACh in the sympathetic ganglion can be radioactively labelled, if the preganglionic fibres are stimulated while the ganglion is perfused with a solution containing radioactive choline. When the ganglion is subsequently perfused with physiological saline containing unlabelled choline, stimulation of preganglionic fibres continues to cause the release labelled ACh. Inhibition of ChE in the ganglion, performed at this stage, brings about an approximately two-fold increase in the amount of radioactive label appearing in the perfusion fluid during stimulation. After the inhibition of ChE, the labelled ACh released cannot be hydrolysed, its choline moiety cannot be re-utilized for the synthesis of new transmitter and the amount of label in the perfusion fluid leaving the ganglion is therefore increased (Collier and MacIntosh, 1969; Collier and Katz, 1974). These experiments indicate that in the presence of active ChE, the ACh is hydrolysed immediately after release, approximately 50% of the choline formed from the released transmitter is taken up and re-utilized for the synthesis of ACh. The view that choline formed from ACh is re-used for transmitter synthesis is supported by observations on the phrenic nerve and diaphragm (Potter, 1970).

5.7 SUMMARY

An over-all scheme of the metabolism of choline in the brain is given in Fig. 5.8.

The main source of choline in the animal body is the liver. Choline is synthesized not as a free compound, but as the choline moiety of phosphatidylcholine. It is

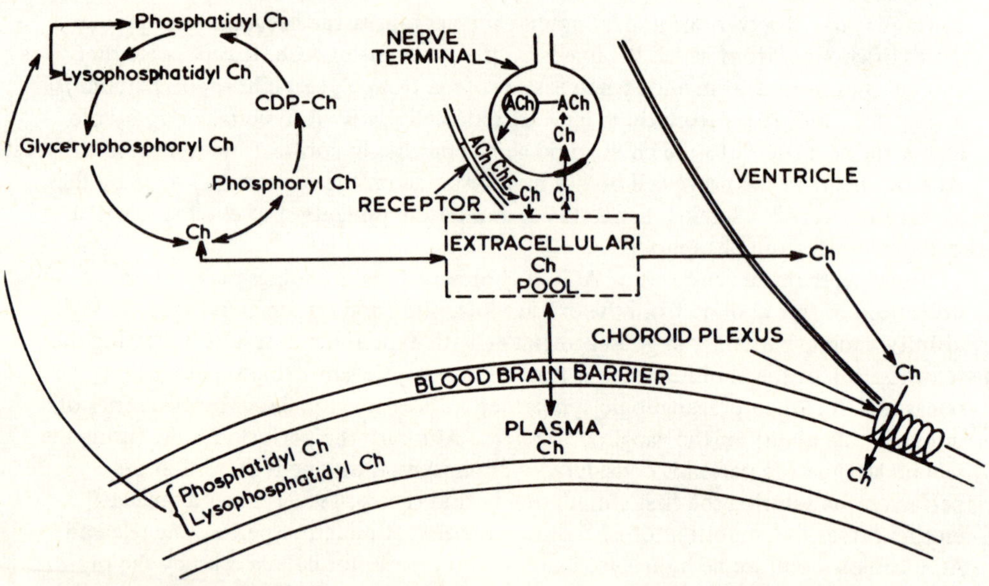

Fig. 5.8 Summary of the metabolism of choline in the brain (after Freeman and Jenden, 1976).

released from phosphatidylcholine mainly via the steps lysophosphatidylcholine to glycerylphosphorylcholine to choline. It is supplied to the brain both as free choline and as choline bound in phospholipids. The ability of the brain to synthesize choline *de novo* is either non-existent or insignificant. At the same time, the brain functions as a producer of free choline: the concentration of free choline in the blood leaving the brain is higher than in the blood coming to the brain.

Most cells are equipped with a low affinity carrier for choline in their surface membranes. In the brain, two carriers have been discovered: 1. a low affinity carrier, with a K_m in the range approximately 40–100 μM, probably present in all neurons and glial cells; 2. a high affinity carrier, with a K_m in the range approximately 0.4–4.0 μM, probably specific for cholinergic nerve terminals. The high affinity carrier is highly dependent on the presence of Na^+, but less so on Cl^-. It is inhibited by ACh, hemicholinium-3 and many drugs. Its activity is stimulated by noradrenaline and prednisolone. The process accomplished by the low affinity carrier is facilitated diffusion. Available evidence is insufficient to allow a decision whether the high affinity carrier catalyses facilitated diffusion or active (uphill) transport. The activity of the high affinity carrier is increased by previous increase in the activity of the neurons or by their previous depolarization. Most probably the high affinity uptake of choline is controlled by the concentration of ACh in the nerve endings.

The synthesis of ACh in the nerve endings is based on the preferential utilization of the choline which is supplied by the high affinity carrier from extracellular fluid. Choline in the extracellular fluid of the brain comes either directly from the free choline of the blood plasma, or from the brain cells, where it has been released from choline containing compounds. The contribution of free choline in the plasma to the synthesis of ACh in the brain is different in different species; it is estimated as 12% in rats, 50% in rabbits, and 80% in mice. Choline produced in synaptic gaps by the hydrolysis of ACh is re-utilized for the synthesis of ACh in presynaptic nerve endings.

AUTHOR'S NOTE

M.J. Dowdall, J.P. Fohlman and D. Eaker (*Nature* **269**, 700–702, 1977) have described the inhibitory effect of presynaptically acting snake venon neurotoxins on the high affinity uptake of choline. G. Ceder and J. Schuberth (*Brain Res.*, **128**, 580–584, 1977) have calculated that 50–60% of choline in mouse brain stem from plasma choline.

6 Organization and control of the synthesis of acetylcholine in presynaptic nerve endings

6.1 INTRODUCTION

The synthesis of ACh occurs in the perikarya of cholinergic neurons, in their neurites and – so far as can be judged from the (not entirely reliable) histochemical demonstration of ChAc within them – also in their dendrites. Both quantitatively and functionally the most important sites of ACh synthesis are the presynaptic portions of cholinergic synapses. In neurochemical literature these portions of the neurites are usually, but somewhat inaccurately, designated as the nerve endings. It should be noted that the presynaptic part of a synapse is not always formed by the ending of the axon. It may be formed also by a dilatation in the course of the axon (*bouton en passant*) (Peters *et al.*, 1970) or, in autonomic postganglionic fibres, by the so-called axonal varicosities (Bennett, 1972). Therefore, when reading that the nerve endings are the main site of the synthesis of synaptic transmitters, one should also include in this term the *bouton en passant* and axonal varicosities, both of which may either constitute, or act as, the presynaptic part of a synapse.

It has been pointed out in Chapter 3.5 that the ACh carried to the nerve endings by axonal transport is unlikely to contribute more than a very minor portion of the total amount of the transmitter which is necessary for the functioning of cholinergic synapses. Most ACh is undoubtedly synthesized in close proximity to the sites from which it is released. The distribution of ChAc in the neurons corresponds to this location of ACh synthesis. When a homogenate of the brain is subjected to subcellular fractionation, the biggest proportion of ChAc is found in the crude mitochondrial fraction. When this fraction is separated into its subfractions by means of sucrose density gradient centrifugation, the largest proportion of ChAc is recovered in the subfraction containing the nerve ending particles (Hebb and Whittaker, 1958; Whittaker, 1965; Tuček, 1967a; see Fig. 6.1). On the basis of experiments involving subcellular fractionation of hypoglossal nuclei and the transection of hypoglossal nerves, Fonnum *et al.* (1973) estimate that the perikarya contain 2%, the axons in the main nerve trunks 42%, and the preterminal axons and their endings in the

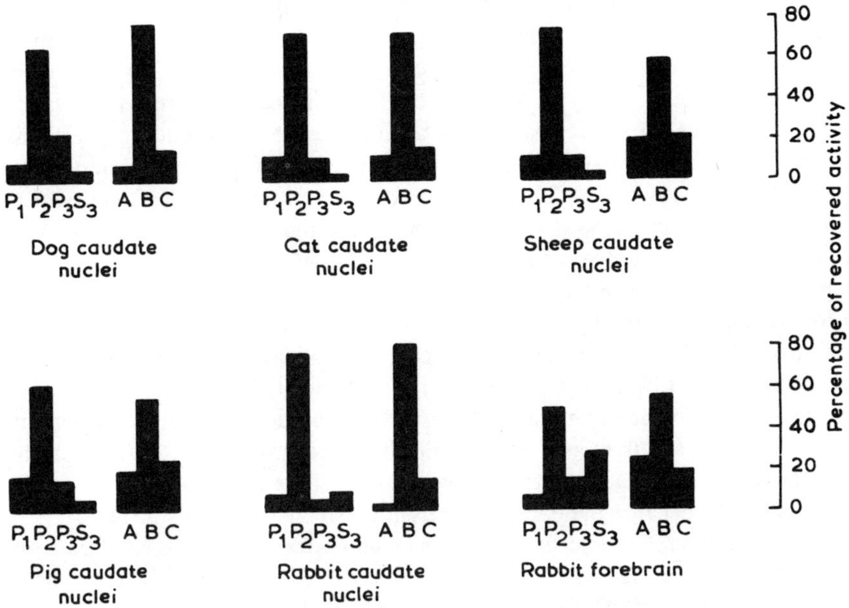

Fig. 6.1 The distribution of ChAc in subcellular fractions of caudate nuclei or of whole brains from several animal species. Enzyme activity in individual fractions is expressed as a percentage of the total activity recovered after fractionation. The crude mitochondrial fraction is denoted by P_2, the fraction of purified nerve endings is denoted by B. See Fig. 4.2 for the description of other fractions (after Tuček, 1967a).

tongue 56% of the total content of ChAc in the cholinergic neurons of the hypoglossal nucleus. All recognized molecular forms of ChAc present in other parts of the neurons are present in the nerve endings (Fonnum and Malthe-Sørenssen, 1973).

A characteristic morphological feature of the presynaptic part of the synapses is the presence of many vesicles with a diameter of 20–100 nm. These so-called synaptic vesicles, first described by De Robertis and Bennett (1954), Palade (1954) and Palay (1954), may be separated into four groups according to their appearance in the electron microscope after fixation with osmic tetroxide or aldehydes (Palay and Chan-Palay, 1973): 1. clear round vesicles (diameter 30–60 nm); 2. small dense-cored vesicles (diameter 30–60 nm); 3. large dense-cored vesicles (diameter 80–100 nm); 4. clear oval vesicles (diameter 20–60 nm). It is generally believed that synaptic vesicles are the storage site of transmitters and that different kinds of vesicles contain different transmitters. The undoubtedly cholinergic engings of motor nerves in skeletal muscles contain clear round vesicles. Presumably all vesicles containing ACh are similar.

The discovery of synaptic vesicles coincided with important developments in the electrophysiology of synaptic transmission. Fatt and Katz (1952), recording the transmembrane potential intracellularly in skeletal muscle fibres, discovered spontaneous transient changes of the resting potential in the area of the neuromuscular junction. These changes were called miniature endplate potentials. They were found to be the consequence of the spontaneous release of discrete quantities (thousands or tens of thousands) of molecules of ACh from the motor nerve endings. Analysis of the postsynaptic potentials elicited by the stimulation of presynaptic nerve fibres revealed that the amount of ACh, released by the nerve impulses, changes in a stepwise manner. The change is as if the total amount of transmitter released were composed of a graded number of smaller amounts of ACh, the so-called ACh quanta, corresponding in size to the amounts of ACh which produce the miniature endplate potentials (del Castillo and Katz, 1954). Further investigations revealed that the quantal mechanism of transmitter release operates at all chemical synapses (reviews Martin, 1966; Katz, 1969, 1971; Hubbard, 1970; Kuno, 1971).

The discovery of vesicles with an unknown function located near the presynaptic membrane, and the simultaneous observation that during synaptic transmission the transmitter is released in quanta, each of which represents thousands of molecules of the transmitter, became the basis of the hypothesis that the transmitter is contained in the synaptic vesicles and during synaptic transmission is released from them into the synaptic cleft (del Castillo and Katz, 1955, 1956; De Robertis and Bennett, 1955; Palay, 1956). The vesicular hypothesis forms the basis of contemporary ideas about the mechanism of transmitter release. It is strongly supported by the findings that the synaptic vesicles isolated from the brain, electric organ or sympathetic ganglia contain ACh (De Robertis *et al.*, 1963; Whittaker *et al.*, 1963, 1964; Whittaker and Sheridan, 1965; Israël *et al.*, 1970; Wilson *et al.*, 1973), and that the transmitter in adrenergic neurons is also contained in storage vesicles (reviews Axelrod and Kopin, 1969; Euler, 1972). In addition, under suitable conditions, stimulation or depolarization of the nerve fibres may change not only the number of synaptic vesicles in the presynaptic endings (De Robertis and Ferreira, 1957; Hubbard and Kwanbunbumpen, 1968; Jones and Kwanbunbumpen, 1968; Ceccarelli *et al.*, 1972, 1973; Heuser and Reese, 1973; Pysh and Wiley, 1974; Zimmermann and Whittaker, 1974a,b; Dunant *et al.*, 1974; Birks, 1974; Boyne *et al.*, 1975), but also the size of the vesicles (Maloshevskii *et al.*, 1975) and the amount of ACh in the vesicles (Zimmermann and Whittaker, 1974a; Boyne *et al.*, 1975; Zimmermann and Denston, 1977b).

The vesicular hypothesis is also supported by observations suggesting that the membranes of the synaptic vesicles are recycled after the release of ACh from the nerve endings (cycle: synaptic vesicles, incorporation into the presynaptic membrane, retrieval of vesicular membrane as coated vesicles, formation of cisternae and then new synaptic vesicles; Heuser and Reese, 1973) and that the stimulation of presynaptic fibres may bring about the translocation of macromolecular substances from the synaptic cleft into the vesicles in the nerve endings (Holtzman *et al.*, 1971; Ceccarelli *et al.*, 1972, 1973; Heuser and Reese, 1973; Zimmermann and Denston, 1977b). In spite of these and other findings, the vesicular hypothesis of transmitter release still remains only a hypothesis more than 20 years after its inception. Convincing proof that the released transmitter originates from synaptic vesicles, that the whole transmitter content of the vesicles is released at once and that the transmitter passes from the vesicles directly into the synaptic cleft has not been presented. On the contrary, observations will be mentioned later which are difficult to reconcile with these assumptions.

Although the problem of ACh storage and release is outside the scope of this book, it will be impossible to avoid mentioning it when we consider the organization of the synthesis of ACh in the presynaptic part of the synapse. Under physiological circumstances the loss of ACh from the nerve endings caused by nerve impulses is rapidly replaced by new synthesis. On the other hand, in the absence of impulse activity the synthesis of new transmitter is regulated so that the store of the transmitter only rarely increases above a certain relatively constant upper limit. It is clear that the synthesis of ACh changes with changes in its release. The interdependence between the synthesis, storage and release of ACh is well documented experimentally; our understanding of the mechanism of this interdependence is surprisingly uncertain.

6.2 LOCALIZATION OF CHOLINE ACETYLTRANSFERASE IN PRESYNAPTIC NERVE ENDINGS

Present views concerning the localization of ChAc in the presynaptic nerve endings are mainly based on experiments with subcellular fractionation of brain homogenates, involving disruption of the separated nerve endings by means of hypo-osmotic shock and further fractionation of their components on sucrose density gradients (see Chapter 4.3.1). These experiments demonstrated that, in general, ChAc is a cytoplasmic enzyme which becomes very easily attached to the membranes. The degree of its affinity to membranes is different in different species. After the fractionation of hypo-osmotically treated nerve endings from guinea pig brain on a density gradient most ChAc was found in the uppermost layer of the gradient, subfraction 0, (see Fig. 4.2), containing the soluble components of the cytoplasm of the nerve endings (Whittaker *et al.*, 1964; Tuček, 1966b). ChAc was found in a similar position on the gradients in experiments with pigeon brain. In experiments with canine, feline or ovine caudate nuclei, however, most ChAc appeared in the layers of the gradients which contained fragments of nerve ending membranes (Tuček, 1966a,b). Big interspecies differences in the affinity of ChAc towards membranes were also found by McCaman *et al.* (1965) using a different fractionation technique.

The binding of ChAc to membranes as observed in experiments with subcellular fractions of brain homogenates of some species does not prove, however, that ChAc is bound to membranes in the living brain of these species. In experiments *in vitro* it is possible to release the membrane-bound ChAc into solution when the ionic strength of the medium and the pH are adjusted to values which are likely to occur in living cells (Fonnum, 1967, 1968; Potter *et al.*, 1968). The binding of ChAc to membranes occurs because the enzyme molecules have a high positive surface charge, whereas the surface charge of the membranes is negative. Species differences in the affinity of ChAc to the membranes can be explained by species differences in the positive surface charge of ChAc (Fonnum, 1970b; Fonnum and Malthe-Sørenssen, 1972, 1973). It is interesting to note that the attachment of ChAc to cell membranes is also indicated by observations on tissues processed for immunofluorescence histochemistry (McGeer *et al.*, 1974).

De Robertis and his colleagues concluded from experiments on the subcellular fractionation of rat brain, that ChAc is located in the synaptic vesicles (De Robertis *et al.*, 1963; De Robertis, 1964; McCaman *et al.*, 1965). Such a conclusion was very attractive for two reasons: it offered an easy answer to the question about the mechanism by which ACh is accumulated in the synaptic vesicles and at the same time it was in perfect accord with the situation existing in adrenergic storage granules. The enzyme catalysing the last step in the synthesis of noradrenaline, i.e. dopamine-β-hydroxylase, is indeed localized inside the granules (review Smith, 1972). It has been shown by Whittaker *et al.* (1964) and Tuček (1966c), however, that the fraction of synaptic vesicles prepared in the way which had been used in the studies from De Robertis' group, is highly contaminated by membranous material. Tuček (1966c) purified synaptic vesicles prepared according to the methods of De Robertis *et al.* (1963) and McCaman *et al.* (1965) by further fractionation on a sucrose density gradient. Little ChAc remained in the layer containing purified synaptic vesicles; most was found in the deeper layers of the gradient containing bigger membrane fragments.

Preliminary histochemical observations of ChAc in the nervous system have not confirmed the localization of ChAc in the synaptic vesicles (Kása *et al.*, 1970; Kása, 1971). According to these observations the enzyme is localized in neuronal cytoplasm; it is never inside the cell organelles (mitochondria, tubules or vesicles), but appears to be partly associated with the external surface of a number of intracellular structures – endoplasmic reticulum, neurotubules, neurofilaments, synaptic vesicles, mitochondria – and with the inner side of the nerve ending surface membrane. The histochemical demonstration of ChAc is a new method which encounters many difficulties. One of the problems is that the incubation has to be performed at a lower ionic strength and pH than is likely to obtain in the cell *in vivo*. Therefore the observations described above cannot be taken as proof that, under physiological conditions, ChAc is bound to the cytoplasmic surface of axonal membranes and organelles. They do, however, provide additional evidence against the view that ChAc is localized inside the synaptic vesicles.

The view that a proportion of ACh is synthesized in the synaptic vesicles and therefore a proportion of ChAc must be localized in these organelles, has been supported by Kaita-Ritchie and Goldberg (1970). In their experiments the synaptosomes from rat brain were incubated in a medium containing [^{14}C] ACh and after the incubation the synaptosomal cytoplasm was separated from the synaptic vesicles. The amount of labelled ACh in the vesicles was only 1.5% of that in the cytoplasm. When, however, the synaptosomes were incubated in the presence of [^{14}C] choline so that the [^{14}C] ACh was formed during the incubation, the content of [^{14}C] ACh in the synaptic vesicles was comparatively higher. It corresponded to 15% of the amount recovered in the cytoplasm, i.e. about 10 times more than in the experiments in which [^{14}C] ACh had been added to the medium. These observations in no way prove that a part of [^{14}C] ACh was produced in the synaptic vesicles. At first sight, they appear to indicate that the ACh which is synthesized directly in the synaptosomes has a better opportunity of getting into the synaptic vesicles than the ACh from the incubation medium. As has, however, been pointed out by MacIntosh and Collier (1976), the exogenous [^{14}C] ACh added to the medium is probably taken up into the cytoplasm of both cholinergic and non-cholinergic synaptosomes (the uptake of ACh not being specific for cholinergic neurons – see Section 6.10), whereas the synthesis of [^{14}C] ACh from [^{14}C] choline occurs in the cytoplasm of cholinergic synaptosomes only. It seems likely that the [^{14}C] ACh from the cytoplasm enters the synaptic vesicles in cholinergic, but not in non-cholinergic nerve endings. The proportion of [^{14}C] ACh in the vesicles will then be higher under conditions in which it is present exclusively in cholinergic synaptosomes (i.e. when it is endogenously synthesized) than when it is present in all synaptosomes. The results of Kaita-Ritchie and Goldberg (1970) can thus be interpreted without assuming any special treatment of endogenously synthesized ACh – although it would be unwise to dismiss such a possibility under other experimental conditions. The problem of the transport of ACh into the synaptic vesicles will be discussed in Section 6.7.

Taken as a whole, the concensus of available evidence concerning the localization of ChAc in the nerve endings strongly supports the view that the enzyme is not enclosed inside cellular organelles and that most of it is probably freely dissolved in the cytoplasm. It has a high affinity towards the membranes – a property which may be of great importance in the organization of the synthesis of ACh in the nerve endings. A feature which is possibly of particular importance to the physiology of nerve endings is the apparent binding of the enzyme to the inner surface of the external membrane of the nerve endings and to the outer surface of synaptic vesicles. The binding of the enzyme to the membranes would be enhanced during activity if this were accompanied by a shift of pH to the acid side in the region of the cell where ChAc is localized. As has been pointed out by Fonnum and Malthe-Sørenssen (1972), the binding of ChAc to the inner surface of the nerve ending membrane might explain the preferential release of newly synthesized ACh (see Section 6.8), because the enzyme would be concentrated in the immediate vicinity of the carrier for choline and of the release sites for ACh. The binding of ChAc to the outer surface of the synaptic vesicles, facilitated by the negative charge of their membranes (Vos *et al.*, 1968; McLaughlin *et al.*, 1973; Bittiger and Heid, 1977), might enable the passage of ACh into the vesicles. At present these considerations are, however, only conjectural and it is not yet possible to say whether the ability of ChAc to bind to the membranes really is important for the function of the synapse.

6.3 FREE, BOUND AND TOTAL ACETYLCHOLINE

The terms free and bound ACh denote two empirically defined pools of ACh in the tissues (review Whittaker, 1969b) and their sum gives the total ACh. The localization of free and bound ACh is not entirely clear. It seems relevant to include basic information about these pools of ACh because this will facilitate consideration of the localization of ACh in the nerve endings and the relation between its synthesis, storage and release. I shall concentrate on the characteristics of free and bound ACh in the brain of mammals and in the electric organ of *Torpedo*, i.e. in those organs in which the two pools of ACh have been mainly studied.

When the brain is carefully homogenized in physiological salt solution containing and inhibitor of ChE, only about 12–25% of the total ACh content of the brain appears in the homogenizing medium (Crossland and Slater, 1968; Beani *et al.*, 1969). The rest of ACh remains bound to the particles of the tissue. The ACh appearing in the solution is called free ACh. The ACh which remains with the particles is called bound ACh (Table 6.1).

Another way to distinguish free and bound ACh is based on their differential susceptibility to hydrolysis by ChE. If the tissue is homogenized in trichloroacetic acid, ChE is immediately inactivated and all ACh is extracted from the tissue giving a value for total ACh. If, however, the tissue is homogenized in physiological salt solution without an inhibitor of ChE, the free ACh is exposed to the action of tissue ChE and hydrolysed whereas the bound ACh is protected from hydrolysis. The homogenate is then acidified by trichloroacetic acid and the bound ACh thus released from the particles can be measured. Free ACh is calculated as the difference between the total and bound ACh (see, e.g., Israël and Tuček, 1974).

Free ACh is generally regarded as ACh which, before the homogenization, was freely dissolved in the cytoplasm of the neurons and their axons. Bound ACh is probably derived mainly from the ACh which is enclosed in the nerve endings undamaged by homogenization, and therefore does not pass into the homogenizing solution and is not exposed to hydrolysis by ChE. In the brain, about one half of the bound ACh may be released from the nerve endings into the medium by mild procedures like repeated freezing and thawing or by exposure to hypo-osmotic conditions (Whittaker, 1959). The same procedures also cause the release of lactate dehydrogenase and of K^+ ions, which are both localized in the cytoplasm. More severe procedures are required to release the other half of the bound ACh – e.g., acidification of the medium to pH 4 or less, or treatment of the homogenate with chloroform, ether etc. The easily released part of bound ACh has been described as the labile fraction and the less easily released part as the stable fraction (Whittaker, 1959). It is assumed that the labile bound ACh corresponds to the ACh which is dissolved in the cytoplasm of the nerve endings, whereas the stable bound ACh most probably represents the ACh which is contained inside the synaptic vesicles.

In the electric organ of *Torpedo*, free ACh constitutes a higher proportion of the total ACh than is the case in the brain (Table 6.1). This is due to the high fragility

Table 6.1 Content of free and bound ACh (nmol/g tissue) in the brain and electric organ

Organ	Total ACh	Free ACh	Bound ACh	Labile bound ACh	Stable bound ACh	Reference
Rat brain	17.7	2.2	15.5			Crossland and Slater (1968)
Guinea pig cerebral cortex	16.7	3.1	14.0	7.3	6.7	Beani *et al.* (1969)
Electric organ of *Torpedo marmorata*	529	260	269			Israël and Tuček (1974)

Data from Crossland and Slater (1968) and Beani *et al.* (1969) have been recalculated to nanomoles on the assumption that in the original studies measurements were expressed in terms of ACh chloride.

of the nerve endings in the electric organ. Most nerve endings become broken during homogenization even if it is performed in an isotonic (0.8 M) medium. As a result, their cytoplasmic ACh (which, in the brain, constitutes the so-called labile bound ACh pool) passes into the medium and becomes part of the free ACh. In addition the synaptic vesicles of the electric organ are released from the nerve endings during isotonic homogenization (Israël *et al.,* 1970), whereas in the brain they are released only when the nerve endings are disrupted by hypo-osmotic treatment (De Robertis *et al.,* 1962, 1963; Whittaker *et al.,* 1963, 1964).

It must be stressed that synaptic vesicles do not constitute a homogeneous compartment and the vesicular ACh therefore does not represent a homogeneous pool. Many observations indicate that there are important differences between cholinergic synaptic vesicles depending on, among other factors, their localization, history and content. It has been suggested that the metabolic turnover of ACh in the vesicles close to presynaptic membranes is much faster than in the vesicles located elsewhere (Barker *et al.,* 1972). This suggestion is based on the observation that, after intraventricular injections of radioactive choline into guinea pig, the specific radioactivity of ACh in the subcellular fraction containing the external membranes of the nerve endings and the synaptic vesicles attached to them (fraction H, see Fig. 4.2) is much higher than in the fraction of purified synaptic vesicles (fraction D). In experiments involving perfusion of the electric organ of *Torpedo*, it has been found that stimulation of its nerve leads to the appearance of a new population of synaptic vesicles, which can be distinguished by electron microscopy (Zimmermann and Denston, 1977a) and isolated by zonal centrifugation (Zimmermann and Denston, 1977b); vesicles in this population released their original content of ACh, but they contain most of the freshly synthesized transmitter. Another indication of the inhomogeneity of synaptic vesicles comes from the observation that zonal centrifugation of homogenates of the electric organ yields fractions of vesicles having different ACh: ATP ratios (Dowdall and Zimmermann, 1974).

Observations on synaptic vesicles isolated from slices of either the electric organ (Marchbanks and Israël, 1971) or the brain (Richter and Marchbanks, 1971b) incubated in the presence of radioactive choline also indicated the inhomogeneity of the vesicles and/or their ACh pool. The vesicles contained a mixture of non-radioactive (old) and radioactive (newly synthesized) ACh. When the vesicles were passed through a Sephadex column, a selective loss of radioactive ACh occurred. At present it seems impossible to decide between two interpretations of this loss. One possibility is that the radioactive ACh was localized in a special population of synaptic vesicles which were more fragile and became broken during the passage through the Sephadex column. This interpretation implies that the vesicles containing newly synthesized ACh are more fragile than those containing old ACh. The other possibility is that the radioactive ACh was localized on the surface of synaptic vesicles and was less firmly connected to them than was the old ACh inside the vesicles. This interpretation leads to the idea that the newly synthesized ACh becomes stabilized in the vesicles only gradually (Marchbanks, 1973, 1975a).

The assumption that in the living neuron the free and labile-bound ACh is freely dissolved in the cytoplasm is mainly based on the ease with which free ACh is released into solution during homogenization, and on the observation that agents releasing the labile bound ACh from the nerve endings also release the cytoplasmically localized K^+ ions and lactate dehydrogenase (Whittaker, 1959, 1969b; Whittaker *et al.*, 1964). That some of the contribution to the free and labile bound pools of ACh comes from the synaptic vesicles or from some other subcellular structure cannot, however, be excluded. It has been mentioned already that the newly synthesized ACh was not retained in synaptic vesicles (and thus was included in the free ACh) during their passage through Sephadex columns (Marchbanks and Israël, 1971; Richter and Marchbanks, 1971b). Synaptic vesicles from the electric organ are osmotically sensitive (Israël *et al.*, 1970; Marchbanks and Israël, 1971; Suszkiw, 1976) and it is hard to imagine that the vesicles from the brain are entirely different in this respect. Therefore it appears likely that the fractionation procedures involving hypo-osmotic treatment of the nerve endings are accompanied by an important loss of ACh from the synaptic vesicles with a concomitant increase in the labile-bound ACh. Conceivably many other procedures, including homogenization itself, can cause a significant escape of the vesicles from the nerve endings (Heuser and Lennon, 1973), and of ACh from the vesicles. It seems important to be aware of the uncertainties about the homogeneity of the free, labile-bound and stable-bound ACh pools when evaluating data from the literature on their metabolic turnover and functional role.

6.4 SURPLUS ACETYLCHOLINE

The term surplus ACh has been used by Birks and MacIntosh (1961) to designate the amount by which the total ACh content in the sympathetic ganglion increases after the inhibition of ChE. As a consequence of the inhibition of ChE, the content of ACh in a perfused cat sympathetic ganglion gradually rises to approximately double the original value, but does not increase any further thereafter (Birks and MacIntosh, 1961; Collier and Katz, 1971). The inhibition of ChE is accompanied by a similar increase of the ACh content to about twice the normal values in the phrenic nerve–diaphragm preparation (Potter, 1970), in the myenteric plexus–longitudinal muscle of the ileum (Hutchinson *et al.*, 1976), and in the perfused chicken heart (Dieterich *et al.*, 1976), but not, however, in frog sartorius muscle (Miledi *et al.*, 1977).

The results of experiments on the formation of surplus ACh in the brain are different *in vivo* and *in vitro*. The content of ACh in the brain is clearly elevated after the administration of ChE inhibitors *in vivo* (Giarman and Pepeu, 1962; Megazzini *et al.*, 1965; Beani *et al.*, 1969; Fonnum and Guttormsen, 1969) and a positive correlation has been found between the degree of ChE inhibition and of ACh increase (Holmstedt *et al.*, 1967). On the other hand, experiments with brain tissue *in vitro* have yielded controversial results. The presence of an inhibitor of ChE in the incubation medium invariably brings about the accumulation of released ACh in the medium; this ACh would be hydrolysed in the absence of the inhibitor. So far as the content of ACh in the tissue is concerned, however, no surplus ACh formation was found in some studies in which a physiological concentration of K^+ was present in the medium (Sattin, 1966; Bhatnagar and MacIntosh, 1967; Bourdois and Szerb, 1972). In some other studies the formation of surplus ACh was observed; for example in rat striatal slices incubated for 3 h the content of ACh was 26% greater when eserine was present in the medium than when it was omitted (Lefresne *et al.*, 1973) and, in cortex slices, eserine increased the content by 82% (Bowers, 1967a). To prevent misunderstanding, it should be stressed that the content of ACh in the brain slices increases considerably during incubation even in the absence of ChE inhibitors (see Section 6.5 and Fig. 6.3); and in speaking about surplus ACh, we are concerned only with that part of the increase of ACh content in the tissue which is dependent on the inhibition of ChE. The reason for the variability of results regarding the surplus ACh in the brain *in vitro* is not clear; perhaps the variability depends on differences in experimental technique, such as differences in the thickness of the tissue slices (and, consequently, differences in the ease with which ACh is washed out from the intercellular space into the medium), and in the degree of tissue damage.

In the myenteric plexus–ileum smooth muscle preparation the surplus ACh is in the form of free ACh (Hutchinson *et al.*, 1976). The increase in brain ACh which occurs *in vivo* after the inhibition of ChE is also mainly attributable to free ACh. The total ACh content in the cerebral cortex of guinea pigs was increased by 41% 20 min after the injection of eserine (1 mg/kg); the content of free ACh was raised by 83%, stable bound by 26% and labile bound by 22% (Beani *et al.*, 1969). The content of ACh in the brain of rats 150 min after the injection of diisopropylphosphorofluoridate (1.8 mg/kg) was increased by 106% (Fonnum and Guttormsen, 1969). Again this increase was mainly based on the change of free ACh; the content of ACh in the particles of the homogenate was elevated by only 18%.

In the sympathetic ganglion the surplus ACh is not released by nerve impulses (Collier and Katz, 1971). The presence of surplus ACh in the phrenic nerve–diaphragm preparation does not result in a higher ACh release during a short stimulation of the phrenic nerve; during prolonged stimulation of the nerve, however, the amount of ACh released decreases more slowly if surplus ACh is present in the tissue. Under these conditions the surplus ACh appears either to replenish the quanta of ACh released by the nerve impulses, or to increase the non-quantal release of ACh during stimulation (Potter, 1970).

It is not clear where the surplus ACh is located. Collier and Katz (1971) proposed that surplus ACh is stored in the presynaptic nerve terminals. Their view was based on the observation that no formation of surplus ACh could be observed in sympathetic ganglia if the ganglia had been decentralized one week before the experiment. The conclusion that the surplus ACh is located in the presynaptic nerve endings may be questioned since the experiment was performed at a time when the activity of ChAc and the synthesis and release of ACh in the ganglion must have been decreased to extremely low values (see Chapter 7.6) and the conditions were therefore entirely different from those in a normal ganglion; e.g., spontaneous release of ACh from the nerve endings was probably completely absent, and it is possible that the pool of surplus ACh is normally formed from just such spontaneously released ACh.

The assumption that the surplus ACh is localized in cholinergic neurons or their endings requires that there is a compartment in cholinergic neurons in which ACh comes into contact with ChE and is hydrolysed in the absence of ChE inhibitors. This would bring about permanent and extremely wasteful hydrolysis of ACh. It seems much more likely that the surplus ACh pool is formed from the ACh which has been released from cholinergic neurons into the extracellular fluid. In the absence of active ChE this ACh may be taken up and accumulated in other neurons, glial cells, muscle fibres, glandular and various other non-neural cells. The accumulation may be accomplished by the carrier-mediated uptake of ACh described in Section 6.10.

After the inhibition of ChE, ACh presumably also accumulates in the extracellular fluid of the brain. Fonnum and Guttormsen (1969) assume that this was the case in their experiments in which diisopropylphosphorofluoridate increased the level of ACh in the brain *in vivo*. The location of surplus ACh in the extracellular fluid of the brain might explain the differences between the formation of surplus ACh in the brain *in vitro* and *in vivo* which were mentioned above. Under conditions *in vitro* most of ACh accumulating in the extracellular fluid will pass into the incubation medium and therefore the amount of surplus ACh in the tissue will be low. Under conditions *in vivo* the released ACh may remain in the extracellular fluid and, because of limitations imposed by the blood–brain barrier, is only slowly removed by the blood. On the other hand, it is evident that in the sympathetic ganglion and perhaps in other organs also the surplus ACh is located intracellularly. The inhibition of intracellular, as well as extracellular, ChE is necessary for ACh accumulation in the sympathetic ganglion (Collier and Katz, 1971). Although the surplus ACh is not released from the sympathetic ganglion by nerve impulses, it is released by perfusion with a high concentration of K^+ ions (Collier and Katz, 1971) or ACh (Collier and Katz, 1975). It is clear that the released ACh originates from intracellular stores.

The fact that the content of ACh in the particulate fractions of brain homogenates including the nerve endings is increased very little after the inhibition of ChE (Beani *et al.*, 1969; Fonnum and Guttormsen, 1969) indicates that ACh in these nerve endings is not in danger of direct contact with ChE and that its concentration inside the nerve endings is not controlled by this enzyme. This point is an important prerequisite for the generally held belief that a proportion of ACh in the nerve endings is freely dissolved in the cytoplasm.

6.5 'RESTING' SYNTHESIS OF ACETYLCHOLINE

Although ACh is the agent mediating the activity of cholinergic neurons in their communication with other cells, the synthesis of ACh in the nerve cells is a permanent process which does not stop even under conditions very closely approaching complete rest. This is well demonstrated by the increase of ACh content in resting tissues which can be observed after the inhibition of ChE (see Section 6.4). The increase indicates an unceasing formation of new ACh in the tissues. Fig. 6.2 shows the increase of ACh content in rat cardiac atria during incubation in a physiological

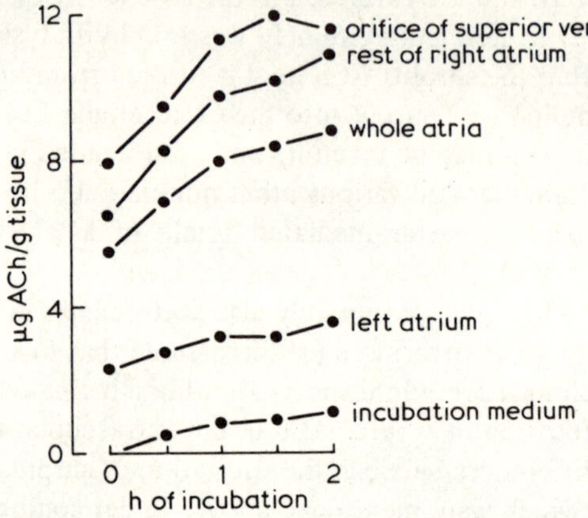

Fig. 6.2 ACh content of individual parts of rat cardiac atria during incubation in a medium containing salts, glucose and eserine. The curves from the top to the bottom correspond to the region around the orifice of the superior vena cava, the rest of the right atrium, the whole atria, the left atrium and the incubation medium. Based on Vlk and Tuček (1964).

salt medium containing glucose and eserine (Vlk and Tuček, 1964). Fig. 6.3 demonstrates the ability of rat striatal slices to increase their ACh content to 9 times the initial values during 30 min incubation in an enriched medium even in the absence of any ChE inhibitor (Sattin, 1966). ACh accumulating in the brain slices during incubation is present as free and labile-bound ACh, both in the presence (Collier *et al.*, 1972) and absence (Sattin, 1966) of eserine.

The unceasing synthesis of ACh is also manifest in observations that the tissue stores of ACh gradually become radioactive if the resting tissue has at its disposal radioactive choline or acetyl–CoA. In the rat diaphragm incubated at rest in the presence of labelled choline, 1/3 of its unlabelled ACh is replaced by labelled ACh within 1 h (Potter, 1970). During incubation of slices of the electric organ in the presence of radioactively labelled choline (Israël *et al.*, 1973), acetate and pyruvate (Israël and Tuček, 1974), the free and bound ACh gradually became radioactive, although the total ACh content remained unchanged (Fig. 4.5). The continuous synthesis of ACh is also revealed by its accumulation in the medium during the

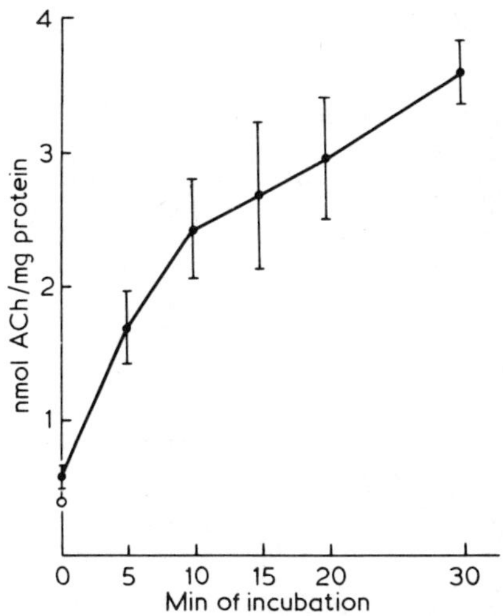

Fig. 6.3 The increase of ACh content in rat striatal slices during 30 min incubation at 37°C. The incubation medium was enriched by compounds like creatine, adenosine, choline, etc. (see original paper for details), but it did not contain any inhibitor of ChE. Filled circles indicate the mean ± S.D. of 6–9 observations. The open circle at time 0 shows the mean ACh content in the striatum immediately after the animal was killed. The difference between the filled and the open circle at time 0 shows the increase of ACh content occurring during the preparation of the slices. According to preliminary experiments, the content of ACh continued to rise until 60–80 min of incubation; by then, it was about 14 times higher than before the incubation (after Sattin, 1966).

incubation of various tissues in the presence of ChE inhibitors. The content of ACh in the medium continues to increase even after its content in the tissue reached its maximum (Mann *et al.*, 1939; Browning and Schulman, 1968; Fig. 6.4).

A part of the resting synthesis of ACh is undoubtedly connected with the random release of single quanta of the transmitter from the presynaptic nerve endings which is revealed by the appearance of miniature endplate potentials on the postsynaptic membrane (Fatt and Katz, 1952). It has been calculated, however, that the spontaneous quantal release of ACh at neuromuscular synapses can provide only a minor part of the total amount of ACh which is released from innervated muscles during incubation *in vitro* (Mitchell and Silver, 1963; Potter, 1970; Fletcher and Forrester, 1975; Katz and Miledi, 1977). Most of the resting release (99%? – Katz and Miledi, 1977) probably occurs as non-quantal molecular leakage of ACh from the nerve fibres; in the area of the neuromuscular junction, the leakage may be revealed by the minute shift of muscle potential occurring after curarization (Katz and Miledi, 1977). In addition to the synthesis of ACh required to replace the spontaneously (quantally and non-quantally) released ACh, it is likely that a part of the

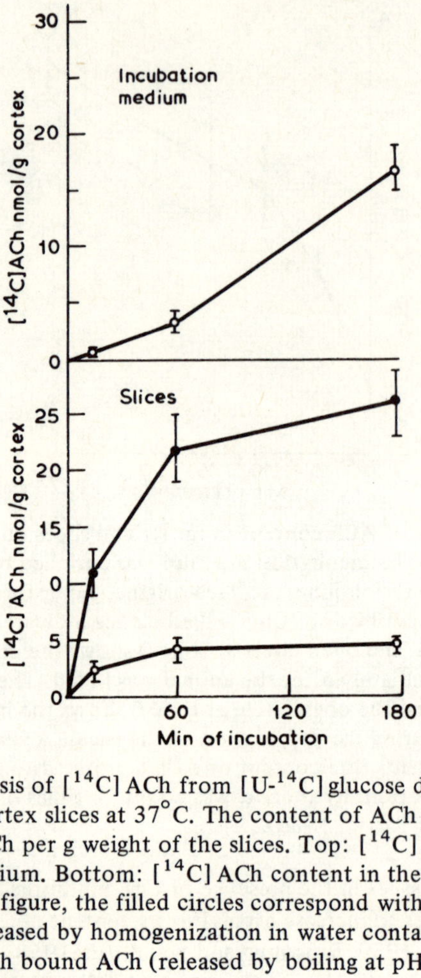

Fig. 6.4 The synthesis of [^{14}C] ACh from [U-^{14}C] glucose during 3 h incubation of rat brain cortex slices at 37°C. The content of ACh is expressed as nmoles of [^{14}C] ACh per g weight of the slices. Top: [^{14}C] ACh content in the incubation medium. Bottom: [^{14}C] ACh content in the slices. In the bottom part of the figure, the filled circles correspond with free and osmotically labile ACh (released by homogenization in water containing eserine), the open circles with bound ACh (released by boiling at pH 4). (After Browning and Schulman, 1968).

resting synthesis of ACh occurs independently of the release of ACh from the cells and is connected with the continuous intracellular metabolic turnover of the transmitter; its intensity has yet to be established.

6.6 ACETYLCHOLINE SYNTHESIS DURING AND AFTER INCREASED SYNAPTIC ACTIVITY

An increase in the release of ACh from the neurons is usually followed by an immediate increase in the synthesis of ACh. In experiments with a blood-perfused sympathetic ganglion the amount of ACh released at rest was such that, with the

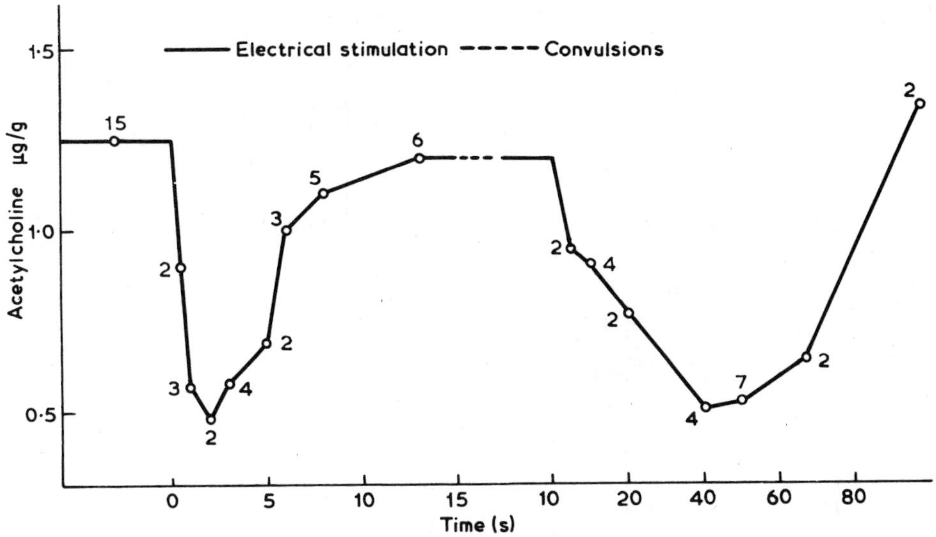

Fig. 6.5 Content of ACh in rat brain (μg ACh/g brain) during electrical stimulation (left) and following convulsions (right). Electrical stimulation was administered by flat electrodes mounted on the head. It lasted 3 sec except for the animals killed at shorter time intervals. The convulsions started after 8–15 sec, i.e. at different time intervals in different animals. For this reason, two time scales are given on the abscissa: on the left, time in sec from the beginning of the stimulation, on the right, time from the beginning of the convulsions. The number of experiments is shown beside the individual points (after Richter and Crossland, 1949).

transmitter content in the ganglion remaining constant, the total ACh content of the ganglion could be expected to turn over once in 8–16 h (Birks and MacIntosh, 1961). On supramaximal stimulation of the preganglionic fibres at 20 Hz the release of ACh was increased so that the total ACh content of the ganglion could be turned over in 10 min. The content of ACh in the ganglion remained unchanged even after 2 h of stimulation. Clearly, the rate of synthesis was adjusted to the rate of release. Similarly, the diaphragm *in vitro* (Potter, 1970) at rest released so much ACh that its total ACh content would be turned over in 134 min. When, however, the phrenic nerve was stimulated at 20 Hz, the release of ACh was augmented so that the amount of ACh released within 5 min corresponded to 34% of the initial ACh content in the diaphragm. The content of ACh in the diaphragm remained unchanged. This implies that the rate of synthesis must have been increased such that the total ACh content of the diaphragm could be turned over in 15 min (Potter, 1970). A classical example of the release-associated increase of the synthesis of ACh in the central nervous system is given in the work of Richter and Crossland (1949; Fig. 6.5). During massive electrical stimulation of the head the content of ACh in the brain of rats was lowered

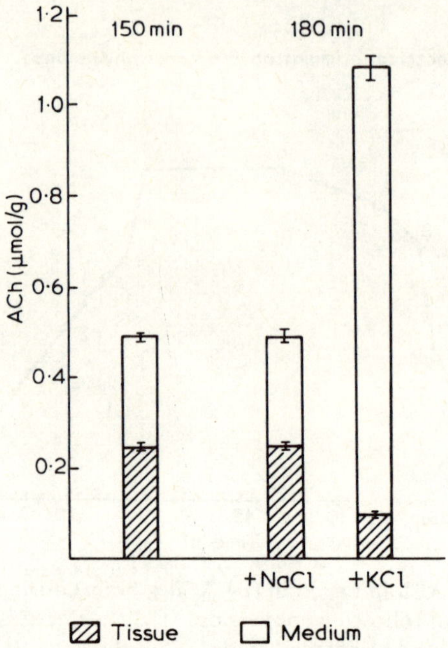

Fig. 6.6 Effect of increased concentration of K^+ ions on the synthesis and content of [^{14}C] ACh in rat striatal slices. The slices were incubated in a physiological medium containing, among other components, KCl 5.6 mM, eserine 0.2 mM, and [2-^{14}C] pyruvate 20 mM. The content of [^{14}C] ACh (expressed in µmoles per g weight) in the slices and in the medium after 150 min of incubation is shown on the left. The concentration of KCl in the medium was then increased to 30 mM, and the incubation continued for another 30 min. The content of [^{14}C] ACh in the slices and in the medium after 30 min of additional incubation in the presence of 30 mM KCl is shown by the column on the extreme right. In the control experiment (middle column), NaCl was added to the medium after 150 min of incubation instead of KCl. The bars indicate S.E.M. (after Lefresne *et al.*, 1973).

by more than 50% within 1 s; after the end of the stimulation it returned to the original level within approximately 10 s.

In biochemical studies on the synthesis of ACh in the brain *in vitro*, the release of ACh is usually stimulated not by electrical pulses, but by an increase of K^+ concentration in the medium. Quastel *et al.* (1936) noted that more ACh was released from brain slices into the medium when the slices were incubated in the presence of an increased concentration of K^+. Mann *et al.* (1939) discovered that in the presence of an elevated concentration of K^+ (27 mM vs. 4 mM) the content of ACh in the incubation medium was augmented, while the content of ACh in the incubated brain tissue was lowered, but the total yield of ACh (tissue + medium) was greatly

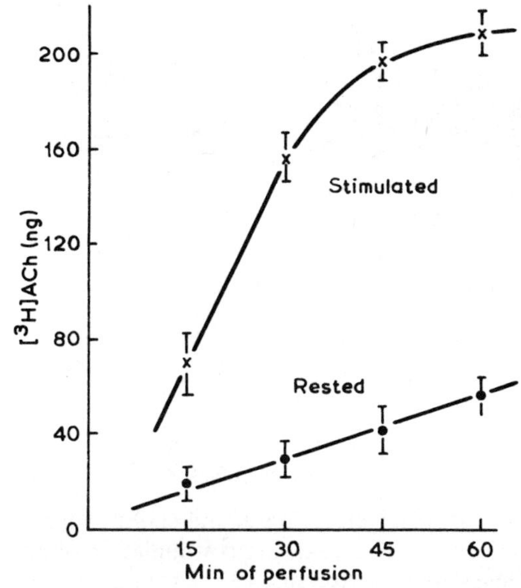

Fig. 6.7 The content of radioactively labelled ACh in the superior cervical ganglion of the cat during perfusion with Locke solution containing [^{3}H] choline. Abscissa: time (min) from the start of perfusion with labelled choline. Ordinate: content of labelled ACh (ng) in the ganglion. Upper curve: during the perfusion, preganglionic fibres were stimulated at 20 Hz. Lower curve: the ganglion was at rest. Individual points are means (± S.E.M.) of 5 experiments (after Collier and MacIntosh, 1969).

increased. This observation has been confirmed many times in various connections (McLennan and Elliott, 1950; Polak and Meeuws, 1966; Browning and Schulman, 1968; Bertels-Meeuws and Polak, 1968; Sharkawi and Schulman, 1969a; Richter and Marchbanks, 1971a,b; Sharkawi, 1972; Molenaar *et al.*, 1973b; Richter, 1976) and is well documented by Fig. 6.6, taken from the study of Lefresne *et al.* (1973). It is assumed that the elevated concentration of K^+ increases the release and, secondarily, the synthesis of ACh by depolarizing the nerve fibres. The synthesis of ACh is not increased by an increased concentration of KCl after the brain tissue was disintegrated (in a brain homogenate) (Sharkawi and Schulman, 1969a). The enhancement of the release and synthesis of ACh by a raised concentration of K^+ is dependent on the presence of Ca^{2+} ions (McLennan and Elliott, 1950; Grewaal and Quastel, 1973; Molenaar *et al.*, 1973a; Richter, 1976). It thus resembles the release of ACh by nerve impulses.

The increased rate of ACh synthesis during augmented synaptic activity is also evident from the effect of nerve stimulation on the incorporation of radioactive precursors into ACh. As has been pointed out in Section 6.5, the store of ACh in an organ or tissue at rest gradually becomes radioactive if the tissue is incubated in the

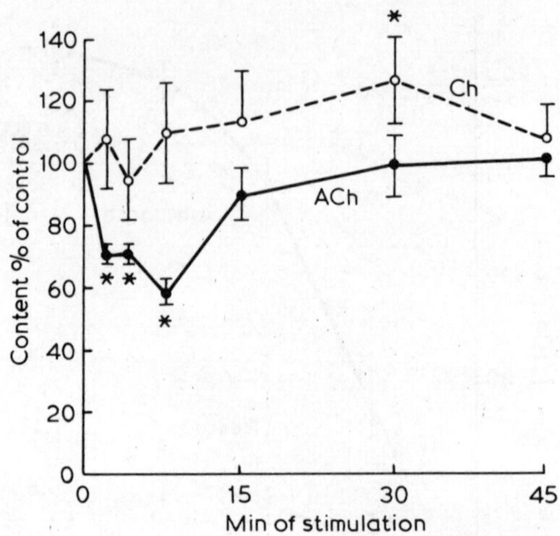

Fig. 6.8 The content of ACh (filled circles) and choline (open circles) in cat superior cervical ganglion during continuous stimulation of preganglionic fibres at 60 Hz. The content of ACh and choline (mean ± S.E.M. of 4–7 experiments) is expressed as a percentage of the content in the contralateral unstimulated ganglion. Asterisks indicate a statistically significant difference ($p < 0.05$) between the experimental and control values (after Friesen and Khatter, 1971).

presence of a radioactive precursor of ACh. The rate of incorporation of radioactive precursors into ACh is very much increased by the stimulation of the appropriate cholinergic nerves (Fig. 6.7 – Collier and MacIntosh, 1969; Potter, 1970).

Some observations give the impression (not fully justified – see below) that the increase of ACh synthesis in response to augmented ACh release starts only after a distinct delay. It has been stated already that the content of ACh in the sympathetic ganglion is not changed after the preganglionic fibres had been stimulated for 2 h at 20 Hz (Birks and MacIntosh, 1961), but it is lowered after 5 min of stimulation (MacIntosh, 1963). When the preganglionic fibres are stimulated at 60 Hz, the content of ACh in the ganglion decreases by 40% within the first 8 min, but it returns to initial values within the next 15 min in spite of continuing stimulation (Fig. 6.8 – Friesen and Khatter, 1971; for a similar finding without quantitative evaluation see also Rosenblueth *et al.*, 1939). Immediately after the end of intensive stimulation the content of ACh in the ganglion regularly shows a transient increase of 30–60% above the resting values (Fig. 6.9 – Friesen and Khatter, 1971; Rosenblueth *et al.*, 1939; Birks and Fitch, 1974; Bourdois *et al.*, 1975). Under suitable conditions the content of ACh in the ganglion may rise above the initial values even before the end of the stimulation (Bourdois *et al.*, 1975). A fall of ACh content soon after the start of the stimulation and a consequent increase can also be observed in the electric organ of *Torpedo* (Israël *et al.*, 1972; Dunnant *et al.*, 1972),

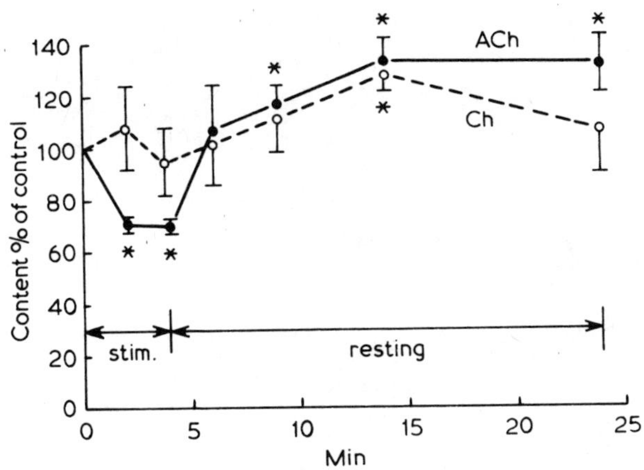

Fig. 6.9 Content of ACh (filled circles) and choline (open circles) in the superior cervical ganglion during 4 min of stimulation of preganglionic fibres at 60 Hz and during 20 min of rest immediately after the end if the stimulation. The content of ACh and choline (mean ± S.E.M.) is expressed as a percentage of the content in the contralateral unstimulated ganglion. Asterisks indicate a statistically significant difference ($p < 0.05$) between the experimental and control values (after Friesen and Khatter, 1971).

1974a, 1977). When the electric organ is stimulated at 5 Hz, its electric response drops sharply during the first minute; then it ceases falling and remains constant for several minutes. Coincident with the drop in the electrical response during the first minute of stimulation the content of ACh falls very steeply; starting from the second minute there follows a transient increase in the ACh content above resting values, but after several minutes a new fall occurs (Fig. 6.10). Later we shall return to the interesting point that these changes of ACh content involve only the free ACh pool.

At first sight the sequence of changes of ACh content in the sympathetic ganglion and electric organ suggests that the synthesis of ACh is very low at the beginning of the stimulation and that it starts to increase only after a certain period of time or after the content of ACh has diminished to a certain low level. This is not necessarily so, however. The point is that the content of ACh in the tissue is the result of a balance between its synthesis and release, and the release of ACh decreases very steeply immediately after the start of repetitive stimulation. In the sympathetic ganglion the decrease of ACh release per nerve impulse at the beginning of repetitive stimulation has been shown by direct measurements (Brown and Feldberg, 1936; Birks and MacIntosh, 1961; Birks and Fitch, 1974), whereas in the electric organ the decrease in the release of ACh is indicated by the fall of the electric response; similar changes of ACh release have been discovered electrophysiologically on the neuromuscular junction (Brooks and Thies, 1962; Hubbard *et al.,* 1969). Even if the

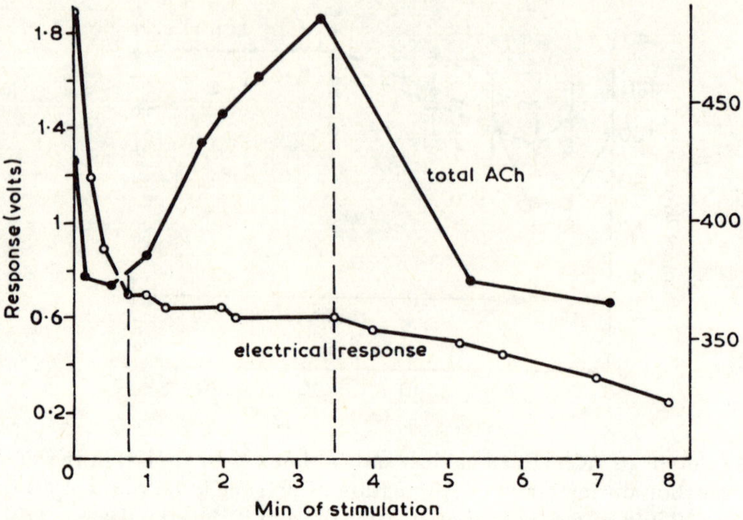

Fig. 6.10 Changes in the electrical response and in the total ACh content of slices of the electric organ of *Torpedo marmorata* during their continuous stimulation by an electric field at 5 Hz. Abscissa: time (min) of stimulation. Ordinate: the scale on the left indicates the size of the electric response in volts, the scale on the right gives the concentration of ACh in nmoles/g (after Dunnant *et al.*, 1974a).

synthesis of ACh increased from the very beginning of the stimulation to a constant high value, the content of ACh might fall in the first stage, while the release per impulse is high, and increased in the second stage, when the release per impulse became low. In order to know the time course of the changes of the synthesis, one must know both the time course of changes in ACh content of the tissue and the time course of changes in the amount of ACh released per impulse. It is most likely that the increased rate of ACh synthesis caused by the stimulation can persist after the stimulation has stopped (Fig. 6.9) and that conditions can occur during intensive stimulation under which the synthesis fails (second fall of ACh content in Fig. 6.10).

In addition to the slow changes in the content of ACh during stimulation which are shown in Fig. 6.10, much faster periodic changes ('rapid oscillations') in the content of ACh in the electrically stimulated electric organ have been discovered recently (Dunant *et al.*, 1974b, 1975, 1977; Israël and Dunant, 1975; Israël *et al.*, 1975). The rapid oscillations have an amplitude of 20–40% of the total ACh content of the tissue at rest and their period is 4–5. It still has to be established whether the oscillations of ACh content mainly reflect periodic variations in the synthesis of ACh, or its release, or both. The oscillations of ACh content are accompanied by similar oscillations of the content of ATP (Israël *et al.*, 1977). Further study of these oscillations may become of utmost importance in the understanding of the control of ACh synthesis.

6.7 THE RELATION OF NEWLY SYNTHESIZED ACETYLCHOLINE TO SYNAPTIC VESICLES

In view of data on the subcellular localization of ChAc (see Section 6.2) it appears most likely that the synthesis of ACh occurs in the cytoplasm of the nerve endings or, more broadly speaking, in their cytoplasmic compartment (possibly including the walls of this compartment). According to the vesicular hypothesis of transmitter release, one has to assume that a newly synthesized molecule of ACh first passes from the cytoplasmic compartment into the synaptic vesicle and only then can it be used for synaptic transmission. How ACh gets into the synaptic vesicles is a mystery. When brain synaptosomes are incubated in the presence of radioactive ACh, the labelled transmitter passes comparatively easily into the labile-bound pool of ACh which is assumed to be freely dissolved in the synaptosomal cytoplasm, but virtually none of it passes into the synaptic vesicles. It does not pass into the vesicles even when these have first been released and isolated from the synaptosomes and afterwards incubated in the presence of labelled ACh, together with ATP and Mg^{2+} to facilitate the transport of the transmitter (Marchbanks, 1968a).

Repeated attempts to achieve selective binding and accumulation of ACh in isolated synaptic vesicles *in vitro* have given little indication of how this process might proceed in the nerve endings *in vivo*. A type of binding of ACh to synaptic vesicles has been observed by Kuriyama *et al.* (1968). The binding occurred, however, in a virtually saltless medium; it was diminished to one half by 5 mM NaCl or KCl and almost completely abolished by the same salts at a concentration of 70 mM. The observed binding seems therefore to be without any physiological importance. Binding of ACh to synaptic vesicles has also been described by Guth (1969) and Burton (1970). The data from their studies cannot be compared quantitatively with what might be happening in the living cells, since in both studies, the vesicles were incubated at extremely low ionic strength, the sucrose with eserine medium containing either 50 μM $CaCl_2$ (Burton) or 3 mM sodium maleate (Guth). Suszkiw (1976) rightly speculated that the vesicles should be first deprived of their own ACh in order to bind the ACh from the medium. He effected the loss of ACh from the vesicles by exposing them to hypo-osmotic conditions; this also caused the loss of ATP from the vesicles and may have damaged them in other ways. With vesicles thus prepared, some accumulation of ACh has been observed – but only in an ion-free medium. In the experiments described by Mattson and O'Brien (1976), the observed binding of external ACh to vesicles corresponded to less than 0.1% of the ACh content recovered in the vesicular fraction of the homogenate.

Available estimates of ACh content in individual synaptic vesicles are surrounded by uncertainty, mainly because it is difficult to assess the loss of ACh during the preparation of the vesicular fraction. Canepa (1964) computed that vesicles with a diameter of 50 nm and with walls 5 nm thick, might contain 45 000 molecules of ACh in the crystalline state. Whittaker and Sheridan (1965) calculated that one synaptic vesicle from the brain could contain 1500 molecules of ACh, if ACh were present in a 0.16 M solution, or 14 000 molecules, if it were adsorbed on the internal surface of the vesicle. On counting the number of vesicles in brain vesicular fractions and on the assumption that 15% of the vesicles were cholinergic, they arrived at an estimate of 2000 molecules of ACh per vesicle. The true proportion of cholinergic vesicles in the total vesicular population is, however, one of the big unknowns in any work of this kind performed on the brain. This problem appears less serious in experiments with synaptic vesicles from sympathetic ganglia, which have yielded an estimate of 1630 molecules of ACh per vesicle (Wilson *et al.*, 1973). The content of ACh in individual synaptic vesicles from the electric organ of *Torpedo* is estimated at 66 000 molecules (Sheridan *et al.*, 1966); the higher value, compared with that for mammalian vesicles, can, for the most part, be explained by the bigger volume of the vesicles and by the higher osmotic concentration of the body fluids in *Torpedo.*

The way in which ACh is retained within the vesicles has not been definitely clarified. At present, the most likely hypothesis appears to be that presented by Whittaker *et al.* (1972). In their view, ACh is bound in the vesicles to an identified acidic protein, vesiculin. The vesicles contain also ATP (Dowdall *et al.*, 1974), which is probably also bound to vesiculin and at the same time provides some of the negative charges required to neutralize the positive charges of ACh. Whittaker *et al.* (1972) suggest that the release of ACh^+ from vesicles undergoing exocytosis is based on ion-exchange with extracellular Na^+.

There is a question, however, as to whether the synaptic vesicles are indeed as important for the release of ACh as is assumed by the vesicular hypothesis. This problem will be mentioned here only briefly because it clearly belongs to the area of ACh storage and release, not of ACh synthesis. The role of synaptic vesicles in transmitter release has recently become the central point of a very active discussion. Strong support for the vesicular hypothesis has been provided by experiments on the *in vivo* incorporation of radioactive choline into the so-called macromolecular and micromolecular fractions of brain synaptosomes. The two fractions were obtained by gel filtration of the material released from brain synaptosomes after their rupture by hypo-osmotic treatment (Aquilonius *et al.*, 1973; Sundwall, 1973). The ACh contained in the macromolecular fraction probably corresponded mainly to the ACh in the synaptic vesicles, and the ACh in the micromolecular fraction probably stemmed mainly from the soluble cytoplasmic ACh. Even at short time intervals after the i.v. injection of labelled choline, the specific radioactivity of ACh in the macromolecular fraction was higher than in the micromolecular one. Similarly the specific radioactivity of ACh in synaptic vesicles isolated by density gradient centrifugation (Molenaar and Polak, 1973) was also higher than in the cytoplasm of the nerve endings as early as one minute after i.v. injection of labelled choline. Analysis of the distribution of radioactive ACh in subcellular fractions of the brain after an intraventricular injection of labelled choline indicated that the synaptic vesicles in the vicinity of the nerve ending membranes contain ACh which is more radioactive than in other synaptic vesicles (Barker *et al.*, 1972). Observations of this kind show that there is rapid metabolic turnover of ACh in synaptic vesicles, as would be expected if it is the vesicular ACh that is released during synaptic activity.

The use of vesicular ACh for synaptic transmission was also inferred from changes in the ACh content of synaptic vesicles in the electric organ during stimulation of its nerve *in vivo* (Zimmermann and Whittaker, 1974a). The content of ACh in synaptic vesicles isolated by zonal centrifugation was lowered by more than one half after the administration of only 500 stimuli to the nerve. An important objection to these experiments has been raised, however, by Dunant *et al.* (1976) who pointed out that the loss of vesicular ACh occurred only when the electric organ was forced to discharge against a high external resistance, i.e. when it was discharged in air and not immersed in sea water.

By perfusing the electric organ with a solution containing sucrose and dextran, it has proved possible to demonstrate that a new population of synaptic vesicles appears in the electric organ when its nerve is stimulated (Zimmermann and Whittaker, 1977; Zimmermann and Denston, 1977a,b). This new population, which is most probably formed by the vesicles which have undergone exocytosis, contains sucrose and dextran taken up from the extracellular fluid. The remarkable feature of the new population of vesicles is that it contains most of the newly synthesized ACh, as would be expected if the vesicles are refilled with new ACh after they have released their original ACh content into the synaptic gap. Another important feature of the observations made by Zimmermann and Denston (1977b) is that the specific radioactivity of ACh in the vesicles isolated from a stimulated electric organ perfused with labelled acetate is higher than the specific radioactivity of total tissue ACh, which indicates the rapid incorporation of newly synthesized ACh into the vesicles.

Other observations, however, indicate that increased synaptic activity brings about considerable changes in the free and labile bound, but not in the stable bound, ACh. The content of total and free ACh in the brain of mice drops considerably during convulsions, but the content of stable-bound ACh is not changed (Kurokawa *et al.*, 1963). During stimulation of the electric organ *in vitro* the content of free ACh undergoes big changes whereas the content of bound ACh remains virtually constant for a long time (Dunant *et al.*, 1972, 1974a, 1977; Israël *et al.*, 1972). Rapid oscillatory changes in the content of ACh in the electric organ during stimulation also involve the free, rather than the bound ACh pool (Dunant *et al.*, 1974b, 1975, 1977; Israël *et al.*, 1975). During electric stimulation of the guinea pig myenteric plexus its ACh content falls due to the reduction of its free ACh (Hutchinson *et al.*, 1976). In experiments with brain slices, incubation in the presence of an increased concentration of K^+ diminishes both the soluble and the vesicular ACh pools (Salehmoghaddam and Collier, 1976).

Findings of this kind do not exclude the vesicular hypothesis, but they do serve as a warning against its uncritical acceptance. The easiest way to reconcile the vesicular hypothesis with the observations just mentioned is to assume that the ACh belonging to the free and labile-bound pools is in fact not freely dissolved in the cytoplasm, but instead, is located in a special population of synaptic vesicles. One has to assume that these vesicles are extremely fragile and do not survive the homogenization and the hypo-osmotic conditions. The extreme fragility of the nerve endings in the homogenate of the brain and the ease with which their ACh (cytoplasmic or vesicular?) passes into the free ACh pool, have been pointed out by Schuberth *et al.* (1970b) and some indications of the fragility of synaptic vesicles have been mentioned in Section 6.3.

It is necessary, however, to admit and consider the possibility of entirely different explanations for the observed phenomena, including the possibility that the ACh released during synaptic transmission originates directly from the cytoplasmic ACh pool. Birks (1974) used this last possibility as the basis on which to explain his finding that stimulation of the sympathetic ganglion may lower the number of synaptic vesicles in synaptic boutons by 75% at a time when the ACh content of the ganglion is not changed. Tauc *et al.* (1974) observed that synaptic transmission from identified cholinergic neurons of squid could be abolished by intraneuronal injection of ChE and the observation was interpreted as an indication that the cytoplasmic ACh is responsible for synaptic transmission. It seems reasonable to assume, however, that a dynamic equilibrium exists in the neurons between their vesicular and extravesicular ACh pools, and that a depletion of the extravesicular ACh by the injected ChE must necessarily affect the vesicular pool of ACh as well. Marchbanks (1975a) suggests that the nerve impulses primarily release the cytoplasmic ACh and the ACh which (he believes) is loosely bound to the surface of the synaptic vesicles. His review (Marchbanks, 1975b) marshals most systematically the objections which can be raised against the vesicular hypothesis of ACh release.

6.8 PREFERENTIAL RELEASE OF NEWLY SYNTHESIZED ACETYLCHOLINE

Collier (1969) achieved radioactive labelling of the store of ACh in the sympathetic ganglion by perfusing the ganglion with radioactive choline and stimulating the preganglionic fibres during the perfusion. Then the perfusion was changed to non-radioactive choline. The preganglionic fibres were again stimulated and the specific radioactivity of the ACh released from the ganglion was measured. It was found that the specific radioactivity of the released ACh was lower than that of the ACh contained in the ganglion. Collier explained this finding as an indication that the nerve impulses cause preferential release of the newly synthesized ACh; therefore the ACh released during the perfusion with non-radioactive choline was of low radioactivity, although the specific radioactivity of the total store of ACh in the ganglion was high.

Birks and Fitch (1974) pointed out that some of the assumptions made by Collier during the calculation of specific radioactivities are controversial. In spite of this, the conclusion that the newly formed ACh is released in preference to the old store of ACh was confirmed by further experimental evidence. It has been found in similarly designed experiments on the rat phrenic nerve–diaphragm preparation that the stimulation of the nerve preferentially releases the ACh which originates from the substrate immediately available to the preparation (Potter, 1970). When slices of brain incubated with labelled choline are stimulated by raised K^+, the ACh released is of a higher specific radioactivity (i.e. more recently synthesized) than the ACh released in the presence of a physiological concentration of K^+ (Richter and Marchbanks, 1971a). Molenaar *et al.* (1973a) observed in experiments with brain slices that the radioactive ACh represented 2.3% of the total ACh content after the slices had been kept in contact with radioactive choline for 5 min; the radioactive ACh represented, however, 8.7% of the ACh which was released into the medium. Preferential release of newly synthesized transmitter has also been confirmed in other studies on brain slices (Lefresne, 1974) and synaptosomes (Guyenet *et al.*, 1975) and can be demonstrated whether the labelled precursor, used to mark the newly synthesized ACh, is choline or acetyl–CoA (Molenaar and Polak, 1976).

Preferential release of newly synthesized transmitter has also been observed in the case in noradrenaline (Kopin *et al.*, 1968) and dopamine (Besson *et al.*, 1969). Its mechanism can be imagined by assuming that the synaptic vesicles in the proximity of the presynaptic membrane undergo repeated cycles of emptying, reconstitution and refilling by the newly synthesized transmitter, whereas the content of transmitter in more distant vesicles remains unused. Other explanations are possible, however; for example, the hypothesis that the newly synthesized ACh is bound to the surface of synaptic vesicles and that the nerve impulses cause preferential release of ACh from the surface of the vesicles (Marchbanks, 1973).

6.9 CONTROL OF THE SYNTHESIS

Experiments performed to examine the effect of increased synaptic activity on the content of ACh in the sympathetic ganglion (Brown and Feldberg, 1936; Birks and MacIntosh, 1961), diaphragm (Potter, 1970), brain (Richter and Crossland, 1949) and other organs indicate that the content of ACh in mammalian tissues is comparatively stable and that the increased release caused by increased activity of cholinergic synapses is rapidly compensated for by increased synthesis. The bigger changes of ACh content caused by the stimulation of the electric organ of *Torpedo* (Dunant *et al.*, 1974a; Zimmermann and Whittaker, 1974a) may be due to an unphysiologically high rate and long duration of stimulation. The fact that the rate of ACh synthesis increases when ACh is released, but that at rest it remains at a low level just necessary to ensure the constant content of ACh, strongly suggests that the control of ACh synthesis is based on a feedback between the content or concentration of ACh at the site of synthesis and the process of synthesis. Opinions differ, however, as to the exact way in which the control is effected. Several hypotheses proposed to explain its mechanism will be discussed here.

The hypothesis which appears to explain most features of the control of ACh synthesis and which is compatible with most experimental findings is the assumption that the control of ACh synthesis in the neurons is based on the law of mass action

(Potter *et al.*, 1968; Glover and Potter, 1971). According to this hypothesis, the synthesis of ACh proceeds until the concentrations of the substrates and products of the reaction reach equilibrium, given by the equilibrium constant (K_{eq}) of the reaction. It is evident *a priori* that the synthesis of ACh in the neurons, controlled by this mechanism, will be influenced by changes both in the concentration of reaction products at the site of synthesis and in the concentration of the substrates. The hypothesis of control by mass action can, therefore, easily incorporate the participation of regulatory mechanisms which affect the supply of substrates (choline and acetyl–CoA).

It is important to consider whether the hypothesis of control by mass action is compatible with what we know about the concentrations of choline, acetyl–CoA, CoA and ACh in the nerve cells. Of particular importance is the question whether the concentration of ACh in the cholinergic neurons is sufficiently high to be considered as the equilibrium concentration in the reaction catalysed by ChAc. The examination of these points is necessarily based on many assumptions. Nevertheless let us ask the question: what concentration of ACh will be in the cholinergic neurons of the brain when the reaction of ACh synthesis has reached equilibrium?

Since $$K_{eq} = \frac{[\text{ACh}] \times [\text{CoA}]}{[\text{Ch}] \times [\text{acetyl–CoA}]},$$

the equilibrium concentration of ACh equals

$$[\text{ACh}] = \frac{K_{eq} \times [\text{Ch}] \times [\text{acetyl–CoA}]}{[\text{CoA}]}$$

In view of lack of data on the concentrations of choline, CoA and acetyl–CoA specifically in cholinergic neurons, it will be assumed that they are the same as in the whole brain. Taking that, for the rat brain, $K_{eq} = 41$ (Glover and Potter, 1971), the concentration of choline at the moment of killing – [Ch] = 27.5 nmol/g (Dross and Kewitz, 1972), the concentration of acetyl–CoA – [acetyl–CoA] = 11 nmol/g (Reynolds and Blass, 1975), and the concentration of CoA – [CoA] = 88.6 nmol/g (Kaplan and Lipmann, 1948; Decker, 1959), the calculation of the equilibrium concentration of ACh gives

$$[\text{ACh}] = \frac{41 \times 27.5 \times 11}{88.6} = 140.0 \text{ (nmol/g)}.$$

This calculation, of course, embraces a number of inaccuracies and uncertainties. One possibility which cannot be excluded is that not only the concentration of ACh, but also the concentrations of other substances in cholinergic neurons may be different from values obtained by biochemical examination of the whole brain. For example, the concentration of choline in the cholinergic neurons may be higher than the average concentration in the whole brain in view of the fact that the cholinergic neurons are equipped with the high affinity carrier for choline (see Chapter 5). On the other hand, the concentration of acetyl–CoA in the cytoplasm of all neurons is almost certainly lower than its concentration in the whole brain, which has been used in the calculation, because acetyl–CoA is more concentrated in the mitochondria (Nicklas *et al.*, 1971).

The real concentration of ACh in cholinergic neurons of the brain is not known. Again, let us make an estimate, based on arbitrary but reasonable assumptions. The content of ACh in the rat brain will be taken as 12 nmol/g weight (Tuček and Diepold, 1963). On the assumption that the neurons represent 1/3 of the weight of the brain (the rest being attributable to glial cells and extracellular fluid), that the ACh is confined to cholinergic neurons, and that cholinergic neurons represent 10% of the total volume of all neurons, the concentration of ACh in the cholinergic neurons will be equal to 12 nmol/g x 30 = 360 nmol/g. Despite the uncertainties associated with this estimate (the main being the proportion of cholinergic neurons in the total neuronal population of the brain), it is evident that, in the light of present knowledge, the estimated equilibrium concentration of ACh (120 nmol/g) and the estimated concentration of ACh in cholinergic neurons (360 nmol/g) do not appear to be vastly different, incompatible values.

In postulating the mass action control of ACh synthesis, it is reasonable to assume that, at rest, ACh is distributed in the cytoplasm of the whole cholinergic neuron, so long as ChAc is present throughout the neuron including the dendrites (for evidence that this is so, see Kása *et al.*, 1970) and so long as the substrates are also distributed throughout the neuron. A higher concentration of ACh in presynaptic nerve endings might be achieved in two ways: by the accumulation of ACh in synaptic vesicles, and by a higher concentration of substrates (most probably choline and perhaps acetyl–CoA also, see later in this chapter) in this part of the neuron.

The hypothesis that ACh synthesis is regulated on the basis of the reaction equilibrium accords well with the results of observations of ACh synthesis by brain tissue *in vitro*. When slices of brain tissue or synaptosomes are incubated in a physiological saline medium containing a suitable energy source, it is regularly found that the content of ACh increases until it reaches a certain limiting value and then remains stable (Fig. 6.4 – Browning and Schulman, 1968; Mann *et al.*, 1939; Sattin, 1966; Bhatnagar and MacIntosh, 1967; Lefresne *et al.*, 1973; Lefresne, 1974). The lack of any further increase in ACh concentration is not due to the exhaustion of the substrates or the sources of energy. Lefresne *et al.* (1973) have shown that brain slices are capable of increasing the synthesis of ACh long after their ACh concentration has reached the plateau value, if the concentration of K^+ in the incubation medium is then increased so that some of the accumulated ACh is released from the tissue into the medium (Fig. 6.6). Lefresne (1974) demonstrated that there is a linear inverse relation between the content of ACh in the brain slices and the rate of synthesis of new ACh in them.

The cessation of further synthesis after the concentration of ACh in the tissue has reached a limiting value, as demonstrated by the above mentioned experiments *in vitro*, might also be explained on the basis of some of the other hypotheses proposed to explain the control of ACh synthesis. They will be discussed later, together with the difficulties that they encounter. It is difficult to explain, in terms of the mass action hypothesis, the difference between the content of ACh found in the brain immediately after killing the animal (and usually accepted as the resting concentration of ACh in the brain) and the limiting value (some 2–14 times greater) which is reached in the course of an incubation even in the absence of ChE inhibitors. Two explanations seem possible (Lefresne, 1974):

(1) The reaction equilibrium *in vitro* is different from that *in vivo* because the intracellular concentrations of substrates are changed under the conditions of incubation.
(2) The value for ACh content found immediately after killing the animal is considerably lower than the true resting state as a result of excitement during killing, ischaemia during the preparation of the tissue, and other unfavourable factors, but the true resting (and equilibrium) values are restored in the course of incubation. Presumably both factors are important.

The idea that the content of ACh found in the brain after killing the conscious animal is lower than the content of ACh which would correspond to the true resting state of brain neurons is supported by at least two types or experimental observation:

(a) that the content of ACh discovered in the brain of animals killed during anaesthesia is higher than in unanaesthetized animals (Richter and Crossland, 1949; Crossland and Merrick, 1954);
(b) that the interruption of the continuity of cholinergic axons in the septum is followed by a transient increase in the content of ACh in the hippocampus containing the terminal parts of these axons (Sethy *et al.*, 1973; Potempska *et al.*, 1975; Rommelspacher and Kuhar, 1975).

In both these experimental situations, the higher ACh content is most probably attributable to the reduction or cessation of impulse flow to the presynaptic nerve endings and to the prevention of its increase during the killing of the animal.

It will be difficult to provide direct and complete experimental proof of the validity of the mass action hypothesis of control of ACh synthesis in the nerve endings. The hypothesis does, however, receive experimental support from observations regarding changes induced in neuronal ACh synthesis and content by changes in the supply of choline and acetyl–CoA. Kuntscherová (1972) observed that the administration of massive doses of choline to rats brings about a significant increase in the content of ACh in several organs including the brain (Fig. 6.11). Her findings have been confirmed by Haubrich *et al.* (1974, 1975c, 1976), Cohen and Wurtman (1975, 1976), Racagni *et al.* (1975), Ulus *et al.* (1977) and Hirsch *et al.* (1977). Eisenstadt and Schwartz (1975) found that the synthesis of ACh in the body of an identified cholinergic neuron in *Aplysia* can be increased by intracellular injections of choline and Treistman and Schwartz (1977) made similar observations on cholinergic axons. It has often been found that the synthesis of ACh changes under conditions which are likely to affect the availability of acetyl–CoA in the neurons; ACh synthesis changes in the same direction as do the presumed changes in the availability of acetyl–CoA (Mann and Quastel, 1940; Endröczi *et al.*, 1967; Gibson

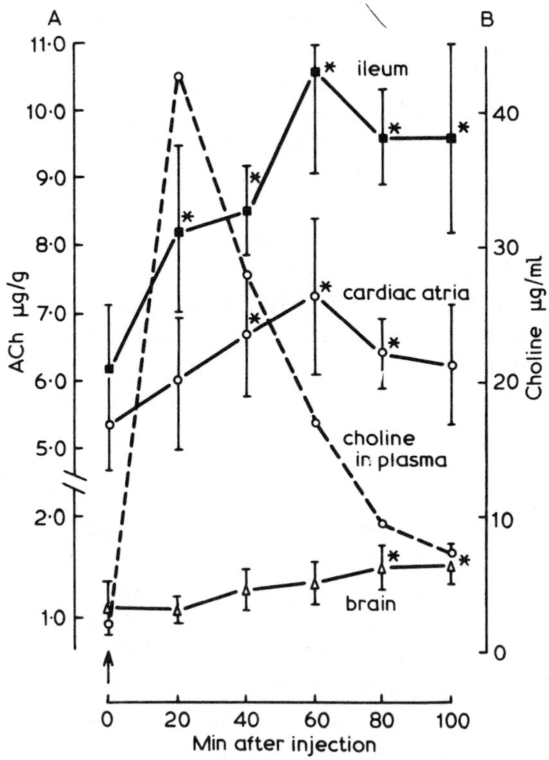

Fig. 6.11 The content of ACh in rat ileum (filled squares), cardiac atria (open circles, solid line) and brain (open triangles) and of choline in the blood plasma (open circles, broken line) following and injection of choline (200 mg/kg body weight, s.c.). Each point represents the mean of 8–10 experiments ± 2 S.E.M. Abscissa: time (min) after injection. Ordinate A: µg ACh/g tissue. Ordinate B: µg free choline/ml blood plasma. The asterisks indicate a statistically significant difference ($p < 0.05$) from control values (after Kuntscherová, 1972).

et al., 1967; Gibson *et al.*, 1975). These experimental observations will be mentioned in more detail later in this chapter.

Besides the hypothesis of mass control, several other hypotheses for the explanations for the mechanism controlling ACh synthesis have been proposed. The alternative hypotheses invoke the possible regulatory role of 1. the availability of the binding sites for ACh, 2. changes in ChAc activity induced by the reaction products (ACh and CoA) or by altered ionic concentrations, and 3. changes in the supply of substrates (choline and acetyl–CoA). All these hypotheses can be reconciled with the hypothesis of the mass action control of ACh synthesis if we assume that the final ACh concentration at the site of ACh synthesis tends to be that corresponding to the reaction equilibrium, but that the position of the equilibrium and the rate at which it is attained depends on the factors encompassed by the alternative hypotheses. The possible regulatory role of these factors will now be discussed in more detail:

Saturation of the binding sites for ACh in the storage space

This factor (MacIntosh, 1963) might play a decisive role in the regulation of synthesis if it were necessary for all ACh to be bound (presumably to vesiculin and ATP in synaptic vesicles). But why does the synthesis stop in the cytoplasm? When brain slices are incubated *in vitro*, synthesis of ACh ceases when its concentration in the tissue reaches a limiting value, although the accumulated ACh is osmotically labile (Sattin, 1966) and, being probably located in the cytoplasm, is unlikely to be bound to saturable sites. Saturation of the binding sites may have a part in the control of ACh synthesis on the basis of the reaction equilibrium, in that, until all binding sites are occupied, the passage of ACh from the compartment of synthesis into the storage compartment postpones the attainment of the equilibrium and ensures further synthesis. When the storage compartment is full, ACh synthesis will decrease because ACh can no longer move away from the compartment of synthesis.

The inhibitory action of ACh on ChAc

This action has been described by many investigators (Berman-Reisberg, 1957; Kaita and Goldberg, 1969; White and Cavallito, 1970a; Glover and Potter, 1971; Morris *et al.*, 1971; Sastry and Henderson, 1972; White and Wu, 1973a; Emson *et al.*, 1974), but it seems that it may be important only at high concentrations of ACh and that, even then, the activity of ChAc would be only partially limited. For example, in the experiments of Kaita and Goldberg (1969) the activity of ChAc from rat brain was lowered by only 45% in the presence of 100 mM ACh while in the experiments of Glover and Potter (1971), the inhibition of ChAc from bovine caudate nuclei did not reach 50% even at an ACh concentration of 200 mM. Rossier and Benda (1977) pointed out that the inhibitory action of ACh on ChAc is much stronger when it is measured in the absence of Cl^- and at an extremely low ionic strength; it seems imperative to check the inhibitory action of ACh on ChAc under conditions closely imitating the ionic composition of intracellular fluid.

The inhibitory action of CoA on ChAc

This action is much stronger than the inhibitory action of ACh (Berman-Reisberg, 1957; White and Cavallito, 1970a; Glover and Potter, 1971; Morris *et al.*, 1971; Sastry and Henderson, 1972; White and Wu, 1973a; Emson *et al.*, 1974) and it might play a role at the concentrations of CoA which are likely *in vivo*. The utilization of acetyl–CoA in the synthesis of ACh will, however, produce only a comparatively small change in the concentration of CoA because the concentration of acetyl–CoA in the brain, and probably in peripheral nerves too, is considerably lower than the concentration of free CoA (Schuberth *et al.*, 1965). The regulatory role of this mechanism also seems improbable for another reason. It would produce the very reverse of what is observed experimentally: increased utilization of ACh would be accompanied by a decrease in the synthesis of ACh because of the increasing concentration of CoA.

In connection with all the suggestions that ACh synthesis in the brain is controlled by changes of ChAc activity, it is worth noting that the inhibitors of ChAc, when administered *in vivo*, decrease the rate of ACh turnover without, however, altering the concentration of ACh in the brain (Haubrich and Wang, 1976; Carson *et al.*, 1976).

Effects of changed ionic environment on the activity of ChAc

Direct effects of the changes of the concentrations of Na^+, K^+, Ca^{2+} and Mg^{2+} on the activity of ChAc are improbable in the range of ionic concentrations likely to occur *in vivo* (Morris and Tuček, 1966). Rossier and Benda (1977) suggest that the activity of ChAc in the nerve endings is regulated by changes in the concentration of Cl^- in its microenvironment. The suggestion is based on their observations that the activity of ChAc is higher in the presence of Cl^- than in the presence of other anions, and that ACh has a strong inhibitory action on ChAc in the absence of Cl^- (at a very low ionic strength of the medium), but only a weak action in the presence of Cl^-. Potter *et al.* (1968) did not, however, find important differences between the activity of ChAc in the presence of several different anions, and the observations regarding the inhibitory action of ACh on ChAc, described by Rossier and Benda (1977), require reinvestigation under conditions resembling those prevailing in the living cells.

High affinity uptake of choline

As has been pointed out in Chapter 5.4, the synthesis of ACh in the nerve endings is probably based on preferential utilization of the choline supplied by the high affinity choline carrier. Not surprisingly, factors altering the high affinity uptake of choline also alter the synthesis of ACh. When the carrier is inhibited by hemicholinium-3, the store of ACh in the tissues is easily exhausted by synaptic activity (Birks and MacIntosh, 1961; Hebb *et al.*, 1964b; Potter, 1970) and the resting synthesis of ACh is diminished (Browning and Schulman, 1968). Similarly, the synthesis of ACh in the synaptosomes is lowered in parallel with the lowering of the high affinity uptake of choline under the influence of the detergent Triton X-100 (Lefresne, 1974). The ability of sympathetic ganglia (Birks, 1963), brain slices (Bhatnagar and MacIntosh, 1967; Collier *et al.*, 1972; Grewaal and Quastel, 1973) and synaptosomes (Haga, 1971; Haga and Noda, 1973; Guyenet *et al.*, 1973a) to synthesize and store ACh is extremely limited in the absence of Na^+. The synthesis of ACh is impaired because the high affinity carrier of choline is Na^+ dependent and, in the absence of Na^+, does not provide enough choline.

These examples show that interference with the supply of choline may reduce the synthesis of ACh. Undoubtedly, an improved supply of choline will increase the synthesis of ACh. This has been shown in the experiments of Kuntscherová (1972) and others demonstrating the increase of ACh stores after the administration of choline *in vivo*. Alterations of ACh synthesis resulting from changes of the high affinity uptake of choline are not contradictory to the hypothesis that the synthesis of ACh is controlled by the law of mass action; the high affinity carrier affects the synthesis of ACh because it changes the concentration of choline at the site of the synthesis and thus alters the equilibrium concentration of ACh.

Although the high affinity carrier of choline can be influenced by many pharmacological agents (Diamond and Kennedy, 1969; Yamamura and Snyder, 1973; Dowdall and Simon, 1973; Guyenet *et al.*, 1973a), it is uncertain what agents affect its activity (and thus the synthesis of ACh) under physiological conditions. An important and very likely possibility is that the high affinity carrier is directly influenced by the ACh in the nerve endings (Whittaker, 1972) and this has been discussed in Chapter 5.4. The possibility is supported by the observations that the high affinity uptake of choline is strongly inhibited by ACh in the incubation medium and that it varies considerably depending on the content of ACh in the nerve endings. A direct action of ACh on the high affinity carrier for choline could provide extremely simple and rapid control of the supply of choline.

Unfortunately, the real importance of the high affinity carrier for choline to the control of ACh synthesis and of factors affecting it, is difficult to evaluate because we do not know if the high affinity carrier mediates facilitated diffusion of choline, without raising its concentration above that in the extracellular fluid, or if it mediates uphill transport (see Chapter 5.4).

Changes in the supply of acetyl–CoA

Acetyl–CoA is present in the nervous tissue in very low concentration and is used for many metabolic purposes; furthermore, for ACh synthesis, it has to be transported from the mitochondrial matrix to the extramitochondrial space. It may therefore be expected that under some circumstances the supply of acetyl–CoA becomes the limiting factor of ACh synthesis. A comparison of the activities of ChAc and the pyruvate dehydrogenase complex (see Chapter 4.3) in the subcellular fraction containing the nerve endings (Tuček, 1967c) also points to such possibility. Both activities are of similar magnitude, although ChAc is present in but a small proportion of the nerve endings and is exclusive to the synthesis of the cholinergic transmitter, whereas the pyruvate dehydrogenase complex is in all nerve endings and is necessary for their energetic metabolism.

It appears that, to date, parallel measurements of the content of ACh and of acetyl–CoA in the brain tissue have been made only in investigations of the effect of thiamine deficiency, and these measurements have yielded contradictory results. In view of the role of thiamine pyrophosphate as the coenzyme of pyruvate dehydrogenase, it would be expected that the synthesis of acetyl–CoA is limited in animals fed on a diet without thiamine. Indeed, Heinrich *et al.* (1973) found that the content of acetyl–CoA and also of ACh was lowered in the brains of thiamine-deficient rats, but Reynolds and Blass (1975) reported that the content of both substances was normal. Earlier data on the content of ACh in the brain of thiamine-deficient animals are also controversial (see Heinrich *et al.*, 1973, for references). The synthesis of ACh is lowered in the brain slices from thiamine-deficient pigeons during incubation *in vitro* (Mann and Quastel, 1940) and thiamine deficiency (or antagonists of thiamine) considerably increase the 'fatiguability' of synaptic transmission in the superior cervical ganglion, presumably by diminishing the supply of ACh for transmission (Perri *et al.,* 1970a,b; Sacchi and Perri, 1973).

Many experimental situations have been described in which the lowered content of ACh seems to be best explained on the basis of a decreased availability of acetyl–CoA for ACh synthesis. Endröczi *et al.* (1967) observed big suckling-dependent changes of free ACh content in the brain of newborn rats, with low values before and high values after suckling. A reduced supply of the acetyl–CoA produced from pyruvate together with a reduced supply of choline may well have been the cause of the diminished ACh content observed by Kuntscherová and Vlk (1968) in the brain of rats after 24 h of starvation, since the content of ACh could be restored by the simultaneous administration of glucose and choline. The lack of the acetyl–CoA produced from pyruvate may have also been responsible for the lowering of the content and synthesis of ACh in the cardiac atria of rats with alloxan diabetes (Kuntscherová and Vlk, 1970). These explanations are based on the quite likely assumption that, in nervous tissue, the pool of acetyl–CoA supporting ACh synthesis is not identical with the total store of acetyl–CoA. This is an important point since the total content of acetyl–CoA is increased in the brain of starving or diabetic rats (Ruderman *et al.,* 1974).

Lefresne *et al.* (1973) observed in experiments with striatal slices that the initial rate of ACh synthesis is dependent on the concentration of pyruvate in the medium. Gibson and Blass (1976) found that the synthesis of ACh in the brain *in vivo* is diminished by hypoglycemia, and Gibson *et al.* (1975) have shown, in brain slices *in vitro*, a beautiful parallelism between changes in the oxidative decarboxylation of pyruvate (induced by bromopyruvate or 2-oxobutyrate) and ACh synthesis.

Taken together, these observations indicate that the availability of acetyl–CoA may be very important for regulating the rate of ACh synthesis in the living neuron. An interesting possibility is that the supply of acetyl–CoA from the mitochondria can be regulated by ionic translocations occurring as a result of nerve impulse activity. Tuček (1967c; see also Polak *et al.,* 1977b) observed that the output of acetyl–CoA from brain mitochondria increased when Ca^{2+} was added to the incubation medium (see Chapter 4.5 and Fig. 4.12) and it has also been shown that the concentration of Ca^{2+} in the presynaptic nerve endings is increased by repetitive impulse activity (Blaustein, 1971; Llinás *et al.,* Babel-Guérin *et al.,* 1977). Although the concentrations of Ca^{2+} used by Tuček (1967c) to increase the output of acetyl–CoA from the isolated mitochondria incubated *in vitro* (0.1 mM and 1.0 mM) were much higher than the concentrations of Ca^{2+} believed to be present in the intracellular fluid, it seems worth considering that the mitochondria in the nerve terminals might be sensitive to lower Ca^{2+} concentrations when they are in their natural intracellular environment. Ca^{2+} could also increase the availability of acetyl–CoA by stimulating the pyruvate dehydrogenase phosphate phosphatase (see Chapter 4.3.2) and thus activating the pyruvate dehydrogenase complex.

Wonnacott and Marchbanks (1976) observed that the content of ACh in brain synaptosomes incubated in the presence of botulinum toxin (to prevent the release of ACh) and high K^+, was higher than in synaptosomes incubated without the toxin, or with the toxin at a low K^+ concentration. From this they concluded that the rate of synthesis of ACh is controlled by depolarization. Although this explanation may be true, the possibility should be considered that the incubation in the presence of high K^+ could have altered the intrasynaptosomal concentrations of substrates (for example by increasing the intrasynaptosomal concentration of Ca^{2+}) and, consequently, the supply of acetyl–CoA from the mitochondria (see above). It has been shown by Kovachich and Haugaard (1977) that the activity of pyruvate dehydrogenase in the brain slices is increased by a high concentration of potassium ions.

6.10 THE ROLE OF THE UPTAKE OF ACETYLCHOLINE IN THE SUPPLY OF TRANSMITTER FOR CHOLINERGIC TRANSMISSION

An important mechanism acting at adrenergic synapse is the uptake of released noradrenaline by presynaptic nerve fibres (see reviews by Brown, 1965; Iversen, 1971; Euler, 1972). Apparently the same molecule of noradrenaline can be used for synaptic transmission many times. This leads to the question whether, at cholinergic synapses, a proportion of ACh required for synaptic transmission can also be provided by its re-uptake and repeated use.

A priori such a situation appears rather improbable, because the released ACh is rapidly hydrolysed by ChE present on the external surface of the presynaptic and postsynaptic membranes. When ChE is inhibited, an energy dependent uptake of ACh, producing an accumulation in the tissue and obeying the kinetics of Michaelis and Menten can, however, be observed in brain slices (Polak and Meeuws, 1966; Schuberth and Sundwall, 1967; Polak, 1969; Liang and Quastel, 1969a,b; Heilbronn, 1969, 1970; Katz *et al.*, 1973; Widlund and Heilbronn, 1974; Kuhar and Simon, 1974), synaptosomes (Potter, 1968), skeletal muscle (Adamič, 1970; Potter, 1970) and sympathetic ganglion (Katz *et al.*, 1973). Its distribution in the tissues, and other features, in addition to the fact that it does not occur unless ChE is inhibited, do not support the view that re-uptake might be important for the economy of ACh in the nerve endings. The system for the active uptake of ACh has no special bearing to the cholinergic neurons. No parallelism was found between the activity of ChAc in different parts of the brain and the uptake of ACh in them (Katz *et al.*, 1973; Kuhar and Simon, 1974). The uptake of ACh in the hippocampus (Kuhar and Simon, 1974) and sympathetic ganglia (Katz *et al.*, 1973) is not changed following degeneration of cholinergic nerve endings in these structures. ACh taken up from the medium into brain cortex slices is not concentrated specifically in certain neurons; instead, it is present in all cells of the slices (Polak, 1969). Potter (1968) observed the uptake of ACh in the subcellular fraction of brain nerve endings, but Widlund and Heilbronn (1974) did not. In the diaphragm the uptake of ACh can be observed both inside and outside the innervated zone of the muscle (Potter, 1970). The ACh which has accumulated from the perfusion fluid in the sympathetic ganglia is not released back into the perfusion fluid by electrical stimulation of the preganglionic nerve fibres and the ACh accumulated in the brain slices is not released by exposing the slices to increased concentration of K^+ (Katz *et al.*, 1973).

Taken together, these experimental observations support the view that the cholinergic nerve endings do not, to any significant degree, re-use released ACh until it has been hydrolysed. The re-utilization of choline produced by the hydrolysis of ACh is discussed in Chapter 5.6, but the re-utilization of acetate for the synthesis of new ACh has not been specially studied; in view of differences between different species and organs in their ability to utilize acetate for ACh synthesis (see Chapter 4) it appears likely that re-use may occur in some species and organs but not in others.

6.11 SUMMARY

Although some ACh is synthesized in all parts of a cholinergic neuron, most of it is produced in close proximity to the sites from which it is released by nerve impulses, i.e. in the terminal parts of the axon and, in some neurons, probably in the *boutons en passant* and in the axonal varicosities as well. The enzyme responsible for the synthesis, ChAc, is mainly dissolved in the cytoplasm of the nerve endings, but a proportion of it is probably adsorbed to the cytoplasmic side of the surface membrane and of other membranes in the nerve endings, including the membranes of the synaptic vesicles. ACh is localized in the cytoplasm and in the synaptic vesicles. It is not clear how the transmitter, synthesized in the cytoplasmic compartment, is transferred to the vesicles. What proportion of the total ACh in the tissue is present in the vesicles is also not clear. It is possible that much of the ACh originally present in the vesicles is released or diffuses from them during the homogenization and fractionation of the tissue. In the synaptic vesicles from the electric organ, ACh is believed to be bound to vesiculin, a specific protein constituent of the vesicles.

Most features of the release of ACh at the synapses are best explained by the vesicular hypothesis, i.e. on the assumption that the nerve impulses cause the release of ACh from the synaptic vesicles. This hypothesis, providing an easy explanation for the fact that ACh is released in discrete quanta, is mainly supported by observations that the amount of vesicular ACh can be altered by stimulation, that the release of old ACh is accompanied by the appearance of newly synthesized ACh in those vesicles which had apparently undergone exocytosis, and that synaptic activity is accompanied by ultrastructural changes indicating exocytosis and recycling of the vesicles. Objections to the vesicular hypothesis of ACh release are mainly based on observations that the nerve impulses more easily produce changes of the so-called free ACh than of the bound ACh; at least some, if not all free ACh is freely dissolved in the cytoplasm, whereas the bound ACh (stable-bound ACh in mammalian preparations) is contained in the synaptic vesicles.

Continuous slow synthesis of ACh proceeds in the cholinergic neurons even under conditions of 'rest'. When the rate of ACh release is increased by nerve impulses, the rate of synthesis is also increased. Recently synthesized ACh is released preferentially during synaptic activity. Several hypotheses have been proposed to explain the mechanism of the control of the synthesis. The control of ACh synthesis is most probably based on the law of mass action, and the resting level of ACh in the compartment of synthesis corresponds to the concentration of ACh to be expected when the synthetic reaction is at equilibrium. Lowering the concentration of ACh in the compartment of synthesis automatically leads to the synthesis of new ACh. According to this hypothesis, the rate of synthesis and the equilibrium concentration of ACh are influenced by changes in the concentrations of the substrates, i.e. acetyl–CoA and choline, at the site of synthesis. The high affinity uptake of choline may represent an additional factor in the mechanism controlling ACh synthesis. Experimental observations indicate that the uptake of choline by the nerve endings is augmented when the concentration of ACh in them is diminished. External (and perhaps also internal) ACh has an inhibitory action on the high affinity carrier of choline. Further investigation is necessary to establish whether the supply of acetyl–CoA for ACh synthesis is influenced by the influx of Ca^{2+} ions into the nerve terminals, as a result of nerve impulses; Ca^{2+} ions might act by causing the activation of pyruvate dehydrogenase phosphate phosphatase and by increasing the permeability of the inner mitochondrial membrane for acetyl–CoA. It has been suggested that the control of ACh synthesis in the nerve endings depends on the inhibitory action of ACh and CoA on ChAc or on the effect of changing ionic concentrations on the activity of ChAc, but these mechanisms do not appear to be of physiological importance.

In contrast to adrenergic synapses, the re-uptake of the released transmitter into the presynaptic nerve endings and its re-utilization for synaptic transmission do not play any role on cholinergic synapses. Observations regarding the re-uptake and re-utilization of choline, which is produced in the synaptic gaps by the hydrolysis of ACh, are described in Chapter 5.

AUTHOR'S NOTE

D.R. Haubrich and T.J. Chippendale (*Life Sci.* **20**, 1465–1478, 1977) have reviewed the problem of the regulation of ACh synthesis in nervous tissue. R.S. Jope and D.J. Jenden (*Life Sci.* **20**, 1389–1392, 1977) have analysed some aspects of the relations between the supply of acetyl–CoA and the transport and acetylation of choline in the crude mitochondrial fraction of rat brain. N. Morel, M. Israël, R. Manaranche and P. Mastour-Frachon (*J. cell Biol.* **75**, 43–55, 1977) and M.J. Dowdall and H. Zimmermann (*Neuroscience* **2**, 405–421, 1977) have isolated pure cholinergic nerve endings from *Torpedo* electric organ and examined some aspects of the synthesis of ACh in them. A. Nagy, G. Várady, F. Joó, Z. Rakonczay and A. Pilc (*J. Neurochem.* **29**, 449–459, 1977) have separated acetylcholine and catecholamine containing synaptic vesicles from brain cortex.

7 Changes in choline acetyltransferase activity during the lifetime of an individual

7.1 INTRODUCTION

It is very likely that measurements of ChAc activity in various organs and tissues removed from animals of the same species at different ages provide reasonably good information about long term changes of ACh synthesis in these organs or tissues during the lifetime of individuals of the species. This chapter does not attempt to review all situations in which the activity of ChAc changes. It summarizes basic information on the changes of ChAc activity related to age (i.e. changes which are associated with normal ontogenetic development and accompany the proliferation, growth, maturation and ageing of cholinergic neurons), to increased or decreased neuronal activity, to the action of hormones and to the damage and regeneration of neurons. A note about the likely influence of the contact with postsynaptic cells on presynaptic ChAc activity is also included.

7.2 CHANGES IN THE ACTIVITY OF CHOLINE ACETYLTRANSFERASE DURING EMBRYONIC DEVELOPMENT AND EARLY POSTNATAL ONTOGENY

Available data on ChAc activity changes in the brain and other organs during embryonic and postnatal development up to maturity (see Table 7.1 for references) are still too fragmentary to permit a generalized picture of the development of cholinergic innervation. During embryonic development ChAc activity appears early in the central nervous system and the periphery. In chick embryos, measurable ChAc activity has been found in the spinal cord after 3.5 days of incubation (Burt, 1968, 1973; Fig. 7.1) and in the cerebral hemispheres and optic lobes after 6 days (Marchisio and Giacobini, 1969). In the rabbit foetus ChAc activity became measurable in the cerebrum after 18 days and in the cerebellum after 21 days of gestation. Guinea pig foetal brain showed activity after 32 days of gestation

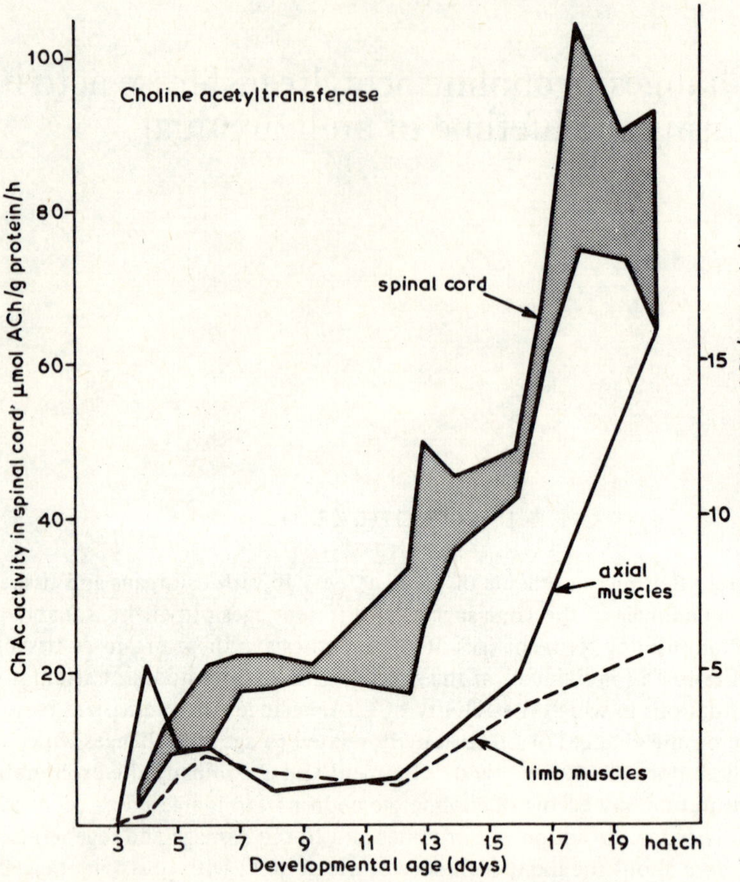

Fig. 7.1 The development of ChAc activity in chick embryos. Dotted area: brachial spinal cord. Continuous line: axial muscles. Broken line: limb muscles. Ordinates: ChAc activity in μmoles ACh/g protein/h in spinal cord (left) and muscles (right). The graph is reprinted from Burt (1973) and is based on observations by Burt (1968) for the spinal cord and by Giacobini (1972) for the muscles.

(Hebb, 1956). In axial and limb muscles of chick embryos ChAc appeared after 4 days of incubation (Giacobini, 1972; Fig. 7.1).

When considering data about the time at which it becomes possible to detect ChAc in various organs, it is necessary to take into account that the findings are dependent on the sensitivity of the methods used for detection and that an inability to measure enzymatic activity before a certain time does not necessarily indicate the absence of the enzyme. Filogamo and Marchisio (1971) assume that, at the early stage of embryonic development, the synthesis of ACh is a property of all neuroblasts, but there is little evidence to support this assumption. Good evidence has

Table 7.1 Studies of ChAc activity during prenatal and early postnatal ontogeny

Organ	Species	Authors	Notes
Whole brain	Rabbit, guinea pig	Hebb (1956)	
	Chick	Burdick and Strittmatter (1965)	
	Man	Mahoney *et al.* (1971)	Also data for the heart, liver, lungs and kidneys; some results differ substantially from comparable findings in the literature
	Rat	Ladinsky *et al.* (1972a)	
	Xenopus laevis	Peng (1976)	
Individual parts of the brain	Rabbit	McCaman and Aprison (1964)	Cortex, caudate nucleus, thalamus, superior colliculus, medulla
	Chick	Marchisio and Giacobini (1969)	Hemispheres, midbrain, optic lobes, cerebellum, medulla, spinal cord
	Chick	Marchisio (1969)	Optic lobes
	Man	Bull *et al.* (1970)	Caudate nucleus, thalamus, corpora quadrigemina, cerebellum, medulla, spinal cord
	Rat	McGeer *et al.* (1971b)	Caudate nucleus
	Rat	Nadler *et al.* (1974)	Hippocampus
	Rat	Sorimachi *et al.* (1974)	Striatum and hippocampus; comparison with choline uptake
	Rat	Coyle and Yamamura (1976)	Whole brain, cortex, midbrain + thalamus, hypothalamus, striatum, medulla + pons
	Rat	Cheney *et al.* (1976c)	Caudate nucleus, nucleus accumbens, nucleus interpeduncularis, raphe dorsalis, locus coeruleus, spinal cord

Table 7.1 (*continued*) Studies of ChAc activity during prenatal and early postnatal ontogeny

Organ	Species	Authors	Notes
Individual parts of the brain	Rat	Singh and McGeer (1977a)	Whole brain, cortex, caudate nucleus + putamen, spinal cord
Spinal cord	Chick	Burt (1968)	
	Chick	Marchisio and Giacobini (1969)	
	Chick	Burt and Narayanan (1970)	
	Man	Bull *et al.* (1970)	
	Rat	Burt (1975)	
	Rat	Kása (1978)	
Brain cell aggregates	Rat and mouse	Honegger and Richelson (1976)	Aggregating cell culture
Sympathetic ganglia	Chick	Marchisio and Consolo (1968)	
	Chick	Doležalová *et al.* (1974)	
	Chick	Sorimachi and Kataoka (1974a)	
	Mouse	Black *et al.* (1971)	
Parasympathetic ganglia	Chick	Sorimachi and Kataoka (1974a)	
	Chick	Chiappinelli *et al.* (1976)	
	Chick	Burt and Narayanan (1976)	
Spinal ganglia	Chick	Marchisio and Consolo (1968)	
	Chick	Doležalová *et al.* (1974)	
Peripheral nerve	Chick	Giacobini (1972)	
Heart atria	Dog	Tuček (1965)	

Table 7.1 (*continued*) Studies of ChAc activity during prenatal and early postnatal ontogeny

Organ	Species	Authors	Notes
Skeletal muscle	Chick	Giacobini (1972)	
	Chick	Giacobini-Robecchi *et al.* (1975)	Effect of botulinum toxin A
	Rat	Tuček (1972)	
	Rat	Diamond *et al.* (1974)	
	Rat	Tuček *et al.* (1976b)	
Iris	Chick	Chiappinelli *et al.* (1976)	
Salivary glands	Rat	Ekström (1976)	

been presented in recent years, however, that the transmitter synthesizing properties of neurons are not fixed at the early stage of their development. In particular, it has been shown that the neurons of sympathetic ganglia, which normally developed adrenergic properties, may become cholinergic under suitable conditions of incubation in cell cultures (Patterson and Chun, 1974; Nurse and O'Lague, 1975; Furshpan *et al.*, 1976; Johnson *et al.*, 1976; Ko *et al.*, 1976; Patterson *et al.*, 1976).

The results of ChAc activity measurements during ontogeny are usually expressed in relation to the weight of protein or tissue; they thus indicate the concentration of the enzyme and not the total amount in the tissue. On this basis, the activity of ChAc appears unchanged if the cholinergic and non-cholinergic components of the tissue grow at the same rate and the content of ChAc, related to the weight or protein content, is not altered. If the non-cholinergic tissue components (e.g. glial cells or non-cholinergic neurons in the brain, or contractile cells in skeletal muscle) grow faster than the cholinergic component the values of ChAc activity expressed per g tissue or per g protein decrease, although the total amount of ChAc in the organ or tissue may remain unchanged or even increase. This is the likely explanation for the transient decrease of ChAc activity in skeletal muscles of chick embryos, which can be observed in the axial muscles after 4, and in the limb muscles after 6, days of incubation (Giacobini, 1972). Even when expressed in relation to the weight of the tissue or to its protein content, however, the activity of ChAc in most parts of the nervous system increases considerably during prenatal development. The increase is not continuous and does not proceed in parallel in different parts of the nervous system and in different organs. The development of ChAc activity in the spinal cord and in the muscles of chick embryos is shown in Fig. 7.1. As in the spinal cord, the activity of ChAc in embryonic chick brain increases most steeply between 16 or 17 and 20 days of incubation (Burdick and Stritmatter, 1965; Marchisio and Giacobini, 1969; Ebel *et al.*, 1974). In comparison with mature animals, the activity of ChAc in the prenatal period is comparatively high in the cerebellum (Hebb, 1956; Marchisio and Giacobini, 1969; Bull *et al.*, 1970) and in the spinal ganglia (Marchisio and Consolo, 1968). The activity (concentration) of ChAc in the rabbit cerebellum reaches a maximum 5–6 days after birth, while in the guinea pig cerebellum peak activity is reached between 45 and 55 days of intrauterine development (Hebb, 1956). Little is known about the prenatal development of ChAc activity in peripheral organs with a cholinergic innervation, with the exception of skeletal muscles.

At the time of hatching the concentration of ChAc in different parts of the chick nervous system was found to decrease; in the spinal cord and in the cerebral hemispheres it fell by more than 50%. It returned to the original level 15 days after hatching; the total content of ChAc in chick brain, although not its activity per unit weight, continued to increase during the rest of the observation period, i.e. up to 60 days (Marchisio and Giacobini, 1969). The postnatal increase of ChAc activity in the brain is very pronounced in the rat, where the activity expressed per unit weight of the brain also shows a steep increase. The activity of ChAc per g weight in the brain of 1 day old rats is only 7%, and that in 20 day old rats 77% of the

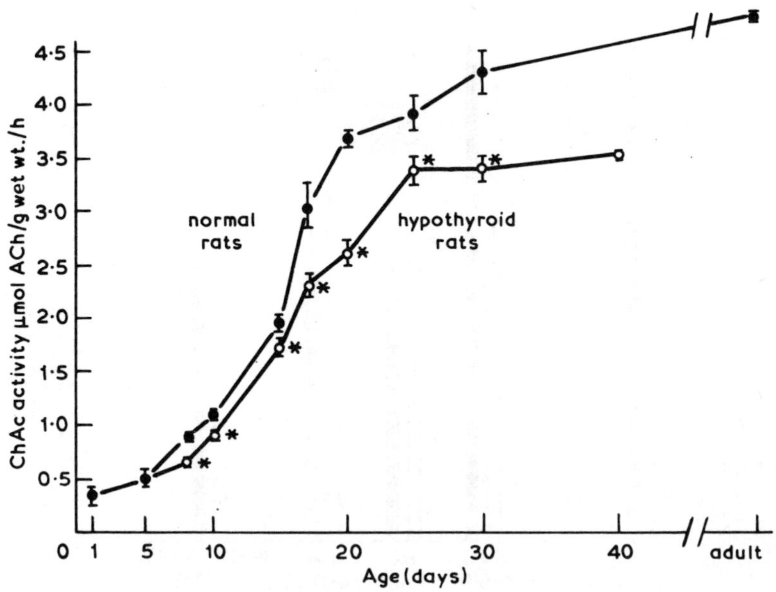

Fig. 7.2 ChAc activity (mean ± S.E.M.) in the brain of rats from the 1st day after birth to adulthood. ●, values found in normal rats; ○, values found in hypothyroid rats; the hypothyroidism was produced by the addition of propylthiouracil to the food of mother rats. The asterisks indicate a significant difference ($p < 0.01$) between normal and hypothyroid animals (after Ladinsky *et al.*, 1972a).

activity in mature animals (Ladinsky *et al.*, 1972a; Fig. 7.2). The activity of ChAc per g tissue in the caudate nuclei of 4 day old rats is 3.8% and in 15 day old rats 56% of the activity in mature animals; ChAc thus approaches adult values more slowly than tyrosine hydroxylase and glutamate decarboxylase (McGeer *et al.*, 1971b). Very steep increases in the specific activity of ChAc, starting 7 days after parturition, have been observed in rat caudate, accumbens and interpeduncular nuclei (Cheney *et al.*, 1976a). The specific activity of ChAc in the lumbar spinal cord of the rat increases more than three fold during the first two weeks of postnatal development and does not substantially change after that (Burt, 1975).

Large postnatal increases of ChAc activity per *g* brain weight are not unique to the rat: immediately after birth, the activity of ChAc per g acetone-dried brain tissue is equal to only 1/3 or 1/2 the adult value in the guinea pig and to 1/4 in the rabbit (Hebb, 1956). When the activity of ChAc per g tissue in various parts of the brain of 3 day old rabbits is expressed as a percentage of the activity in adult animals, the activities are: cerebral cortex, 23%; caudate nuclei, 16%; superior colliculi, 24%; thalamus, 38%; and medulla, 62% (McCaman and Aprison, 1964). The activity of

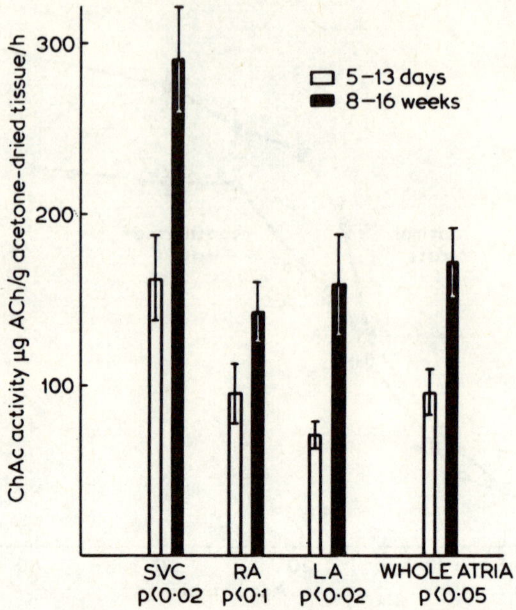

Fig. 7.3 Comparison of ChAc activity in various parts of the cardiac atria in dogs aged 5–13 days and 8–16 weeks. SVC, the area around the orifice of the superior vena cava; RA, the rest of the right atrium; LA, the left atrium. The bars indicate S.E.M. The statistical significance of the difference between the values for younger and older animals is indicated on the bottom of the graph (after Tuček, 1965).

ChAc in the medulla is already approaching adult values on day 6 of life. The postnatal increase of ChAc activity is accompanied by an increase of the activity of the high affinity choline carrier (Sorimachi *et al.*, 1974). The concentration of ACh in the brain of newborn rats is 1/2 to 1/4 of that in adults (Welsh and Hyde, 1944b; Crossland, 1951).

These data indicate that the postnatal maturation of the mammalian central nervous system is accompanied not only by an increase in volume of cholinergic neurons, but also by a substantial increase in their ability to synthesize and store ACh. A similar increase can also be observed in the peripheral nervous system and in peripheral organs with a cholinergic innervation. The activity of ChAc in parasympathetic ciliary ganglia increases steeply up to 10 days, and more slowly up to 28 days, after hatching (Sorimachi and Kataoka, 1974a). Big prenatal and postnantal increases of ChAc activity have been observed in the sympathetic ganglia of mice and chicks (Black *et al.*, 1971, Sorimachi and Kataoka, 1974a; Doležalová *et al.*, 1974). In the chick spinal ganglion the activity of ChAc (related to the whole ganglion) increases 9-fold on the second day after hatching and does not change after that (Doležalová *et al.*, 1974). In mouse sciatic nerve the activity of ChAc per mm nerve increases more than 5 times

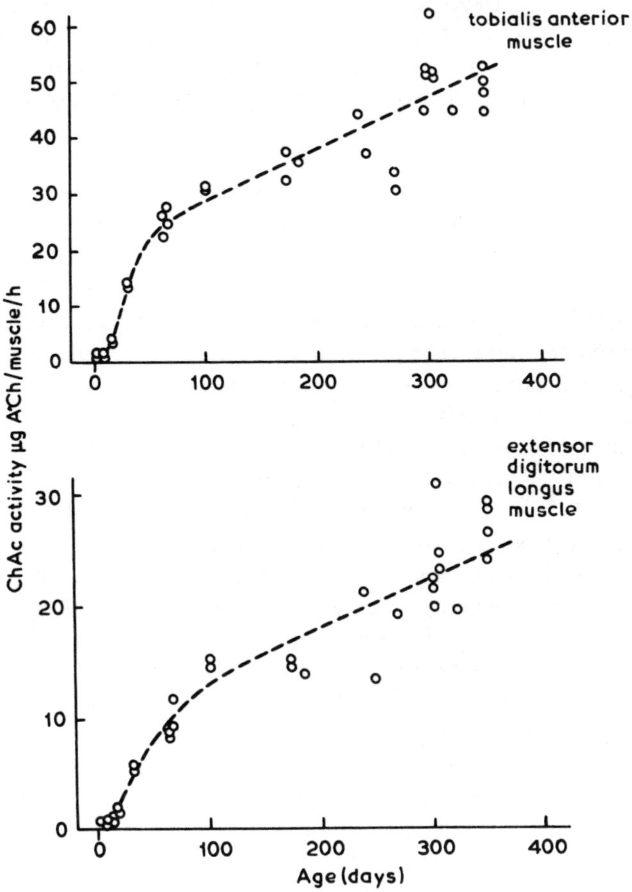

Fig. 7.4 Postnatal development of total ChAc activity in the tobialis anterior muscle and extensor digitorum longus muscle of rats (after Tuček, 1972).

between 2 and 36 weeks of age (Jablecki and Brimijoin, 1975). Fig. 7.3 shows the increase in ChAc activity in the cardiac atria of dogs between 1 and 16 weeks of age (Tuček, 1965).

Postnatal development of rat skeletal muscles is accompanied not only by a big increase in the weight of the muscles, but also by a big increase in ChAc activity (Fig. 7.4). The total ChAc activity in the rat tibialis anterior muscle is 309 times, and in the extensor digitorum longus muscle 231 times, higher at the age of 353 days than at the age of 30 hours (Tuček, 1972). The steepest increase of ChAc activity in the muscles occurs during the first 60 days after birth. During some periods the activity of ChAc in the muscles (attributable mainly to ChAc in the intramuscular branches and endings of the motor nerve – Tuček, 1973a) increases faster than does the weight of the muscles (Tuček, 1972; Tuček *et al.*, 1976b). The activity of ChAc in rat muscles also increases during the period when the animals are regarded as quite 'mature': between 3 and 9 months of age it increases in the extensor digitorum longus muscle by 50% and in the soleus muscle by 55% (Tuček and Gutmann, 1973).

7.3 CHOLINE ACETYLTRANSFERASE ACTIVITY CHANGES IN OLD AGE

Data on ChAc activity changes in old age are very scarce (see Table 7.2 for references). Only men and rats have been studied. In men, the activity of ChAc is reduced in many parts of the central nervous system after the age of 50 (McGeer and McGeer, 1975, 1976). The highest changes occur in the cerebral cortex, where as much as 50% of the ChAc seems to be lost (McGeer and McGeer, 1975). In rats, the activity of ChAc in the caudate nuclei has been found to fall at the age of 29 months, but it does not change in the rest of the brain (McGeer *et al.*, 1971a). The activity of ChAc (per g acetone-dried tissue) in the sciatic nerve of rats aged 26–28 months is about 73%, and in the cardiac atria about 64%, of the activity in rats aged 8–10 months; no difference between the two age groups has been found in the cardiac ventricles and in the gastrocnemius muscle (Verkhratsky, 1970). The total ChAc activity in the limb muscles falls considerably, however; in the extensor digitorum longus muscle of rats at the age of 28–29 months the total activity of ChAc is 41%, and in the soleus muscle 40%, of that at the age of 9 months (Tuček and Gutmann, 1973; Fig. 7.5). At the same time, the activity in the diaphragm is virtually unchanged. The fall in ChAc activity is greater than the fall in the number of muscle fibres; apparently, neuromuscular junctions in the limb muscles of old rats possess a reduced amount of enzyme for the synthesis of ACh. The difference between the diaphragm, where ChAc activity does not change, and the limb muscles is probably connected with the difference in their functional activity. In view of its respiratory function, the diaphragm is continually activated and this activation seems to ensure that the motorneurons of the phrenic nerve maintain their ChAc synthesis at a high level.

7.4 THE EFFECT OF NEURONAL ACTIVITY AND INACTIVITY ON CHOLINE ACETYLTRANSFERASE

Although it seems very likely that a long term increase or decrease of the activity of cholinergic neurons is accompanied by an increase or decrease in their ChAc activity, unequivocal experimental evidence supporting this contention is rather limited. The relation between the activity of the neurons and their ChAc content has been most thoroughly investigated in parasympathetic neurons innervating the salivary glands. Parasympathetic decentralization (preganglionic parasympathetic denervation) of the parotid gland decreases its ChAc activity by approximately one

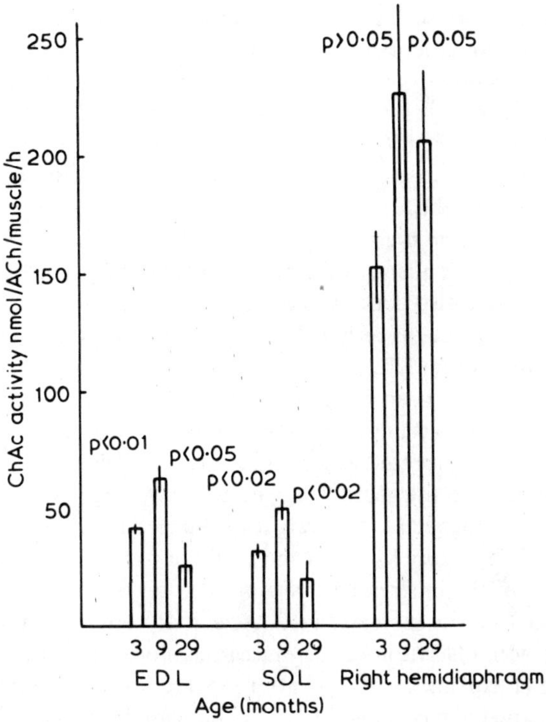

Fig. 7.5 Total ChAc activity in extensor digitorum longus muscle (EDL), soleus muscle (SOL) and right hemidiaphragm of rats aged 3, 9, and 29 months. The bars indicate S.E.M. The values of p shown in the graph indicate the statistical significance of the difference between 3 and 9 month old and between 9 and 29 month old animals (after Tuček and Gutmann, 1973).

Table 7.2 Studies of ChAc activity in old age

Organ	Species	Authors	Notes
Brain	Rat	McGeer *et al.* (1971a)	Data for caudate nucleus and for the rest of the brain
	Man	McGeer and McGeer (1975, 1976)	Many areas of the brain
Peripheral nerve	Rat	Verkhratsky (1970) Jablecki and Brimijoin (1975)	
Heart	Rat	Verkhratsky (1970)	
Skeletal muscle	Rat	Tuček and Gutmann (1973)	

quarter (Nordenfelt, 1967; Ekström and Holmberg, 1972b). It is impossible to decide to what degree the decrease of ChAc activity is caused by the reduction of the impulse activity in parasympathetic ganglionic neurons and postganglionic nerve fibres, and to what degree it is due to the loss of the trophic influence of preganglionic fibres on ganglionic nerve cells; it is certainly not caused by the loss of ChAc from the preganglionic fibres, since these fibres do not enter the gland. In some salivary glands of some mammalian species the activity of ChAc is clearly increased after surgical or chemical sympathectomy (Nordenfelt, 1965; Ekström, 1972); this increase may be explained on the assumption that the sympathetic denervation is followed by an increased frequency of nerve impulses in parasympathetic nerves (Ekström, 1972), but it is also conceivable that the increase in ChAc activity is a result of axonal sprouting of terminal parasympathetic axons in the sympathetically denervated gland (Nordenfelt, 1965).

The activity of ChAc has been found to increase in the parotid glands of rats fed with voluminous dry diet containing much cellulose (Ekström, 1974). This increase of ChAc activity has been interpreted as a consequence of higher impulse activity in parasympathetic nerve fibres to the gland; it might also have been associated with the increase in the volume of the gland (the weight of the gland increased by 48% at a time when the activity of ChAc rose by 17%) and could have been the consequence of the retrograde influence of the innervated tissue on the presynaptic nerve endings, as is discussed in Section 7.8. The increases of ChAc activity observed in the partotid gland after chronic administration of the muscarine blocking agent piperidinethyldiphenylacetamide (Ekström, 1974) and after repeated teeth amputations (Ekström, 1977a) have been explained as being due to the increased impulse activity in secretory nerves. After the activity of the parotid glands had been increased by ligation of the ducts of all other big salivary glands, its weight increased within four weeks by 52% and its ChAc activity by 32% (Ekström, 1975). ChAc activity in the parotid gland was reduced in rats kept on a liquid diet (Ekström, 1973) or treated with pilocarpine; presumably, this reduction was a result of diminished reflex stimulation of the gland (Ekström, 1977b).

The ChAc activity in the intramuscular branches and endings of motor nerves in skeletal muscles is also probably influenced by changes in neural impulse activity. In the soleus muscle immobilized for 7–10 days, the activity of ChAc corresponds to only 50% or so of the activity in the contralateral control muscle (Snyder *et al.*, 1973; Tuček *et al.*, 1976b; Fig. 7.6). It is possible, however, that in these experiments the immobilization did not produce a true decrease of ChAc activity in the muscles, but that it only arrested the growth of the muscles and the increase of ChAc activity by which the growth of the muscles is usually accompanied. Tenotomy is followed by a decrease of ChAc activity in the muscles (Diamond *et al.*, 1974), while the so-called compensatory muscle hypertrophy, produced by the tenotomy of synergistic muscles, is accompanied by an increase in ChAc activity (Snyder *et al.*, 1973). The compensatory hypertrophy and the accompanying increase of ChAc activity have been interpreted as a consequence of an increase in the activity of

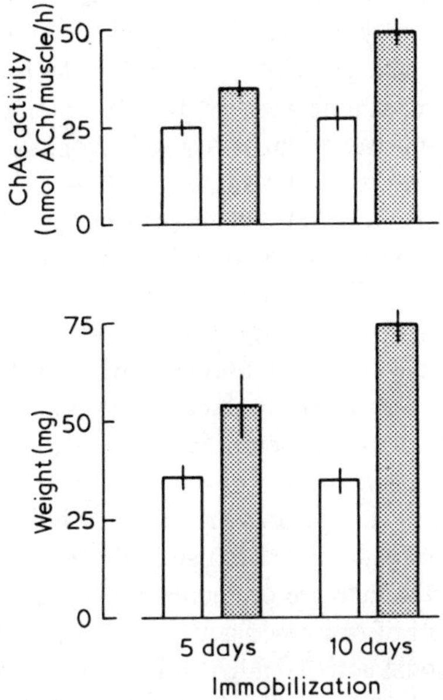

Fig. 7.6 The effect of the immobilization of the limb on the total ChAc activity and on the weight of rat soleus muscle. The immobilization lasted 5 or 10 days. Columns represent mean values ± S.E.M. Immobilized limb, white columns; contralateral control limb, dotted columns (based on Tuček *et al.,* 1976b).

the muscle and its motor nerve, but in reality the hypertrophy of the muscle after the tenotomy of its synergists develops because the muscle is stretched by its antagonists (Gutmann *et al.*, 1971; Macková and Hník, 1973).

Unilateral denervation of the diaphragm brings about an increase in ChAc activity in the innervated half of the diaphragm; the increase is probably associated with the higher respiratory frequency appearing after denervation (Ekström, 1975). The increase in the activity of ChAc observed in the soleus muscle of castrated male rats after the administration of testosterone (Tuček *et al.*, 1976b) and the increase in ChAc activity in the extensor digitorum longus muscle, observed after the administration of tetanus toxin (Tonge *et al.*, 1975), have been also explained as consequences of increased impulse activity in corresponding motor nerve fibres. As pointed out in Section 7.3, the continuous activity of the phrenic nerve and diaphragm may be responsible for the fact that ChAc activity in the diaphragm remains unchanged in old animals, although the activity of ChAc in their limb muscles decreases (Tuček and Gutmann, 1973; Fig. 7.5). On the other hand, long-term endurance exercise on the treadmill does not increase ChAc activity in the limb muscles (Crockett *et al.*, 1976).

Increased activity of the nerve fibres to adrenal glands, evoked by repeated exposure of animals to stress, brings about an increase of ChAc activity in the adrenal (Goldberg and Welch, 1972; Welch and Goldberg, 1973), but a single exposure to stress does not affect it (Welch and Goldberg, 1973). An increase of ChAc activity in the adrenals and in the sympathetic ganglion has also been described after the administration of reserpine and was thought to result from the increase in the impulse activity of preganglionic sympathetic fibres (Oesch, 1974). The increase of ChAc activity after reserpine has not, however, been confirmed in a more recent study (Hendry, 1976). An attempt to produce a change in the activity of ChAc in cortical visual areas by changing their functional activity has been made by Maletta and Timiras (1968). No change of ChAc activity was observed in the superior colliculus, lateral geniculate body or visual cortex of adult rats which were kept in darkness for 3 weeks. On the other hand, in rats kept in darkness from birth to 3 weeks of age, the activity of ChAc in the superior colliculus was lowered by 64% and in the lateral geniculate body by 52%; it was unchanged in the cerebral cortex. Surgical removal of one eye in chicks resulted in changes in ChAc activity in some areas of the brain, but only after an extremely long delay (Marchisio, 1969).

The mechanism ensuring the increase or decrease of ChAc synthesis in cholinergic neurons during their increased of decreased activity has yet to be elucidated. Conceivably, the change of neuronal activity might influence the synthesis of ChAc in two ways. First, the change of ChAc synthesis might be based on the coupling between the electrically induced movement of ions across the membranes of the dendrites, neuronal somas and, perhaps, the axons of cholinergic nerve cells, and the processes controlling the synthesis of nucleic acids and proteins in them. Second, the change in the activity of cholinergic neuron might mainly act by producing a change in the postsynaptic effector cell; the change in its functional state would then bring about an alteration in the retrograde transsynaptic information, reaching the soma of the presynaptic cholinergic neuron; this, in turn, would produce a change in neuronal synthesis of nucleic acids and proteins. The first possibility is evident and certainly plays the leading role. The second possibility may appear too complicated, but some examples of the role of retrograde transsynaptic influences in the control of ChAc synthesis are given in Section 7.8.

7.5 ENDOCRINE INFLUENCES ON THE SYNTHESIS OF ACETYLCHOLINE AND THE ACTIVITY OF CHOLINE ACETYLTRANSFERASE

The relations between the endocrine balance of the organism and the synthesis of ACh in the nervous system have been investigated less than it would seem desirable, although some findings clearly indicate that an excess or a lack of some hormones may considerably change the synthesis of ACh in certain parts of the nervous system. The content of ACh and the activity of ChAc in the brain have been lowered

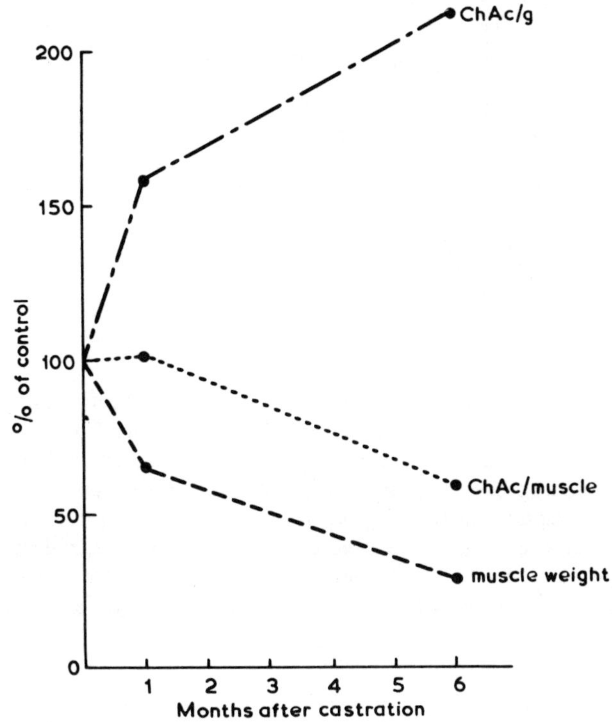

Fig. 7.7 The effect of castration on the activity of ChAc and on the weight of the levator ani muscle in male rats. The castration was performed at the age of one month; the time after castration in months is on the abscissa. The upper curve indicates the activity of ChAc per g weight of the muscle, the middle curve – total ChAc activity in the muscle, the lower curve – the weight of the muscle. All values are expressed as a percentage of values found in control (non-castrated) rats of the same age (after Gutmann *et al.*,1969).

in rats treated by the anti-thyroid drug propylthiouracil (Ladinsky *et al.*, 1972a; Fig. 7.2). The administration of triiodothyronine restored the activity of ChAc in the brain to normal levels. In rats treated by triiodothyronine during the first two weeks of their life, the activity of ChAc in the brain stem was increased by 40% (Rastogi *et al.*, 1977). In adult rats, experimental hyperthyroidism produced by the administration of dried thyroid gland was not accompanied by a change in the content of ACh, but brain homogenates from treated animals showed a significant increase in their ability to synthesize ACh in a saline medium with glucose (Tuček and Diepold, 1963). It is not clear whether this increase was the result of an increase in the activity of ChAc, a greater availability of acetyl–CoA, or an improved supply of choline.

After an injection of insulin, the content of free (Welsh, 1943) and total ACh

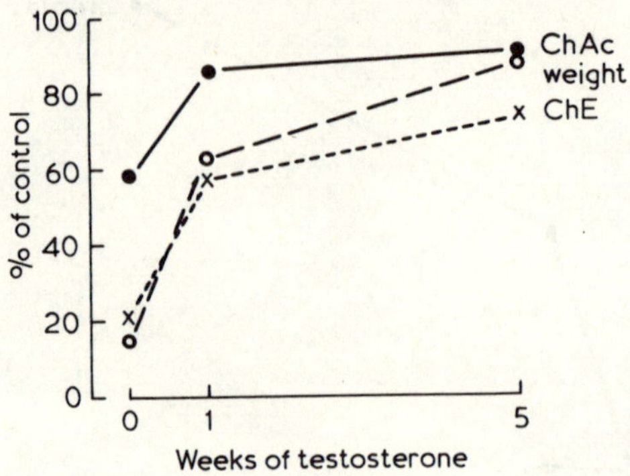

Fig. 7.8 The effect of testosterone on the activity of ChAc and ChE in the levator ani muscle of castrated male rats and on its weight. The castration was performed at the age of one month. All rats were killed as 14 months; testosterone was administered during the last week or the last five weeks of their life. Abscissa: duration of testosterone administration in weeks. Ordinate: enzyme activities (measured as moles ACh synthesized or hydrolysed/muscle/h) and muscle weight, expressed as a percentage of the values found in control (non-castrated) rats of the same age (after Tuček *et al.*, 1976a).

(Crossland *et al.*, 1955) in the rat brain is reduced. During alloxan diabetes the content of ACh in the brain is not changed, but it is diminished in the cardiac atria; the ability of the atria to synthesize ACh during incubation *in vitro* is also lowered (Kuntscherová and Vlk, 1970). The administration of the glucocorticoid, dexamethasone to newborn rats decreased the activity of ChAc in their superior cervical sympathetic ganglia (Ciaranello and Axelrod, 1975). This reduction was caused by a slowing in the development of preganglionic sympathetic neurons. The administration of cortisone to rats did not alter the activity of ChAc in the muscles, although it produced muscular atrophy (Diamond *et al.*, 1974). Repeated administrations of noradrenaline to rat lateral cerebral ventricels were followed by an increase in the activity of ChAc in virtually the whole brain (Singer *et al.*, 1971).

The activity of ChAc in various organs is usually very similar in both sexes. In the brain of female rats the activity of ChAc in the preoptic suprachiasmal region of the hypothalamus exceeds that in males (Libertun *et al.*, 1973). The activity of ChAc in this area was lowered in female rats injected by testosterone immediately after birth. The administration of testosterone thus probably inhibited the development of cholinergic neurons in this area. The activity of ChAc in the anterior part of the hypothalamus undergoes cyclic changes during the oestrous cycle (Kobayashi *et al.*, 1963).

Testosterone clearly influenced the activity of ChAc in experiments with the levator ani muscle of male rats (Gutmann *et al.*, 1969; Tuček *et al.*, 1976a). The levator ani is a striated muscle, the development of which is androgen-dependent. Prenatally it also develops in female rats, but postnatally it virtually disappears. In males its development is arrested by castration, whereas the administration of testosterone stimulates its growth. The activity of ChAc in the levator ani muscle is also lower in castrated than in control rats (Gutmann *et al.*, 1969; Fig. 7.7), but control levels can be rapidly restored by the administration of testosterone (Tuček *et al.*, 1976a; Fig. 7.8). In normal (non-castrated) males, testosterone increases the activity of ChAc neither in the levator ani muscle (Tuček *et al.*, 1976a), nor in the limb muscles (Tuček *et al.*, 1976b). In castrated male rats the activity of ChAc in the soleus muscle was slightly but statistically significantly increased by testosterone (Tuček *et al.*, 1976b). The levator ani muscles is a target organ for testosterone and contains receptor for adrogens (Jung and Baulieu, 1972). It is likely that testosterone acts primarily on the muscle and that the muscle fibres secondarily stimulate the development of their motor nerve endings by a retrograde transsynaptic mechanism. One cannot exclude, however, some other mechanisms of testosterone action; the hormone could directly affect the spinal motoneurons for the levator ani muscle, or it might act on higher nerve centres, perhaps in the hypothalamus, and these in turn might alter the activity of spinal motoneurons for the levator ani muscle, and increase their ChAc synthesis. The much smaller increase in ChAc activity, observed in the soleus muscle of castrated rats after testosterone administration, is perhaps a result of the general increase of motor activity (Asdell *et al.*, 1962).

7.6 CHANGES IN THE SYNTHESIS OF ACETYLCHOLINE CAUSED BY TRANSECTION AND WALLERIAN DEGENERATION OF CHOLINERGIC AXONS

The content of ACh and the activity of ChAc in organs with a cholinergic innervation are diminished or entirely lost after denervation. This is the result of the destruction of cholinergic axons and their postsynaptic endings. Changes in ChAc activity in the peripheral stump of a rabbit nerve following its transection are shown in Fig. 7.9 (Tucek, 1974). The first day after the interruption of the nerve, there is just a small decrease of ChAc activity at the proximal end of the peripheral nerve stump. This change is probably a consequence of continuing proximo–distal transport of the enzyme (see Chapter 3.4.2 and Fig. 3.8). The activity of ChAc does not change on the second day, but during the third day it falls steeply throughout the segment of the peripheral nerve stump taken for examination. After 9 and 30 days the activity of ChAc in the peripheral nerve stump represents less than 1% of the activity in corresponding segments of the control nerve. The steep fall of ChAc 70 h after the transection of the nerve corresponds to the loss of axonal integrity, which has been found by Gutmann and Holubář (1950) to occur in most axons of the rabbit nerve 72 h after neurotomy.

A question frequently discussed in studies of Wallerian degeneration is whether

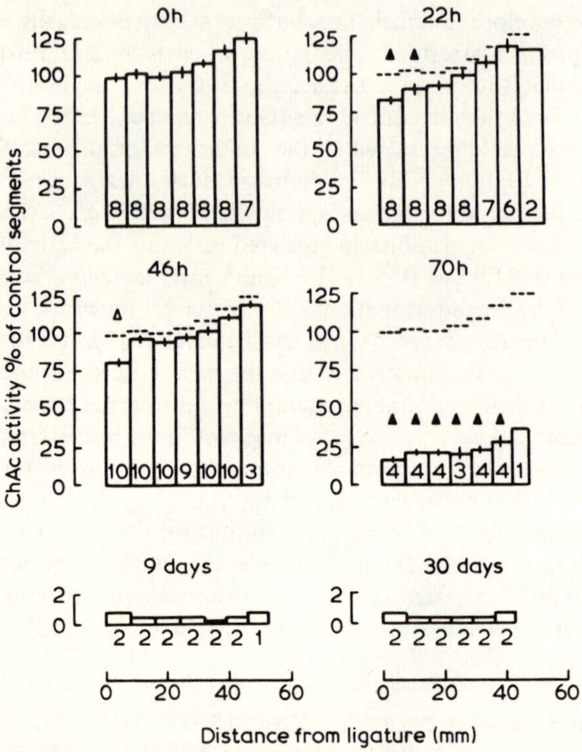

Fig. 7.9 The activity of ChAc in the peripheral stump of rabbit peroneal nerve during 30 days after nerve ligation and transection. The activity was measured in a series of 8 mm long segments from the proximal end of the peripheral nerve stump. The distance (mm) of individual segments from the site of nerve transection is shown at the bottom of the figure; the segment nearest to the ligature is on the left. The activity of ChAc is expressed as a percentage of the activity (mean ± S.E.M.) found in control segments. Numerals at the bottom of the columns give the number of observations. Broken horizontal lines show the activity in the segments at time 0. The triangles indicate the statistical significance of the difference between the activity at a given time after the interruption of the nerve and the activity in the same segment at time 0; △, $p < 0.05$; ▲, $p < 0.005$ (after Tuček, 1974).

the degeneration occurs simultaneously in the whole peripheral nerve stump, or whether the degenerative change spreads proximo–distally (see Gutmann and Holubář; 1950; Lubińska, 1964; Zhabotinskii, 1965; Joseph, 1973; Donat and Wiśniewski, 1973). It may be seen from Fig. 7.9 that in the seven 8 mm long nerve segments examined (constituting a stretch of 56 mm from the proximal end of the peripheral nerve stump), the activity of ChAc decreased in all within the same time interval, between 46 and 70 h, after nerve interruption. Consequently, degenerative changes either occur simultaneously in the whole peripheral nerve stump, or they spread very fast, so that the spreading can be detected only by using very short time intervals for investigation.

The activity of ChAc in the interrupted nerve falls very early if the nerve is deprived of the blood supply (Tuček *et al.*, 1975, 1978b; see Chapter 3.4.5 and Fig. 3.12). In ischaemic isolated segements of the nerve *in vivo* examined 22 h after nerve sections, the total ChAc activity had been diminished by 50% but total AChE activity had not been changed. Evidently, ChAc is an earlier victim of axonal necrosis than AChE; perhaps it is a general rule that axoplasmic enzymes are affected by degenerative changes sooner than the enzymes bound to the membranes.

In earlier investigations, a fall of ChAc activity in degenerating rabbit nerves to values lower than 1% of controls was found by Hebb (1962). Nachmansohn *et al.* (1946) and Berry and Rossiter (1958) described the complete disappearance of the enzyme. Whereas the activity of ChAc in degenerating nerves falls to extremely low values, the content of ACh in peripheral stumps of interrupted nerves decreases less than the enzyme. 5 days after the interruption of a rabbit nerve the content of ACh in its peripheral stump had decreased to 20% of control values, but was still close to this level 15 days later (Evans and Saunders, 1967). A similar change was also found in a cat nerve after a single lesion, but in an isolated segment of a cat nerve (i.e. in a segment separated both from the neuronal perikarya and the peripheral organs), the content of ACh decreased to only 2% of control values (Evans and Saunders, 1967). It is not clear by what mechanism the continued connection of the degenerating nerve to the peripheral organs can influence the decrease of the ACh level in the nerve. In MacIntosh's (1941) experiments, 3–25% of ACh content was retained in the peripheral stump of cat phrenic, hypoglossal and sciatic nerves 5–8 days after section. In experiments on sectioned pigeon oculomotor nerve, 19–36% of ACh remained in the peripheral stump after 3–10 days (Pilar *et al.*, 1973); in degenerating guinea pig sciatic nerve, however, the content of ACh was close to zero 4 days after nerve section (Muralt and Schulthess, 1944).

Changes of ACh and ChAc during the degeneration of frog nerves differ markedly from those observed in mammals. This is partly due to the fact that Wallerian degeneration proceeds much more slowly in poikilothermic than in homoiothermic animals. The main reason for the differences, however, seems to reside in the fact that frog Schwann cells start to participate directly in ACh metabolism during nerve degeneration. This was first suggested by the observation of the reappearance of miniature endplate potentials in denervated frog muscles (Birks *et al.*, 1960; see also Miledi and Stefani, 1970, and Bevan *et al.*, 1973, 1976). In intact neuromuscular junctions, miniature endplate potentials are caused by the spontaneous quantal release of ACh from the nerve endings (see Chapter 6). In denervated frog muscles, miniature endplate potentials reappear after a period of electric silence, at a time when the motor terminals have degenerated and the postsynaptic membrane of the muscle endplate is in contact with a Schwann cell. Since the miniature endplate potentials in denervated muscles are cholinergicly-evoked, Schwann cells adjacent to the endplates have to be regarded as the source of ACh quanta. The release of ACh from frog Schwann cells can be stimulated electrically (Dennis and Miledi, 1974a). In denervated muscles of the rat, reappearance of miniature endplate potentials is observed only extremely rarely (Miledi and Slater, 1968). Although this might be connected with the fact that, in denervated rat muscles, Schwann cells retract from contact with the postsynaptic membrane, differences between ChAc changes in degenerating frog and mammalian nerves suggest that an involvement in ACh metabolism is a specific feature of Schwann cells in degenerating frog (as opposed to mammalian) nerves.

In frog nerves, the decrease of ChAc activity as a result of Wallerian degeneration is preceded by an increase (Tuček *et al.*, in preparation). The maximum increase (by about 20%) was observed 15 days after nerve section and the steep decrease of ChAc activity only started 30 days after nerve section. Even at a time when the axons were completely degenerated and the nerves consisted almost entirely of bands of Schwann cells, the activity of ChAc per mm length of the degenerated nerves did not fall below 20% of activity in control nerves. The increase of ChAc activity in the peripheral nerve stump during the first month after nerve section indicates that the synthesis of new ChAc is taking place in the part of the nerve separated from the neuronal perikarya. The Schwann cells are again the most likely location of the synthesis of new ChAc. Changes of ACh content in degenerating frog nerves also differ from those in mammalian nerves. During the first two weeks after nerve section, the content of ACh in the peripheral stump of a frog nerve does not fall below 50% of the control value; indeed, at 3 and 10 days after nerve section it increases 50% above control values (Umrath *et al.*, 1966; see also Hellauer and Umrath, 1939). Erratic values of ACh content in degenerating frog sciatic nerve, fluctuating between 10% and 330% of controls, have been observed by Miledi *et al.* (1977). Some irregularities observed in the time course of changes during degeneration of frog nerves may perhaps reflect a large individual variation in the rate of development of degeneration in frogs.

The decrease of ACh synthesis, caused by Wallerian degeneration of cholinergic axons, has been observed not only in peripheral nerves, but also in many other parts of the nervous system. In sympathetic ganglia, transection of preganglionic fibres is followed by decreases in ACh content (MacIntosh, 1938), in the ability of the ganglia to synthetize ACh (Feldberg, 1943) and in the activity of ChAc (Hebb and Waites, 1956). In cat lumbosacral sympathetic ganglia the activity of ChAc decreases by 98% after preganglionic denervation (Buckley *et al.*, 1967b); the residual enzymatic activity is located in the perikarya of some (about 14%) of the cells of the sympathetic ganglion. In the cerebral cortex, the activity of ChAc decreased by 83% after it was undercut (Hebb *et al.*, 1963). In the hippocampus it is possible to reduce the activity of ChAc to a small percentage of normal values by electrolytic destruction of septal nuclei, which are the source of cholinergic axons reaching the hippocampus (Fig. 5.5 – Kuhar *et al.*, 1973; Oderfeld-Nowak *et al.*, 1973, 1974). A similar localized decrease of ChAc activity may be achieved in the interpeduncular nuclei by the electrocoagulation of the habenula (Kataoka *et al.*, 1973).

Denervation of peripheral organs is also followed by profound changes in the synthesis of ACh. In the parotid glands, ChAc activity decreases considerably after parasympathetic postganglionic denervation (Nordenfelt, 1963, 1967); some residual activity is probably attributable to the preservation of some stray cholinergic fibres reaching the gland (Ekström and Holmberg, 1972a; Alm and Ekström, 1976). Cold-destruction of periarterial nerves travelling to the intestine in the mesentery does not measurably affect the activity of ChAc in the intestinal wall, but cold-destruction of the nerve tissue in the intestinal wall causes the disappearance of ChAc (Filogamo and Marchisio, 1970). No data seem to be available regarding ChAc changes in the heart following damage to its nerve supply; the content of ACh in the cardiac atria is reduced by about 25% after right-sided vagotomy and by about 25% after left-sided vagotomy (Tuček and Vlk, 1962). Parasympathetic denervation causes the virtually complete disappearance of ChAc (Ehinger *et al.*, 1966) and ACh (Ehinger *et al.*, 1970) in the iris and of ACh in the corneal epithelium (Fitzgerald and Cooper, 1971). In the electric organ of *Electrophorus electricus,* ChAc activity was decreased by 50% 1 week after nerve section and was undetectable after 3 months (Rosenberg *et al.*, 1964).

In mammalian skeletal muscles, the ACh content 4–8 weeks after denervation, is reduced to 10–15% (Bhatnagar and MacIntosh, 1960), 6–13% (Hebb, 1962), 4–9% (Hebb *et al.*, 1964a) or 2.2% (Potter, 1970) of control values. Recent observations thus fail to confirm the earlier claim that the content of ACh is increased in denervated muscles (Chenykaeva, 1943). Denervation of mammalian skeletal muscles is followed by disappearance of their miniature endplate potentials (Miledi and Slater, 1968, 1970); the amount of ACh which can be released from the muscle by direct electrical stimulation is considerably lowered (Krnjević and Straughan, 1964; Stewart and Martin, 1966; Alkon *et al.*, 1970). At the same time, however, the spontaneous release of ACh from the whole muscle is diminished by only about 50% (Mitchell and Silver, 1963) or even less (Krnjević and Straughan, 1964). The large spontaneous release of ACh from denervated muscles and the regular finding of a residual ACh content in these muscles even several weeks after denervation indicate that, in addition to the pool of ACh in motor nerve fibres, there is a second pool of ACh in skeletal muscles which is not destroyed by Wallerian degeneration and which is the source of the spontaneous resting release after denervation.

Data on ChAc activity changes in muscles after denervation are in good agreement with the idea of two pools of ACh in skeletal muscles. In rat diaphragm, the activity of ChAc 6 weeks after denervation corresponds to 4% (Hebb *et al.*, 1964a) or 2.5% (Potter, 1970) of control values. In rat sternomastoid muscle, 8% of ChAc activity is preserved in its neural part 6.5 days after denervation (Israël, 1970). The fall of ChAc activity in rat limb muscle after denervation proceeds in two stages (Tucek, 1968a, 1973a; Fig. 7.10). A rapid exponential fall of ChAc activity occurs in the muscles during the first 72–96 h after nerve section, the activity decreasing

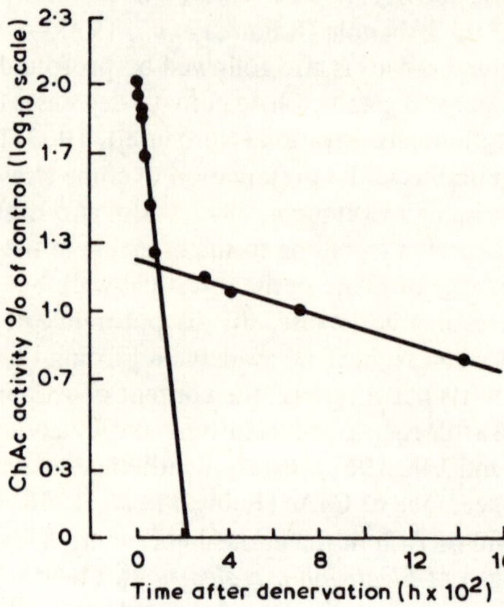

Fig. 7.10 ChAc activity in rat soleus muscle after denervation. Abscissa: time after denervation, expressed in hundreds of hours. Ordinate: decadic logarithm of the percentage of ChAc activity remaining in the muscle (in comparison with the contralateral control muscle) at the given time after denervation. The value 2.0 corresponds to 100%, 1.0 corresponds to 10% (after Tuček, 1973a).

by 80–90%. A slow decrease follows thereafter. 7 months after denervation, the activity of ChAc in rat tibialis anterior muscle was 3.4%, and in the extensor digitorum longus, 3.3% of the activity in the contralateral control muscles (Tuček, 1973a). There is little doubt that the ChAc disappearing during the period of rapid fall represents the enzyme which is localized in the motor nerve terminals and in intramuscular nerve branches. The remaining 10–20% of the enzyme represents a different pool, the localization of which has not been clarified.

The following possibilities seem to be particularly worth considering in an attempt to explain the localization of the pool of ChAc remaining in skeletal muscles after denervation:

(a) The presence of ChAc in some, perhaps vasomotor, nerve fibres which reach the muscle by a route other than the main nerve supply. This possibility does not seem likely, as autonomic nerve fibres going to skeletal muscle are contained in their motor nerves (Tiegs, 1953) and the content of ACh in the muscles is not affected by sympathectomy (Bhatnagar and MacIntosh, 1960).

(b) The presence of ChAc in muscle fibres themselves. This possibility is supported by observations that ChAc is present in a low concentration in the so-called aneural parts of the muscles (Hebb *et al.*, 1964a; McCaman *et al.*, 1967; Israël, 1970; Flood *et al.*, 1970; Potter, 1970). Recent findings that ACh is also present in aneural parts of frog muscle and that a low level of ACh remains both in neural and aneural parts of frog muscles after denervation (Miledi *et al.*, 1977) also support the idea that ACh is present within the muscle fibres. On the other hand, spontaneous release of ACh from the denervated diaphragm can be observed only in zones which, in the normal diaphragm, contain motor nerve endings (Mitchell and Silver, 1963). Denervation causes the same percentage lowering of ChAc activity in the 'neural' and 'aneural' zones of the diaphragm (Hebb *et al.*, 1964a; Potter, 1970); this raises the doubt as to whether the 'aneural' part of the muscle is indeed free of nerve fibres and endings. It has been suggested earlier that ACh is synthesized in the muscle cells of intestinal smooth muscle (Feldberg and Lin, 1950), but recent investigations (Paton and Zar, 1968; Schmidt *et al.*, 1969; Filogamo and Marchisio, 1970) contradict this view. The release of ACh from non-innervated stimulated embryonic chick heart has been strongly suggested by experimental observations described by Coraboeuf *et al.* (1970). Apparently, the localization of a proportion of ChAc in the muscle fibres is a possibility, which has not been proved, but which plausibly explains some experimental findings.

(c) The localization of ChAc in Schwann cells. The occurrence of ChAc and ACh in Schwann cells of degenerating frog nerves has been discussed earlier in this chapter. There are no data which directly indicate that ChAc and ACh are also present in Schwann cells of degenerating mammalian nerves. As already mentioned, ChAc activity in degenerated mammalian nerves falls below 1% of the original value (Hebb, 1962; Tuček, 1974). It might be argued that the synthesis of ChAc in Schwann cells was responsible for the delayed increase of ChAc activity in denervated mouse muscles, which was described by M. McCaman (1966). Since this delayed increase, which was not confirmed in other studies (Tuček, 1973a), was accompanied by an increase in the weight and protein content of the muscles (McCaman and McCaman, 1965), it is more likely that it was caused by muscle reinnervation. The presence of ChAc in intramuscularly localized Schwann cells in frogs may be responsible for the comparatively high residual ChAc content in denervated frog muscles (Tuček *et al.*, in preparation).

(d) The possibility that the synthesis of ACh in denervated muscles, ascribed to the activity of ChAc, is in fact due to the activity of carnitine acetyltransferase (White and Wu, 1973c; see Chapter 2.5.4). It is unlikely that carnitine acetyltransferase could be responsible for all residual ACh synthesis in denervated muscles and for the spontaneous release of ACh from them, but its quantitative contribution to the synthesis of ACh in denervated mammalian muscles requires examination. In denervated frog muscles, it is not responsible for more than 50% of their high residual ACh synthesis (Tuček *et al.*, in preparation).

The post-denervation decrease of ChAc in a skeletal muscle occurs earlier if the motor nerve is interrupted near the muscle (Emmelin *et al.*, 1966; Tuček, 1968b, 1973a). A similar dependence of the time course of various presynaptic and postsynaptic denervation changes on the length of the peripheral nerve stump has been observed many times (Luco and Eyzaguirre, 1955; Vial, 1955; Gutmann *et al.*, 1955; see review Lubińska, 1975) and has usually been taken to mean that the longer the peripheral nerve stump, the longer the time during which it is capable of supplying the trophic factors, necessary for the preservation of normal structure and function of the nerve endings and muscle fibres. In the light of direct measurements of ChAc activity in the peripheral nerve stump (Tuček, 1974), it seems likely that the delayed fall of ChAc in denervated muscles connected with long peripheral nerve stumps is attributable to the prolonged supply of some factors other than ChAc, postponing degenerative destruction of the nerve endings.

7.7 CHOLINE ACETYLTRANSFERASE IN REGENERATING NEURONS

The ability of cholinergic neurons whose axons form peripheral nerves to restore their processes after structural damage is evident from observations of the reinnervation of the muscles and other organs. On the other hand, the ability of central cholinergic neurons to regenerate their processes inside the central nervous system, while suspected, had not been clearly demonstrated until the elegant experiments of Svendgaard *et al.*, (1976). In these experiments, the iris was transplanted into the brain and its innervation from interrupted axons of brain nerve cells was observed. It has been found that the regenerative capacity of central cholinergic neurons is not greatly inferior to that of their peripheral counterparts when given similar conditions for the growth of regenerating axons.

Most studies regarding ChAc in regenerating neurons have been performed on peripheral nerves. During the first days after nerve interruption, ChAc activity at the end of the central nerve stump increases. In experiments on goat sciatic nerve, the increase of ChAc spread over a distance of 3 cm from the site of nerve interruption and reached its maximum 6–7 days after neurotomy (Hebb and Silver, 1963). The content of ACh proximally to the site of nerve interruption also increases during the first 5 days after nerve interruption (Evans and Saunders, 1967). The main reason of the increase of ChAc and ACh content above the site of interruption of a nerve is undoubtedly the arrest of their proximo–distal transport (see Chapter 3). The increase may also be partly due to the sprouting of axons at the site of interruption.

Hebb and Silver (1963) working on the goat sciatic nerve found that when the nerve section was repeated more proximally 1 week after a distal nerve section, ChAc again accumulated above the proximal section. When, however, the proximal section was performed 3–4 weeks after the distal section, no increase of ChAc above the proximal section occurred. 4 weeks after the interruption of the sciatic nerve, the activity of ChAc in the corresponding ventral spinal roots was diminished; the area of diminished ChAc activity spread from the spinal cord to the periphery, so that 12 weeks after the section of the sciatic nerve ChAc activity was reduced in the whole central nerve stump by 30–40%. The decrease of ChAc activity in the central nerve stump at long time intervals after nerve section has been confirmed by many investigators. ChAc activity in the central stump of rabbit hypoglossal nerve was reduced 1 week after nerve section, by 37% (Frizell and Sjöstrand, 1974b) and after 4 weeks by 50% (Fonnum *et al.*, 1973); in mouse sciatic nerve 3–8 mm above the site of interruption, it was decreased by 49% 3 weeks after nerve interruption (Jablecki and Brimijoin, 1975).

These observations suggest that the supply of ChAc from neural perikarya to the axons remains low for several weeks after the interruption of the nerve. This is probably a consequence of diminished ChAc synthesis in the bodies of the nerve cells. Fonnum *et al.* (1973) found that the activity of ChAc in the nucleus of the hypoglossal nerve is considerably reduced 2 and 4 weeks after the interruption of the nerve. This finding contrasts with the fact that the amount of proteins in nerve cell bodies is increased during the period of regenerative axonal growth (Brattgård *et al.*, 1957), but it corresponds to Watson's (1974) concept that the synthesis of enzymes responsible for the production of transmitters is dependent on the functional contact of axonal terminals with postsynaptic cells (see Section 7.8). According to this concept, the synthesis of ChAc in regenerating cholinergic neurons would be expected to be low until the time when the regenerating axons start to form synapses with the effector cells. Discordant observations have been made by Jablecki and Brimijoin (1975): although the content of ChAc in the central stumps of mouse sciatic nerves is diminished 10–80 days after nerve interruption, the amount of enzyme transported proximo–distally is not changed and the rate of its transport is increased. In adrenergic nerves, axonal trauma has been found to cause a depression in the synthesis and storage of amine storage granule (Karlström and Dahlström, 1973).

The activity of ChAc in regenerated axons remains low for long periods of time. 4 weeks after neurotomy, the activity of ChAc in the rabbit vagal nerve 20 mm distal to the site of the interruption corresponds to 60% of control values (Frizell and Sjöstrand, 1974a). In cat nerves it corresponds to 17% of control values after 20 and 46 weeks of regeneration (Carlsson *et al.*, 1971a). When examined 1.5 years after nerve section, the activity of ChAc in the goat sciatic nerve was found to have returned to control levels (Hebb and Silver, 1963). The low ChAc level observed in the nerves a long time after their regeneration is probably connected with the fact that the diameter of regenerated axons remains low for a long period (Gutmann and Sanders, 1943) and the axons therefore contain less axoplasm than the axons in control nerves.

The relation between the restitution of ChAc activity in reinnervated organs and the resumption of synaptic transmission has not yet been studied in detail. The increase of ChAc activity in the nerve precedes the increase of the weight of the reinnervated muscle and the restitution of its function, evaluated according to its locomotor activity and electromyogram (Carlsson *et al.*, 1971a). During reinnervation of the muscles, the synapses are preferentially restored in the area where they were located before denervation. In accordance with this the increase of ChAc activity in the muscle, which accompanies its reinnervation, is also found in the area which originally contained the motor endplates, even when the regenerating nerve stump had been sutured into the aneural part of the muscle (Israël, 1970).

When the synaptic contact between the motor nerve ending and the muscle fibre is restored, it is first of all accompanied by the restoration of miniature endplate potentials, indicating the spontaneous quantal release of ACh. In the initial stage of reinnervation, nerve stimulation is not able to produce endplate potentials; somewhat later, the endplate potentials are subliminal and do not bring about the appearance of muscle action potentials (Dennis and Miledi, 1974b, c; Bennett *et al.*, 1973). Transmission is fully restored only later. Presumably, the initial insufficiency of neuromuscular transmission is mainly caused by the fact that the nerve impulses cannot spread to the terminal branches of motor axons or spread only to some of them (Miledi, 1960; Dennis and Miledi, 1974b,c). No experimental data are available which enable a quantitative judgement to be made about the ability of the nerve endings to synthetize ACh during this transient period of reinnervation. The activity of ChAc in rat muscle, which was considerably reduced during the period of denervation, increased after reinnervation, but it did not reach the level of the control muscle and remained at about 80% of the control value for many weeks (Carlsson *et al.*, 1971b). Similarly, ChAc activity in parasympathetically denervated parotid gland remains below normal for as long as a year after its reinnervation (Ekström and Emmelin, 1974).

7.8 RETROGRADE TRANSSYNAPTIC INFLUENCES ON THE ACTIVITY OF CHOLINE ACETYLTRANSFERASE IN CHOLINERGIC NEURONS

Functional contact of neurons with their target cells is of the utmost importance for the development and function of the neurons and for their restitution after structural damage (for review see Hamburger, 1955; Prestige, 1970; Watson, 1974; Price, 1974; Smith and Kreutzberg, 1976). This generally accepted view is mainly based on the results of experiments in which developing neurons have been deprived of their peripheral innervation fields or in which regenerating axons have been prevented from re-establishing synaptic contacts with the corresponding effector cells. It is very likely that the nerve cell bodies continuously receive information from their axonal endings and that the pattern of their metabolism varies depending on the presence or absence of functional contacts with the target cells (see review by Watson, 1974); some observations included in this chapter suggest that the neurons are influenced not only by the presence or absence of synaptic contacts, but also by the alterations of the functional state of postsynaptic cells. Chemical agents carrying the information from axonal endings probably reach the nerve cell bodies thanks to the mechanisms of retrograde axonal transport. Their nature has not been identified; in sympathetic neurons, postsynaptic cells probably influence their presynaptic neurons by supplying them with the nerve-growth factor. This section reviews observations indicating that the contact with postsynaptic cells also influences the activity of ChAc in cholinergic neurons and their axonal terminals.

The importance for the synthesis of ChAc in the neurons of synaptic contacts with the target cells or, under some circumstances, of the mere presence of other cells, is well seen in experiments with neuronal cell cultures. When a cell suspension from mouse embryonic spinal cord is cultivated in the presence of embryonic myotubes, the activity of ChAc in the mixed culture increases 7 times faster than it does in spinal cord cells cultivated alone (Giller *et al.*, 1973). Similarly, ChAc activity in aggregating cell cultures of chick embryonic neural retinal cells, incubated as a mixture with cells from the optic lobe or from the telencephalon, is higher than in aggregating cultures of cells from the three sources incubated separately (Adler and Teitelman, 1974). It is tempting to explain the increase of ChAc activity in mixed cell cultures by the formation of cholinergic synapses, but it is not certain that this is the correct explanation. When sympathetic neurons are cultivated in the presence of non-neural cells from sympathetic ganglia, the synthesis of ACh in the culture is 100–1000 times higher than in the neurons cultivated alone (Patterson and Chun, 1974). In this case, the formation of synaptic contacts is unlikely, but the cultivation of sympathetic neurons with non-neural cells stimulates the development of cholinergic properties in cells which would otherwise be adrenergic (Patterson *et al.*, 1976).

In experiments *in vivo*, the formation of neuro–effector synapses in chick iris has been found to coincide with a 200–fold increase in the activity of ChAc in the iris: this suggests that the formation of neuromuscular junctions triggers the synthesis of ChAc in the nerve cells (Chiappinelli *et al.*, 1976). The dependence of ChAc activity in the preganglionic nerve terminals of sympathetic ganglia, on the intactness of ganglionic neurons has been found in many experiments in which the number of ganglionic neurons was altered by various experimental procedures. Partial destruction of sympathetic ganglionic neurons by 6-hydroxydopamine or by antiserum against the nerve-growth factor prevents the normal developmental increase of ChAc activity in the preganglionic nerve terminals in the sympathetic ganglia (Black *et al.*, 1972). Similarly, the extirpation of salivary glands and iris from chick embryos at an early stage of development, resulting in a decrease in the number of adrenergic neurons in the superior cervical ganglion, causes a decrease in the activity of ChAc in the ganglion, i.e. in the terminals of preganglionic cholinergic fibres (Dibner *et al.*, 1977). On the other hand, the activity of ChAc in the sympathetic ganglion is considerably increased after the administration of the nerve-growth factor, which is known to increase the number of adrenergic neurons (Thoenen *et al.*, 1972). Presumably, variations of ChAc activity observed in these experiments on sympathetic ganglia reflect variations in the number of cholinergic synapses present.

The activity of ChAc in an organ may be altered, however, not only by evoking a change in the number of cholinergic synapses, but also by evoking a change in the functional state of postsynaptic cells. This has been demostrated in studies on the activity of ChAc in the levator ani muscle of rats after either castration or the administration of testosterone (Gutmann *et al.*, 1969; Tuček *et al.*, 1976a). The levator ani has been shown to contain specific androgen binding receptors (Jung and

Baulieu, 1972). The effect of castration on the activity of ChAc in the levator ani muscle may be seen from Fig. 7.7. One month after castration, the weight of the muscle is 35% lower in castrated than in control rats, but the activity of ChAc does not differ in the two groups. Five months later, however, the weight of the muscle is reduced by 71% and the activity of ChAc by 41%. The administration of testosterone brings about the rapid restitution of muscle weight and ChAc activity (Fig. 7.8).

Changes in the levator ani muscle weight and ChAc activity after castration and testosterone administration are not accompanied by changes in the number of muscle fibres and, consequently, there are no changes in the number of neuromuscular synapses (Tuček *et al.*, 1976a). The adrenergic innervation of male accessory sex organs, evaluated by their content of noradrenaline, has been found to be affected by castration and administration of testosterone in the same way (Wakade and Kirpekar, 1973; Sjöstrand and Swedin, 1976; Kvist and Sjöstrand, 1976) as the cholinergic innervation of the levator ani muscle, evaluated by its ChAc activity. Although one may speculate about other explanations of the effects of castration and testosterone on ChAc activity, the assumption that the development of cholinergic nerve endings adapts to the development of postsynaptic cells innervated by them seems most likely. Such an assumption is supported by the observation of a direct relation between the diameter of the muscle fibre, the size of its motor endplate, the frequency of the miniature endplate potentials in it, and the number of quanta which are released by one nerve impulse (Kuno *et al.*, 1971). The adaptation of presynaptic nerve terminals to the changing state of the postsynaptic cell may well depend on the retrograde trophic influence of the postsynaptic cell on the presynaptic neuron, but this is a matter for further investigation.

Although this section is devoted to retrograde transsynaptic influences on ChAc in cholinergic neurons, it seems appropriate to ask the question whether the metabolism of ACh in cholinergic neurons is also subject to anterograde trophic transsynaptic influences, i.e. to trophic influences from the cells by which cholinergic neurons are innervated. Such influences are best revealed by changes after denervation. In cholinergic ciliary ganglion neurons, the level of ACh has been found to fall to unmeasurably low levels 11 days after the transection of preganglionic nerve fibres (Pilar *et al.*, 1973). The loss of ACh stores strongly suggests the loss of ACh synthesis in the denervated ciliary ganglion. It does not seem, however, that the ability to synthesize ACh is invariably lost in cholinergic neurons deprived of innervation: as already mentioned in Section 7.4, preganglionic parasympathetic denervation reduced the activity of ChAc in the parotid gland by only 25%, which is far from a complete arrest of ACh synthesis.

7.9 SUMMARY

Prenatal and early postnatal development of the central nervous system and of peripheral organs receiving a cholinergic innervation is accompanied by a marked increase in their ChAc activity. This increase is based not only on the growth of cholinergic neurons, but also on the elevation of the concentration of ChAc in them. Transient decreases of ChAc activity, observed in some tissues during development, may be caused by the fact that during certain periods the non-cholinergic components of these tissues develop faster than the cholinergic ones. In old age the activity of ChAc in cholinergic neurons generally diminishes.

The activity of ChAc in the neurons is very probably influenced by their functional activity. This is suggested by observations on salivary glands, adrenal glands and skeletal muscles, but the relation between functional activity of the neurons and ChAc synthesis in them requires a more searching investigation. Changes of ChAc activity depending on hormonal influences have been well demonstrated in the brain during hypothyroidism (a decrease) and after the administration of noradrenaline into the brain ventricles (an increase); a sex-dependent difference in ChAc activity has been found in the preoptic suprachiasmal area of the hypothalamus. Androgenic hormones influence the activity of ChAc (and general development) of the levator ani muscle.

A big decrease of ChAc activity leading to its virtually complete disappearance is observed during Wallerian degeneration of peripheral nerves in homoiothermic animals. In frog nerves, Wallerian degeneration of the axons is accompanied by the formation of ChAc in Schwann cells. The post-denervation decrease of ChAc activity in skeletal muscles proceeds in two stages. During the first, rapid stage the enzyme disappears from intramuscular branches and terminals of the motor nerve, while the occurrence of the second, slow stage of ChAc decrease points to the existence of a second pool of ChAc in the muscles; its localization is not clear. The activity of ChAc in the axons is diminished during regeneration and for a long time after the regeneration has been completed.

ChAc activity in cholinergic neurons and their axonal terminals is greatly influenced by the formation of synaptic contacts with postsynaptic cells. Experiments on hormonally induced changes in the levator ani muscle indicate that ChAc activity in cholinergic nerve terminals is also dependent on the functional state of postsynaptic cells. The mechanism of the retrograde transsynaptic influence of the postsynaptic on the presynaptic cell has not been clarified.

AUTHOR'S NOTE

Ontogenetic changes of ChAc activity have been described for neuronal and glial cell enriched fractions from rat brains by Y. Nagata, T. Nanba and M. Ando (*Neurochem. Res.* **1**, 299–312, 1976) and for the neurointermediate lobe of the rat pituitary by M.R.G.P. Gallardo, M.A. Cannata and J.H. Tramezzani (*J. neural Transmiss.* **41**, 93–98, 1977). The development of ChAc activity in a sympathetic ganglion has been shown to be slowed down after spinal transection (R.W. Hamill, E.M. Bloom and I.B. Black, *Brain Res.* **134**, 269–278, 1977) and after chemical destruction of the peripheral sympathetic system (E.M. Johnson, M.T. Caserta and

L.L. Ross, *Brain Res.* **136**, 455–464, 1977). High ChAc activity has been found in the adrenals of old animals (D.J. Reis, R.A. Ross and T.H. Joh, *Brain Res.* **136**, 465–474, 1977). Factors affecting the development of cholinergic properties and/or ChAc activity in neural cells cultivated *in vitro* have been analysed by P.H. Patterson and L.L.Y. Chun (*Develop. Biol.* **60**, 473–481, 1977), L.F. Reichardt and P.H. Patterson (*Nature* **270**, 147–151, 1977), D. Ross, M. Johnson and R. Bunge (*Nature* **267**, 536–539, 1977), J.H. Greenberg and B.K. Schrier (*Develop. Biol.* **61**, 86–93, 1977), E.L. Giller, J.H. Neale, P.N. Bullock, B.K. Schrier and P.G. Nelson (*J. cell Biol.* **74**, 16–29, 1977) and D. Schubert, S. Heinemann and Y. Kidikoro (*Proc. natn. Acad. Sci. U.S.A.* **74**, 2579–2583, 1977). Prolonged ganglionic blockade has been shown to diminish the activity of ChAc in the rat parotid gland (J. Ekstrom and B. Lindmark, *J. Physiol., Lond.*, **271**, 31–32P, 1977).

8 Conclusion

In previous chapters I have tried to give a survey of what is known about basic cellular aspects of the synthesis of ACh in cholinergic neurons of vertebrates. An attempt to select the most important and best documented findings and to summarize them in the concluding chapter would lead to unnecessary repetition. Let us devote the last chapter to the consideration of the opposite question: what are the weak points, and the most important gaps and uncertainties in the present understanding of the biosynthesis of ACh as the transmitter of cholinergic neurons? Stressing those aspects which we do not understand may help us to get a clearer picture of those that we do understand.

The use of radioisotopic methods for the measurement of ChAc activity brought about enormous progress in the investigation of the enzyme (Chapter 2). Further studies of ChAc will undoubtedly lead to the complete elucidation of the structure of its active centre and of the whole molecule of ChAc. A question of exceptional importance to the physiology of the cholinergic neuron, and to the understanding of its development and adaptation to changing requirements concerns the mechanisms controlling the synthesis of ChAc. Chapter 7 contains data indicating that the synthesis of ChAc in the neurons undergoes changes dependent on age, neuronal activity, the presence of functional contact with postsynaptic cells and axonal injury or regeneration, but the mechanisms responsible are as yet completely unknown. Despite some relevant and very interesting recent experimental observations, little is known with certainty about the factors which decide that a certain neuron will become cholinergic and another one will not.

Although it is almost certainly a much simpler problem, the mechanism by which ChAc is transported from the body of the neuron to the presynaptic nerve ending has not been clarified. We can give a detailed description of the transport (Chapter 3), but we are unable to explain the underlying molecular mechanism. This is true both for the slow transport, which is probably responsible for the supply of ChAc to the nerve endings, and for the fast transport, which is probably important for cholinergic synaptic transmission mainly because it supplies material for the synaptic vesicles.

Thanks to the use of radioisotopic methods we have at our disposal abundant experimental evidence about the supply of substrates for the synthesis of ACh (Chapters 4 and 5). The findings pointing to pyruvate as the main precursor of the acetyl groups of ACh in the brain and those showing the importance of the high affinity carrier for choline appear to be of particular significance in this area. Among the unresolved questions concerning the supply of acetyl groups for the synthesis of ACh, the problem of transport of acetyl–CoA from the mitochondrial matrix to the cytoplasmic compartment appears to be the most important. Even if it subsequently proves that, in other mammals, pyruvate is not as important a source of the acetyl groups of ACh as it is in the rat brain, the question of the mechanism of supply of intramitochondrial acetyl–CoA for the extramitochondrial synthesis of ACh will remain since acetyl–CoA is also generated intramitochondrially from the other likely sources of the acetyl groups of ACh. It is difficult to estimate how much acetyl–CoA is available in the presynaptic nerve endings for the synthesis of ACh; it seems desirable to know this since the supply of acetyl–CoA might be one of the factors limiting or controlling the synthesis of ACh.

Unclarified problems also remain with regard to the supply of the second substrate for the synthesis of ACh–choline. Data on the preferential utilization, for the synthesis of ACh, of the choline supplied by the high affinity uptake form an important contribution to the general understanding of the synthesis of ACh in cholinergic neurons. The basic nature (active transport vs. facilitated diffusion) of the high affinity uptake of choline has still to be established, however. The intracellular concentration of choline in the neurons is not established, nor is it clear how readily available the choline is for the synthesis of ACh; it is therefore difficult to assess the extent to which the supply of choline can be the limiting or controlling factor in the synthesis of ACh. The relation between the large supply of bound choline to the brain and the preferential utilization of free choline for the synthesis of ACh is also unclear. Is the free choline produced from the bound form in the nerve cells or in the glia? Is it then released into the extracellular fluid, from which is it taken up by the nerve endings?

A number of problems remain in our understanding of the organization and control of ACh synthesis in the nerve endings (Chapter 6). It seems certain that the synthesis occurs in the cytoplasmic compartment of cholinergic neurons, mainly in presynaptic axonal endings. Does it proceed diffusely throughout the cytoplasm of the whole presynaptic ending, or in only a certain area of it; alternatively, does it proceed mainly on the walls of the cytoplasmic compartment? The questions of how ACh gets into the synaptic vesicles and how the assumed concentration gradient between the vesicles and the neighbouring cytoplasm is formed are, as yet, unanswered. The steepness of this gradient is also uncertain. The findings concerning the preferential release of free ACh have led to a more critical evaluation of the vesicular hypothesis of ACh release, but other studies of the ultrastructure and biochemistry of the synapses have produced important arguments in its favour. In my view, the apparent contradiction between the vesicular hypothesis and the finding that the nerve impulses preferentially release the free ACh may be explained on assumption that the free ACh is not homogeneous and that it is contained not only in the cytoplasm, but also in a population of labile synaptic vesicles. It is evident that we need to learn more about what happens to the newly synthesized molecules of ACh, how the synaptic vesicles become filled with them, and at what stage in the life cycle of synaptic vesicles this filling or refilling occurs. These points are closely connected with the problem of the mechanism by which the synthesis of ACh is controlled. The hypothesis, discussed in Chapter 6, that the control of ACh synthesis is based on the maintenance of the reaction equilibrium, suffers from uncertainty about the true concentrations of acetyl–CoA, CoA, choline and ACh at the site of synthesis and requires direct experimental verification.

These are just some of the gaps in the present knowledge about the organization of ACh synthesis at the level of a single cholinergic neuron. Looking at the nervous system as a whole, the most conspicuous gap regarding the synthesis of ACh seems to be the lack of information as to which neurons in the central nervous system – apart from a few well-established groups – synthesize ACh as their transmitter. Detailed topography of cholinergic neurons in the brain will undoubtedly be worked out after the development of reliable histochemical methods for ChAc. Then it will also become possible to identify what properties, apart from the possession of the same transmitter, are common to cholinergic neurons, what their functional roles in the central nervous system have in common, and in what respects their position and role differ from those of other types of neurons. Very important contributions to the physiology and pathophysiology of cholinergic neurons can be expected from the elaboration of methods permitting the measurement of the metabolic turnover of ACh in individual parts of the nervous system or even in single nerve cells. It is to be hoped that the pharmacologists will find ways of influencing the synthesis of ACh for therapeutic purposes.

This, however, brings us to areas outside the scope of this book, which had a much more limited goal – to describe the synthesis of ACh at the level of the single cell. The reader most certainly will have realized that even this is a difficult task, and I cannot but apologize for the defects which I was unable to avoid while trying to describe this rapidly developing and most interesting area of our knowledge.

References

Aas, M. (1971), Organ and subcellular distribution of fatty acid activating enzymes in the rat. *Biochim. biophys. Acta.*, **231**, 32–47.

Aas, M. and Bremer, J. (1968), Short-chain fatty acid activation in rat liver. A new assay procedure for the enzymes and studies on their intracellular localization. *Biochim. biophys. Acta.*, **164**, 157–166.

Adamič, Š. (1970), Accumulation of acetylcholine by the rat diaphragm. *Biochem. Pharmac.*, **19**, 2445–2451.

Adamič, Š. (1970), [^{3}H]choline entry and [^{3}H]acetylcholine formation in leech segmental ganglia. *Biochem. Pharmac.*, **24**, 1763–1766.

Adler, R. and Teitelman, G. (1974), Aggregates formed by mixtures of embryonic neural cells: activity of enzymes of the cholinergic system. *Dev. Biol.*, **39**, 317–321.

Alkon, D.L., Schmidt, D.E., Green, J.P. and Szilagyi, P.I.A., (1970), The release of acetylcholine from the innervated and denervated diaphragm. *J. Pharmac. exp. Ther.*, **174**, 346–349.

Alkonyi, I. and Sándor, A. (1969), β-methyl-δ-keto-$\Delta\alpha\beta$-hexenoic acid and mesityl oxide as acetyl donors in the enzymic synthesis of acetylcholine. *FEBS Letters*, **5**, 338–340.

Allman, D.W., Galzigna, L., McCaman, R.E. and Green, D.W. (1966), The membrane systems of the mitochondrion. IV. The localization of the fatty acid oxidizing system. *Archs. Biochem. Biophys.*, **117**, 413–422.

Allred, J.B. and Guy, D.G. (1969), Determination of coenzyme A and acetyl–CoA in tissue extracts. *Analyt. Biochem.*, **29**, 293–299.

Alm, P. and Ekström, J. (1976), Uncharted cholinergic nerves in the rabbit parotid gland. *Q. Jl. exp. Physiol.*, **61**, 127–132.

Amano, T., Richelson, E. and Nirenberg, M. (1972), Neurotransmitter synthesis by neuroblastoma clones. *Proc. natn. Acad. Sci. U.S.A.*, **69**, 258–263.

Anderson, N.G. (1956), Techniques for the mass isolation of cellular components. In: *Physical Techniques in Biological Research* Vol. 3, (Oster, G. and Pollister, A.W. eds.), pp. 299–392. Academic Press, New York.

Ansell, G.B. and Spanner, S. (1967), The metabolism of labelled ethanolamine in the brain of the rat *in vivo*. *J. Neurochem.*, **14**, 873–885.

Ansell, G.B. and Spanner, S. (1968a), The long term metabolism of the ethanolamine moiety of rat brain myelin phospholipids. *J. Neurochem.* **15**, 1371–1373.

Ansell, G.B. and Spanner, S. (1968b), The metabolism of [Me-^{14}C] choline in the brain of the rat *in vivo. Biochem. J.*, **110**, 201–206.

Ansell, G.B. and Spanner, S. (1970), The origin and turnover of choline in the brain. In: *Drugs and Cholinergic Mechanisms in the CNS* (Heilbronn E. and Winter, A., eds), pp. 143–162, Almqvist and Wiksell, Stockholm.

Ansell, G.B. and Spanner, S. (1971), Studies on the origin of choline in the brain of the rat. *Biochem. J.*, **122**, 741–750.

Ansell, G.B. and Spanner, S. (1975), The origin and metabolism of brain choline. In: *Cholinergic Mechanisms* (Waser, P.G., ed.), pp. 117–129, Raven Press, New York.

Appleton, H.D., La Du, B.N., Levy, B.B., Steele, J.M. and Brodies, B.B. (1953), A chemical method for the determination of free choline in plasma. *J. biol. Chem.*, **205**, 803–813.

Aprison, M.H., Shea, P.A. and Richter, J.A. (1974), Methodology for a radioenzymatic assay of acetylcholine and choline – from the living animal to the measurement in extracts of CNS tissues. In: *Choline and Acetylcholine: Handbook of Chemical Assay Methods,* (Hanin, I., ed.), pp. 63–80, Raven Press. New York.

Aquilonius, S.-M., Schuberth, J. and Sundwall, A. (1970), Choline in the cerebrospinal fluid as a marker for the release of acetylcholine. In: *Drugs and Cholinergic Mechanisms in the CNS* (Heilbronn, E. and Winter, A., eds), pp. 399–410. Almqvist and Wiksell, Stockholm.

Aquilonius, S.-M., Nyström, B., Schuberth, J. and Sundwall, A. (1971), Cerebrospinal fluid choline in extrapyramidal disease. *Acta pharmac. tox.*, **29**, 3.

Aquilonius, S.-M., Flentge, F., Schuberth, J., Sparf, B. and Sundwall, A. (1973), Synthesis of acetylcholine in different compartments of brain nerve terminals *in vivo* as studied by the incorporation of choline from plasma and the effect of pentobarbital on this process. *J. Neurochem.*, **20**, 1509–1521.

Aquilonius, S.-M., Ceder, G., Lying-Tunell, U., Malmlund, H.O. and Schuberth, J. (1975), The arteriovenous difference of choline across the brain of man. *Brain Res.*, **99**, 430–433.

Artenie, V. (1968), Choline acetyltransferase of the nervous tissue of animals (Russ.). *Usp. biol. khim.*, **9**, 129–140.

Asdell, S.A., Doornenbal, H. and Sperling, G.A. (1962), Sex steroid hormones and voluntary exercise in rats. *J. Reprod. Fert.*, **3**, 26–32.

Atweh, S.F. and Kuhar, M.J. (1976), Effects of anesthetics and septal lesions and stimulation on ^{3}H-acetylcholine formation in rat hippocampus. *Eur. J. Pharmac.*, **37**, 311–319.

Atweh, S., Simon, J.R. and Kuhar, M.J. (1975), Utilization of sodium-dependent high affinity choline uptake *in vitro* as a measure of the activity of cholinergic neurons *in vivo Life Sci.*, **17**, 1535–1544.

Axelrod, J. and Kopin, I.J. (1969), The uptake, storage, release and metabolism of noradrenaline in sympathetic nerves. In: *Mechanisms of Synaptic Transmission* (Akert, K. and Waser, P.G. eds), *Progress in Brain Res.*, Vol. 31, pp. 21–32, Elsevier, Amsterdam.

Babel-Guérin, E., Boyenval, J., Droz, B., Dunant, Y. and Hassig, R. (1977), Accumulation of calcium in cholinergic axon terminals after nerve activity. Localization by electron miscroscope radioautography at the nerve-electroplaque junction of *Torpedo. Brain Res.*, **121**, 348–352.

Bachhawat, B.K., Robinson, W.G. and Coon, M.J. (1955), The enzymatic cleavage of β-hydroxy-β-methylglutaryl coenzyme A to acetoacetate and acetyl coenzyme A. *J. biol. Chem.*, **216**, 727–736.

Baker, R.R. and Dowdall, M.J. (1976), Some properties of choline acetyltransferase isolated from the electric organ of *Torpedo marmorata*: specificity for choline analogues and inhibition by certain amines and amino acids. *Neurochem. Res.*, **1**, 153–169.

Balázs, R., Magyar, K. and Richter, D. (1964), The operation of the tricaboxylic acid cycle in brain mitochondrial preparations. In: *Comparative Neurochemistry* (Richter, D., ed), pp. 225–248, Pergamon Press, Oxford.

Balfour W.E. and Hebb, C. (1952), Mechanisms of acetylcholine synthesis. *J. Physiol.* (Lond.), **118**, 94–106.

Banks, P. and Mayor, D. (1972), Intra-axonal transport in noradrenergic neurons in the sympathetic nervous system. *Biochem. Soc. Symp.* **36**, 133–149.

Banns, H.E. (1976), A study of the molecular sizes and stability of choline acetyltransferase. *J. Neurochem.*, **26**, 967–971.

Banns, H., Hebb, C. and Mann, S.P. (1977), The synthesis of ACh from acetyl–CoA, acetyl-dephospho–CoA and acetylpantetheine phosphate by choline acetyltransferase. *J. Neurochem.*, **29**, 433–437.

Barker, L.A. (1976a) Subcellular aspects of acetylcholine metabolism. In: *Biology of Cholinergic Function* (Goldberg, A.M. and Hanin, I. eds), pp. 203–238. Raven Press, New York.

Barker, L.A. (1976b) Modulation of synaptosomal high affinity choline transport. *Life Sci.*, **18**, 725–732.

Barker, L.A. and Mittag, T.W. (1975) Comparative studies of substrates and inhibitors of choline transport and choline acetyltransferase. *J. Pharmacol. exp. Ther.*, **192**, 86–94.

Barker, P.J., Fincham, N.J. and Hardwick, D.C. (1968), The availability of carnitine acetyltransferase in mitochondria from guinea pig liver and other tissues. *Biochem. J.*, **110**, 739–746.

Barker, L.A., Dowdall, M.J. and Whittaker, V.P. (1972), Choline metabolism in the cerebral cortex of guinea pigs. *Biochem. J.*, **130**, 1063–1075.

Barlow, R.B. and Dixon, R.O.D. (1973), Choline acetyltransferase in the nettle *Urtica dioica L. Biochem. J.*, **132**, 15–18.

Barondes, S.H. (1969), Axoplasmic transport. In: *Handbook of Neurochemistry* (Lajtha, A. ed)., Vol. 2, pp. 435–446, Plenum Press, New York.

Barondes, S.H. and Samson, F.E. (1967) Axoplasmic transport. *Neurosciences Res. Progr. Bull.*, **5**, 307–370.

Barth, C., Sladek, M. and Decker, K. (1971), The subcellular distribution of short-chain fatty acyl–CoA synthetase activity in rat tissues. *Biochim. biophys. Acta*, **248**, 24–33.

Barth, C., Sladek, M. and Decker, K. (1972), Dietary changes of cytoplasmic acetyl–CoA synthetase in different rat tissues. *Biochim. biophys. Acta*, **260**, 1–9.

Bartley, J., Abraham, S. and Chaikoff, I.L. (1965), Concerning the form in which acetyl units produced in mitochondria are transferred to the site of *de novo* fatty acid synthesis in the cell. *Biochem. biophys. Res. Commun.*, **19**, 770–776.

Beani, L., Bianchi, C., Megazzini, P., Ballotti, L. and Bernardi, G. (1969), Drug induced changes in free, labile and stable acetylcholine of guinea pig brain. *Biochem. Pharmac.*, **18**, 1315–1324.

Beattie, D.S. (1968), The submitochondrial distribution of the fatty acid oxidizing system in rat liver mitochondria. *Biochem. biophys. Res. Commun.*, **30**, 57–62.

Beattie, D.S. and Basford, B.F. (1965), Brain mitochondria. III. Fatty acid oxidation by bovine brain mitochondria. *J. Neurochem.* **12**, 103–111.

Beattie, D.S. and Basford, R.E. (1966), Brain mitochondria. V. Incorporation of fatty acids into phospholipids in bovine brain mitochondria. *J. biol. Chem.*, **241**, 1419–1423.

Beenakkers, A.M.T. and Henderson, P.T. (1967), The localization and function of carnitine acetyltransferase in the flight muscles of the locust. *Eur. J. Biochem.*, **1**, 187–192.

Ben-Ari, Y., Zigmond, R.E., Shute, C.C.D. and Lewis, P.R. (1977), Regional distribution of choline acetyltransferase and acetylcholinesterase within the amygdaloid complex and stria terminalis system. *Brain Res.*, **120**, 435–445.

Bennett, M.R. (1972), *Autonomic Neuromuscular Transmission.* Cambridge University Press, Cambridge.

Bennett, M.R., McLachlan, E.M. and Taylor, R.S. (1973), The formation of synapses in reinnervated mammalian striated muscle. *J. Physiol.* (Lond.), **233**, 481–500.

Berman-Reisberg, R. (1957), Properties and biological significance of choline acetylase. *Yale J. Biol. Med.*, **29**, 403–435.

Berman, R., Wilson, I.B. and Nachmansohn, D. (1953), Choline acetylase specificity in relation to biological function. *Biochim. biophys. Acta*, **12**, 315–324.

Berry, J.F. and Rossiter, R.J. (1958), Chemical studies of peripheral nerve during Wallerian degeneration. VIII. Acetic thiokinase and choline acetylase. *J. Neurochem.*, **3**, 59–64.

Berry, J.F. and Whittaker, V.P. (1959), The acyl-group specificity of choline acetylase. *Biochem. J.* **73**, 447–458.

Bertels-Meeuws, M.M. and Polak, R.L. (1968), Influence of antimuscarinic substances on *in vitro* synthesis of acetylcholine by rat cerebral cortex. *Brit. J. Pharmac.*, **33**, 368–380.

Besson, M.J., Cheramy, A., Feltz, P. and Glowinski, J. (1969), Demonstration of release of newly synthesized dopamine from dopamine-containing terminals in the striatum of the rat. *Proc. natn. Acad. Sci. U.S.A.*, **62**, 741–748.

Bevan, S., Miledi, R. and Grampp, W. (1973), Induced transmitter release from Schwann cells and its suppression by actinomycin D. *Nature New Biol.*, **241**, 85–86.

Bevan, S., Grampp, W. and Miledi, R. (1976), Properties of spontaneous potentials at denervated motor endplates of the frog. *Proc. R. Soc.* B, **194**, 195–210.

Bhatnagar, S.P. and MacIntosh, F.C. (1960), Acetylcholine content of striated muscle. *Proc. Canad. Fed. biol. Soc.*, **3**, 12–13.

Bhatnagar, S.P. and MacIntosh, F.C. (1967), Effects of quaternary bases and inorganic cations on acetylcholine synthesis in nervous tissue. *Can. J. Physiol. Pharmac.*, **45**, 249–268.

Bird, E.D. and Iversen, L.L. (1974), Huntington's chorea. Post-mortem measurement of glutamic acid decarboxylase, choline acetyltransferase and dopamine in basal ganglia. *Brain* **97**, 457–472.

Birks, R.I. (1963), The role of sodium ions in the metabolism of acetylcholine. *Can. J. Biochem. Physiol.* **41**, 2573–2597.

Birks, R.L. (1974), The relationship of transmitter release and storage to fine structure in a sympathetic ganglion. *J. Neurocytol.*, **3**, 133–160.

Birks, R. and MacIntosh, F.C. (1961), Acetylcholine metabolism of a sympathetic ganglion. *Can. J. Biochem. Physiol.*, **39**, 787–827.

Birks, R.I. and Fitch, S.J.G. (1974), Storage and release of acetylcholine in a sympathetic ganglion. *J. Physiol.* (Lond.), **240**, 125–134.

Birks, R., Katz, B. and Miledi, R. (1960), Physiological and structural changes at the amphibian myoneural junction, in the course of nerve degeneration. *J. Physiol. (Lond.)*, **150**, 145–168.

Bisby, M.A. (1976), Axonal transport. *Gen. Pharmac.*, **7**, 387–394.

Bishop, M.R., Sastry, B.V.R., Schmidt, D.E. and Harbison, R.D. (1976), Occurrence of choline acetyltransferase and acetylcholine and other quaternary ammonium compounds in mammalian spermatozoa. *Biochem. Pharmac.*, **25**, 1617–1622.

Bittiger, H. and Heid, J. (1977), The subcellular distribution of particle-bound negative charges in rat brain. *J. Neurochem.*, **28**, 917–922.

Bjǿrnstad, P. and Bremer, J. (1966), *In vivo* studies on pathways for the biosynthesis of lecithin in the rat. *J. Lipid Res.*, **7**, 38–45.

Black, E.C., Robertson, A.C. and Parker, R.R. (1961), Some aspects of carbohydrate metabolism in fish. In: *Comparative Physiology of Carbohydrate Metabolism in Heterothermic Animals* (Martin, A.W. ed.), pp. 89–124, University of Washington Press, Seattle.

Black, I.B., Hendry, I.A. and Iversen, L.L. (1971), Trans-synaptic regulation of growth and development of adrenergic neurones in a mouse sympathetic ganglion. *Brain Res.*, **34**, 229–240.

Black, I.B., Hendry, I.A. and Iversen, L.L. (1972), The role of postsynaptic neurons in the biochemical maturation of presynaptic cholinergic nerve terminals in a mouse sympathetic ganglion. *J. Physiol.* (Lond.), **221**, 149–159.

Blaustein, M.P. (1971), Preganglionic stimulation increases calcium uptake by sympathetic ganglia. *Science*, **172**, 391–393.

Blažka, P. (1958), The anaerobic metabolism of fish. *Physiol. Zoöl.*, **31**, 117–128.

Bligh, J. (1952), The level of free choline in plasma. *J. Physiol. (Lond.)*, **117**, 234–240.

Bligh, J. (1953), The role of the liver and the kidneys in the maintenance of the level of free choline in plasma. *J. Physiol.* (Lond.), **120**, 53–62.

Bourdois, P.S. and Szerb, J.C. (1972), The absence of 'surplus' acetylcholine formation in prisms prepared from rat cerebral cortex. *J. Neurochem.*, **19**, 1189–1193.

Bourdois, P.S., McCandless, D.L. and MacIntosh, F.C. (1975), A prolonged after-effect of intense synaptic activity on acetylcholine in a sympathetic ganglion. *Can. J. Physiol. Pharmac.*, **53**, 155–165.

Bowers, M.B. (1967a), Factors influencing maintenance and release of acetylcholine in rat cortical brain slices. *Int. J. Neuropharmac.*, **6**, 399–403.

Bowers, M.B. (1967b) Choline in cerebrospinal fluid. *Life Sci.*, **6**, 1927–1933.

Bowery, N.G. and Neal, M.J. (1975), Failure of denervation to influence the high affinity uptake of choline by sympathetic ganglia. *Brit. J. Pharmac.*, **55**, 278P.

Boyne, A.F., Bohan, T.P. and Williams, T.H. (1975), Changes in cholinergic synaptic vesicle populations and the ultrastructure of the nerve terminal membranes of *Narcine brasiliensis* electric organ stimulated to fatigue *in vivo J. cell Biol.*, **67**, 814–825.

Bradford, H.F. (1968), Carbohydrate and Energy Metabolism. In: *Applied Neurochemistry* (Davison, A.N. and Dobbing, J., eds), pp. 222–250. Blackwell, Oxford.

Brattgård, S.-O., Edstrom, J.-E. and Hyden, H. (1957), The chemical changes in regenerating neurons. *J. Neurochem.*, **1**, 316–325.

Bray, J.J. and Austin, L. (1969), Axoplasmic transport of ^{14}C proteins at two rates in chicken sciatic nerve. *Brain Res.*, **12**, 230–233.

Bray, J.J., Kon, C.M. and Breckenridge, B.M. (1971), Reversed polarity of rapid axonal transport in chicken motoneurons. *Brain Res.*, **33**, 560–564.

Brdiczka, D., Pette, D., Brunner, G. and Miller, F. (1968), Kompartimentierte Verteilung von Enzymen in Rattenlebermitochondrien. *Eur. J. Biochem.*, **5**, 294–304.

Brdiczka, D., Gerbitz, K. and Pette, D. (1969), Localization and function of external and internal carnitine acetyltransferases in mitochondria of rat liver and pig kidney. *Eur. J. Biochem.*, **11**, 234–240.

Bremer, J. and Greenberg, D.M. (1960), Biosynthesis of choline *in vitro Biochim. biophys. Acta* **37**, 173–175.

Bremer, J. and Greenberg, D.M. (1961), Methyl transfering enzyme system of microsomes in the biosynthesis of lecithin (phosphatidylcholine). *Biochim. biophys. Acta* **46**, 205–216.

Bremer, J., Figard, P.H. and Greenberg, D.M. (1960), The biosynthesis of choline and its relation to phospholipid metabolism. *Biochim. biophys. Acta*, **43**, 477–488.

Bressler, R. and Katz, R.I. (1965), The effect of carnitine on the rate of incorporation of precursors into fatty acids. *J. biol. Chem.*, **240**, 622–627.

Brooks, V.B. and Thies, R.E. (1962), Reduction of quantum content during neuromuscular transmission. *J. Physiol. (Lond.)*, **162**, 298–310.

Brown, G.L. (1965), The release and fate of the transmitter liberated by adrenergic nerves. *Proc. R. Soc. B.*, **162**, 1–9.

Brown, G.L. and Feldberg, W. (1936), The acetylcholine metabolism of a sympathetic ganglion. *J. Physiol. (Lond.)*, **88**, 265–283.

Browning, E.T. (1971), Free choline formation by cerebral cortical slices from rat brain. *Biochem. biophys. Res. Commun.*, **45**, 1586–1590.

Browning, E.T. (1972), Fluorometric enzyme assay for choline and acetylcholine. *Analyt. Biochem.*, **46**, 624–638.

Browning, E.T. (1976), Acetylcholine Synthesis: substrate availability and the synthetic reaction. In: *Biology of Cholinergic Function* (Goldberg, A.M. and Hanin, I. eds), pp. 187–201, Raven Press, New York.

Browning, E.T. and Schulman, M.P. (1968), [^{14}C] Acetylcholine synthesis by cortex slices of rat brain. *J. Neurochem.*, **15**, 1391–1405.

Brownstein, M.J., Saavedra, J.M., Axelrod, J., Zeman, G.H. and Carpenter, D.O. (1974), Coexistence of several putative neurotransmitters in single identified neurons of *Aplysia. Proc. natn. Acad. Sci. U.S.A.*, **71**, 4662–4665.

Brownstein, M., Kobayashi, R., Palkovits, M. and Saavedra, J.M. (1975) Choline acetyltransferase levels in diencephalic nuclei of the rat. *J. Neurochem.*, **24**, 35–38.

Buckley, B.M. and Williamson, D.H. (1973), Acetoacetate and brain lipogenesis: developmental pattern of acetoacetyl–coenzyme A synthetase in the soluble fraction of rat brain. *Biochem. J.* **132**, 653–656.

Buckley, G., Consolo, S., Giacobini, E. and McCaman, R. (1967a) A micromethod for the determination of choline acetylase in individual cells. *Acta physiol. scand.*, **71**, 341–347.

Buckley, G., Consolo, S., Giacobini, E. and Sjöqvist, F. (1967b), Choline acetylase in innervated and denervated sympathetic ganglia and ganglion cells of the cat. *Acta physiol. scand.* **71**, 348–356.

Bull, G. and Oderfeld-Nowak, B. (1971), Standardization of a radiochemical assay of choline acetyltransferase and a study of the activation of the enzyme in rabbit brain. *J. Neurochem.*, **18**, 935–941.

Bull, G., Feinstein, A. and Morris, D. (1964), Sedimentation behaviour and molecular weight of choline acetyltransferase. *Nature* (Lond.), **21**, 1326.

Bull, G., Hebb, C. and Ratković, D. (1970), Choline acetyltransferase activity of human brain tissue during development and maturity, *J. Neurochem.*, **17**, 1505–1516.

Buniatian, H., Hovhannissian, V.S. and Aprikian, G.V. (1965), The participation of *N*-acetyl-L-aspartic acid in brain metabolism. *J. Neurochem.*, **12**, 695–703.

Burdick, C.J. and Strittmatter, C.F. (1965), Appearance of biochemical components related to acetylcholine metabolism during the embryonic development of chick brain. *Archs. Biochem. Biophys.*, **109**, 293–301.

Burešová, M. and Tuček, S. (1977), Cessation of axonal transport of acetylcholinesterase after administration of cycloheximide. *Brain Res.*, **124**, 379–384.

Burgen, A.S.V., Burke, G. and Desbarats-Schonbaum, M.L. (1956) The specificity of brain choline acetylase. *Brit. J. Pharmac.*, **11**, 308–312.

Burnstock, G. (1976), Do some nerve cells release more than one trnasmitter? *Neuroscience,* **1**, 239–248.

Burt, A.M. (1968), Acetylcholinesterase and choline acetyltransferase activity in the developing chick spinal cord. *J. exp. Zool.* **169**, 107–112.

Burt, A. (1969), The histochemical demonstration of choline acetyltransferase activity in the spinal cord of the rat. *Anat. Rec.*, **163**, 162.

Burt, A.M. (1971), The histochemical localization of choline acetyltransferase. In: *Histochemistry of Nervous Transmission* (Eränkö, O., ed), *Progress in Brain Res.*, Vol. 34, pp. 327–335, Elsevier, Amsterdam.

Burt, A.M. (1973), Choline acetyltransferase and neuronal maturation. In: *Neurobiological Aspects of Maturation and Aging* (Ford, D.H. ed), *Progress in Brain Res.*, Vol. 40, pp. 245–252, Elsevier, Amsterdam.

Burt, A.M. (1975), Choline acetyltransferase and acetylcholinesterase in the developing rat spinal cord. *Exp. Neurol.*, **47**, 173–180.

Burt, A.M. and Narayanan, C.H. (1970), Effect of extrinsic neuronal connections on development of acetylcholinesterase and choline acetyltransferase activity in the ventral half of the chick spinal cord. *Expl Neurol.*, **29**, 201–210.

Burt, A.M. and Narayanan, C.H. (1976), Choline acetyltransferase, choline kinase, and acetylcholinesterase activities during the development of the chick ciliary ganglion. *Expl. Neurol.*, **53**, 703–713.

Burt, A.M. and Silver, A. (1973a), Non-enzymatic imidazole-catalysed acyl transfer reaction and acetylcholine synthesis. *Nature New Biol.*, **243**, 157–159.

Burt, A.M. and Silver, A. (1973b) Histochemistry of choline acetyltransferase: a critical analysis. *Brain Res.*, **62**, 509–516.

Burton, R.M. (1970), Chemical constituents which can bind acetylcholine. In: *Drugs and Cholinergic Mechanisms in the CNS* (Heilbronn, E. and Winter, A., eds), pp. 271–290, Almqvist and Wiksell, Stockholm.

Busch, H. (1955), Studies on the metabolism of pyruvate-2-C^{14} in tumor-bearing rats. *Cancer Res.*, **15**, 365–374.

Byers, M.R. (1974), Structural correlates of rapid axonal transport: evidence that microtubules may not be directly involved. *Brain Res.*, **75**, 97–113.

Canepa, F.G. (1964), Acetylcholine quanta. *Nature* (Lond.), **201**, 184–185.

Carlini, E.A. and Green, J.P. (1963), Acetylcholine activity in the sciatic nerve. *Biochem. Pharmac.*, **12**, 1367–1376.

Carlsson, C.-A., Bolander, P. and Sjöstrand, J. (1971a), Changes in axonal transport during regeneration of feline ventral roots. *J. neurol. Sci.*, **14**, 75–93.

Carlsson, C.-A., Bolander, P. and Sjöstrand, J. (1971b), Biochemical and histochemical changes in the feline gastrocnemius muscle during regeneration of ventral roots. *J. neurol. Sci.*, **14**, 95–105.

Carroll, P.T. and Buterbaugh, G.G. (1975a), Regional differences in high affinity choline transport velocity in guinea pig brain. *J. Neurochem.*, **24**, 229–232.

Carroll, P.T. and Buterbaugh, G.G. (1975b) High affinity choline transport in guinea pig brain and the effect of norepinephrine. *J. Neurochem.*, **24**, 917–924.

Carroll, P.T. and Goldberg, A.M. (1975), Relative importance of choline transport to spontaneous and potassium depolarized release of ACh. *J. Neurochem.*, **25**, 523–527.

Carson, V.G., Jenden, D.J., Cho, A.K. and Green, R. (1976), Effects of the choline acetyltransferase inhibitor 3′ chloro-4-stilbazole on brain acetylcholine metabolism. *Biochem. Pharmac.*, **25**, 195–199.

Ceccarelli, B., Hurlbut, W.P. and Mauro, A. (1972), Depletion of vesicles from frog neuromuscular junctions by prolonged tetanic stimulation. *J. cell Biol.*, **54**, 30–38.

Ceccarelli, B., Hurlbut, W.P. and Mauro, A. (1973), Turnover of transmitter and synaptic vesicles at the frog neuromuscular junction. *J. cell Biol.*, **57**, 499–524.

Chakrin, L.W. and Shideman, F.E. (1968), Synthesis of acetylcholine from labeled choline by brain. *Int. J. Neuropharmac.,* **7**, 337–349.

Chakrin, L.W. and Whittaker, V.P. (1969), The subcellular distribution of (*N*-Me-^{3}H)acetylcholine synthesized by brain *in vivo. Biochem. J.,* **113**, 97–107.

Chakrin, L.W., Shideman, F.E. and Marrazi, A.S. (1968), The *in vivo* synthesis and release of tritium-labeled acetylcholine by cat cerebral cortex. *Int. J. Neuropharmac.,* **7**, 351–358.

Chang, C.C. and Lee, C. (1970), Studies on the (^{3}H)choline uptake in rat phrenic nerve–diaphragm preparations. *Neuropharmac.,* **9**, 223–233.

Chao, L.-P. (1975), Subunits of choline acetyltransferase(EC 2.3.1.6). *J. Neurochem.,* **25**, 261–266.

Chao, L.-P. and Wolfgram, F. (1972), Spectrophotometric assay for choline acetyltransferase. *Analyt. Biochem.,* **46**, 114–118.

Chao, L.P. and Wolfgram, F. (1973), Purification and some properties of choline acetyltransferase (EC 2.3.1.6) from bovine brain. *J. Neurochem.,* **20**, 1075–1081.

Chao, L.-P. and Wolfgram, F. (1974), Activation, inhibition and aggregation of choline acetyltransferase (EC 2.3.1.6). *J. Neurochem.,* **23**, 697–701.

Chaplin, E.R., Goldberg, A.L. and Diamond, I. (1976), Leucine oxidation in brain slices and nerve endings. *J. Neurochem.,* **26**, 701–707.

Chappell, J.B. (1968), Systems used for the transport of substrates into mitochondria. *Brit. med. Bull.,* **24**, 150–157.

Cheney, D.L. and Costa, E. (1977), Pharmacological implication of brain acetylcholine turnover measurements in rat brain nuclei. *Ann. Rev. Pharmac.,* **17**, 369–386.

Cheney, D.L., Gubler, C.J. and Jaussi, A.W. (1969), Production of acetylcholine in rat brain following thiamine deprivation and treatment with thiamine antagonists. *J. Neurochem.,* **16**, 1283–1291.

Cheney, D.L., Lefevre, H.F. and Racagni, G. (1975a), Choline acetyltransferase activity and mass fragmentographic measurement of acetylcholine in specific nuclei and tracts of rat brain. *Neuropharmac.,* **14**, 801–809.

Cheney, D.L., Costa, E., Hanin, I., Racagni, G. and Trabucchi, M. (1975b), Acetylcholine turnover rate in brain of mice and rats: effects of various dose regimens of morphine. In: *Cholinergic Mechanism* (Waser, P.G., ed.), pp. 217–228, Raven Press, New York.

Cheney, D.L., Costa, E., Hanin, I., Trabucchi, M. and Wang, C.T. (1975c), Application of principles of steady-state kinetics to the *in vivo* estimation of acetylcholine turnover rate in mouse brain. *J. Pharmac., exp. Ther.,* **192**, 288–296.

Cheney, D.L., Costa, E., Racagni, G. and Zsilla, G. (1976a) Cholinergic and adenylate cyclase systems in rat brain nuclei during development. In: *Brain Dysfunction in Infantile Febrile Convulsions* (Brazier, M.A.B. and Coceani, F., eds), pp. 41–53, Raven Press, New York.

Cheney, D.L., Racagni, G. and Costa, E. (1976b) Distribution of acetylcholine and choline acetyltransferase in specific nuclei and tracts of rat brain. In: *Biology of Cholinergic Function,* (Goldberg, A.M. and Hanin, I., eds), pp. 655–659, Raven Press, New York.

Cheng, S.-C. (1971a), CO_2 fixation in the nervous tissue. *Int. Rev. Neurobiol.*, **14**, 125–157.

Cheng, S.-C. (1971b) The tricarboxylic acid cycle. In: *Handbook of Neurochemistry*, Lajtha, A., ed.), Vol. 9, pp. 283–315, Plenum Press, New York.

Cheng, S.-C. (1972), Pyruvate metabolism in the lobster nerve as affected by the partial pressure of carbon dioxide: observations on the synthesis of acetylcholine and on metabolic compartmentation. *J. Neurochem.*, **19**, 461–471.

Cheng, S.-C. and Nakamura, R. (1970), A study on the tricarboxylic acid cycle and the synthesis of acetylcholine in the lobster nerve. *Biochem. J.*, **118**, 451–455.

Chenykaeva, E.Yu. (1943), Content of acetylcholine in embryonic and denervated muscles of the rabbit (Russ.). *Izv. A.N. SSSR, ser, biol.*, **1**, 35–38.

Chiappinelli, V., Giacobini, E., Pilar, G. and Uchimura, H. (1976), Induction of cholinergic enzymes in chick ciliary ganglion and iris muscle cells during synapse formation. *J. Physiol.* (Lond.), **257**, 749–766.

Choi, R.L., Freeman, J.J. and Jenden, D.J. (1975), Kinetics of plasma choline in relation to turnover of brain choline and formation of acetylcholine. *J. Neurochem.*, **24**, 735–741.

Chojnacki, T., Korzybski, T. and Ansell, G.B. (1964), The methylation of natural and unnatural analogues of ^{32}P-labelled phosphatidylethanolamine by brain and liver tissue. *Biochem. J.*, **90**, 18P–19P.

Chuang, H.Y.K., Mohammad, S.F. and Mason, R.G. (1976), Acetylcholinesterase, choline acetyltransferase, and the postulated acetylcholine receptor of canine platelets. *Biochem. Pharmac.*, **25**, 1971–1977.

Ciaranello, R.D. and Axelrod, J. (1975), Effects of dexamethasone on neurotransmitter enzymes in chromaffin tissue of the newborn rat. *J. Neurochem.*, **24**, 775–778.

Cleland, W.W. (1963), The kinetics of enzyme-catalyzed reactions with two or more substrates or products. I. Nomenclature and rate equations. *Biochim. biophys. Acta*, **67**, 104–137.

Cleland, W.W. (1970), Steady state kinetics. In: *The Enzymes* (Boyer, P.D., ed.), Vol. 2, pp. 1–65, Academic Press, New York.

Clinkenbeard, K.D., Sugiyama, T., Moss, J., Reed, W.D. and Lane, M.D. (1973), Molecular and catalytic properties of cytosolic acetoacetyl coenzyme A thiolase from avian liver. *J. biol. Chem.*, **248**, 2275–2284.

Clinkenbeard, K.D., Reed, W.D., Mooney, R.A. and Lane, M.D. (1975), Intracellular localization of the 3-hydroxy-3-methylglutaryl coenzyme A cycle enzymes in liver. *J. biol. Chem.*, **250**, 3108–3116.

Coggeshall, R.E., Dewhurst, S.A., Weinreich, D. and McCaman, R.E. (1972), Aromatic acid decarboxylase and choline acetylase activities in a single identified 5-HT containing cell of the leech. *J. Neurobiol.*, **3**, 259–265.

Cohen, E.L. and Wurtman, R.J. (1975), Brain acetylcholine: Increase after systemic choline administration. *Life Sci.*, **16**, 1095–1102.

Cohen, E.L. and Wurtman, R.J. (1976), Brain acetylcholine: control by dietary choline. *Science*, **191**, 561–562.

Collier, B. (1969), The preferential release of newly synthesized transmitter by a sympathetic ganglion. *J. Physiol.* (Lond.), **205**, 341–352.

Collier, B. and Ilson, D. (1977), The effect of preganglionic nerve stimulation on the accumulation of certain analogues of choline by a sympathetic ganglion. *J. Physiol.* (Lond.), **264**, 489–509.

Collier, B. and Katz, H.S. (1971), The synthesis, turnover and release of surplus acetylcholine in a sympathetic ganglion. *J. Physiol.* (Lond.), **214**, 537–552.

Collier, B. and Katz, H.S. (1974), Acetylcholine synthesis from recaptured choline by a sympathetic ganglion. *J. Physiol.* (Lond.), **238**, 639–655.

Collier, B. and Katz, H.S. (1975), Studies upon the mechanism by which acetylcholine releases surplus acetylcholine in a sympathetic ganglion. *Brit. J. Pharmac.*, **55**, 189–197.

Collier, B. and MacIntosh, F.C. (1969), The source of choline for acetylcholine synthesis in a sympathetic ganglion. *Can. J. Physiol. Pharmac.*, **47**, 127–135.

Collier, B., Poon, P. and Salehmoghaddam, S. (1972), The formation of choline and of acetylcholine by brain *in vitro*. *J. Neurochem.*, **19**, 51–60.

Collier, B., Lovat, S., Ilson, D., Barker, L.A. and Mittag, T.W. (1977), The uptake, metabolism and release of homocholine: studies with rat brain synaptosomes and cat superior cervical ganglion. *J. Neurochem.*, **28**, 331–339.

Comline, R.S. (1946), Synthesis of acetylcholine by non-nervous tissue. *J. Physiol.* (Lond.), **105**, 6P.

Consolo, S., Ladinsky, H., Peri, G. and Garattini, S. (1972), Effects of central stimulants and depressants on mouse brain acetylcholine and choline levels. *Eur. J. Pharmac.*, **18**, 251–255.

Consolo, S., Ladinsky, H. and Bianchi, S. (1975), Decrease in rat striatal acetylcholine levels by some direct- and indirect-acting dopaminergic antagonists. *Eur. J. Pharmac.*, **33**, 345–351.

Cooke, W.J. and Robinson, J.D. (1971), Factors influencing choline movements in rat brain slices. *Biochem. Pharmac.*, **20**, 2355–2366.

Coraboeuf, E., Le Douarin, G. and Obrecht-Courtis, G. (1970), Release of acetylcholine by chick embryo heart before innervation. *J. Physiol.* (Lond.), **206**, 383–395.

Costa, E., Cheney, D.L. and Racagni, G. (1976), Steady state and dynamics of putative neurotransmitters in tel-diencephalic nuclei: a study using multiple ion detection. In: *Drugs and Central Synaptic Transmission* (Bradley, P.B. and Dhawan, B.N., eds), pp. 37–48, MacMillan Press, London.

Cottrell, G.A. (1976), Does the giant cerebral neurone of *Helix* release two transmitters: ACh and serotonin? *J. Physiol.* (Lond.), **259**, 44P–45P.

Coyle, J.T. and Yamamura, H.I. (1976), Neurochemical aspects of the ontogenesis of cholinergic neurons in the rat brain. *Brain Res.*, **118**, 429–440.

Crockett, J.L., Edgerton, V.R., Max, S.R. and Barnard, R.J. (1976), The neuromuscular junction in response to endurance training. *Expl. Neurol.*, **51**, 207–215.

Crossland, J. (1951), The use of liquid air in the extraction of acetylcholine. *J. Physiol.* (Lond.), **114**, 318–324.

Crossland, J. and Merrick, A.J. (1954), The effect of anaesthesia on the acetylcholine content of brain. *J. Physiol.* (Lond.), **125**, 56–66.

Crossland, J. and Slater, P. (1968), The effect of some drugs on the 'free' and 'bound' acetylcholine content of rat brain. *Brit. J. Pharmac.*, **33**, 42–47.

Crossland, J., Elliott, K.A.C. and Pappius, H.M. (1955), Acetylcholine content of brain during insulin hypoglycemia. *Am. J. Physiol.*, **183**, 32–34.

Cuénod, M., Boesch, J., Marko, P., Perisic, M., Sandri, C. and Schonbach, J. (1972), Contributions of axoplasmic transport to synaptic structures and functions. *Int. J. Neurosci.*, **4**, 77–87.

Currier, S.F. and Mautner, H.G. (1974), On the mechanism of action of choline acetyltransferase. *Proc. natn. Acad. Sci. U.S.A.*, **71**, 3355–3358.

Currier, S.F. and Mautner, H.G. (1976), Evidence for a thiol reagent inhibiting choline acetyltransferase by reacting with the thiol group of coenzyme A forming a potent inhibitor. *Biochem. biophys. Res. Commun.*, **69**, 431–436.

D'Adamo, A.F. and D'Adamo, A.P. (1968), Acetyl transport mechanisms in the nervous system. The oxoglutarate shunt and fatty acid synthesis in the developing rat brain. *J. Neurochem.*, **15**, 315–323.

D'Adamo, A.F. and Haft, D.E. (1965), An alternate pathway of α-ketoglutarate catabolism in the isolated, perfused rat liver. I. Studies with DL-glutamate-2 and -5-^{14}C. *J. biol. Chem.*, **240**, 613–617.

D'Adamo, A.F., Gidez, L.I. and Yatsu, F.M. (1968), Acetyl transport mechanisms. Involvement of *N*-acetyl aspartic acid in *de novo* fatty acid biosynthesis in the developing rat brain. *Expl. Brain Res.*, **5**, 267–273.

Dahlström, A. (1967a), The transport of noradrenaline between two stimultaneously performed ligations of the sciatic nerves of rat and cat. *Acta physiol. scand.*, **69**, 158–166.

Dahlström, A. (1967b), The intraneuronal distribution of noradrenaline and the transport and life span of amine storage granules in the sympathetic adrenergic neuron. *Naunyn-Schmiedeberg's Archs. Pharmakol.*, **257**, 93–115.

Dahlström, A. (1971), Axoplasmic transport (with particular respect to adrenergic neurons). *Phil. Trans. R. Soc. Ser. B.* **261**, 325–358.

Dahlström, A. and Häggendal, J. (1970), Axonal transport of amine storage granules in sympathetic adrenergic neurons. In: *Biochemistry of Simple Neuronal Models* (Costa, E. and Giacobini, E., eds), *Adv. Biochem. Psychopharmacol.*, Vol. **2**, pp. 65–93, Raven Press, New York.

Dahlström, A. and Heiwall, P.O. (1975), Intra-axonal transport of transmitters in mammalian neurons. *J. Neural Transmiss.*, Suppl. **12**, 97–114.

Dahlström, A.B., Evans, C.A.N., Häggendal, C.J., Heiwall, P.-O. and Saunders, N.R. (1974a), Rapid transport of acetylcholine in rat sciatic nerve proximal and distal to a lesion. *J. neural Transmiss.*, **35**, 1–11.

Dahlström, A., Häggendal, J., Heilbronn, E., Heiwall, P.-O. and Saunders, N.R. (1974b), Proximodistal transport of acetylcholine in peripheral cholinergic neurons. In: *Dynamics of Degeneration and Growth in Neurons* (Fuxe, K., Olson, L. and Zotterman, Y., eds), pp. 275–289, Pergamon Press, Oxford.

Dahlström, A., Heiwall, P.-O., Häggendal, J. and Saunders, N.R. (1975a), Effect of antimitotic drugs on the intraaxonal transport of neurotransmitters in rat adrenergic and cholinergic nerves. *Ann. N.Y. Acad. Sci.*, **253**, 507–516.

Dahlström, A., Heiwall, P.-O. and Larsson, P.A. (1975b), Comparison between the effect of colchicine and lumicolchicine on axonal transport in rat motor neurons. *J. Neural Transmiss.*, **37**, 305–311.

Dale, H.H. (1935), Pharmacology and nerve-endings. *Proc. R. Soc. Med.*, **28**, 319–332.

Dale, H.H. (1953), *Adventures in Physiology*, p. 636, The Wellcome Trust, London.

Das, N. and Srere, P.A. (1972), Exchange of methyl protons of acetyl coenzyme A catalyzed by adenosine triphosphate citrate lyase. *Biochemistry*, **11**, 1534–1537.

Dauterman, W.C. and Mehrotra, K.N. (1963), The *N*-alkyl group specificity of choline acetylase from rat brain. *J. Neurochem.*, **10**, 113–117.

Davison, P.F. (1970), Axoplasmic transport: physical and chemical aspects. In: *The Neurosciences, Second Study Program*, (Schmitt, F.O., ed), pp. 851–857, The Rockefeller University Press, New York.

Dawson, R.M.C. (1956), Liver glycerylphosphorylcholine diesterase. *Biochem. J.*, **62**, 689–693.

Decker, K. (1959), *Die aktivierte Essigsäure*, F. Enke Verlag, Stuttgart.

De Duve, C., Wattiaux, R. and Baudhuin, P. (1962), Distribution of enzymes between subcellular fractions in animal tissues. *Adv. Enzymol.*, **24**, 291–358.

Del Castillo, J. and Katz, B. (1954), Quantal components of the endplate potential. *J. Physiol.*, (Lond.), **124**, 560–573.

Del Castillo, J. and Katz, B. (1955), Local activity at a depolarized nerve–muscle junction. *J. Physiol.*, (Lond.), **128**, 396–411.

Del Castillo, J. and Katz, B. (1956), Biophysical aspects of neuromuscular transmission. *Progr. Biophys. biophys. Chem.*, **6**, 121–170.

Dennis, M.J. and Miledi, R. (1974a), Electrically induced release of acetylcholine from denervated Schwann cells. *J. Physiol.*, (Lond.), **237**, 431–452.

Dennis, M.J. and Miledi, R. (1974b), Non-transmitting neuromuscular junctions during an early stage of endplate reinnervation. *J. Physiol,*, (Lond.), **239**, 553–570.

Dennis, M.J. and Miledi, R. (1974c), Characteristics of transmitter release at regenerating frog neuromuscular junctions. *J. Physiol.*, (Lond.), **239**, *571–594.*

Denton, R.M., Randle, P.J., Bridges, B.J., Cooper, R.H., Kerbey, A.L., Pask, H.T., Severson, D.L., Stansbie, D. and Whitehouse, S. (1975), Regulation of mammalian pyruvate dehydrogenase. *Molec. cell Biochem.*, **9**, 27–53.

De Robertis, E.D.P. (1964), *Histophysiology of synapses and neurosecretion.* Pergamon Press, Oxford.

De Robertis, E. and Bennett, H.S. (1954), Submicroscopic vesicular component in the synapse. *Fed. Proc. Fedn. Am. Socs. exp. Biol.*, **13**, 35.

De Robertis, E.D.P. and Bennett, H.S. (1955), Some features of the submicroscopic morphology of synapses in frog and earthworm. *J. biophys. biochem. Cytol.*, **1**, 47–58.

De Robertis, E. and Ferreira, A.V. (1957), Submicroscopic changes of the nerve endings in the adrenal medulla after stimulation of the splanchnic nerve. *J. biophys. biochem. Cytol.*, **3**, 611–614.

De Robertis, E., Rodríguez de Lores Arnaiz, G. and Pellegrino de Iraldi, A. (1962), Isolation of synaptic vesicles from nerve endings of the rat brain. *Nature* (Lond.), **194**, 794–795.

De Robertis, E., Rodriguez de Lores Arnaiz, G., Salganicoff, L., Pellegrino de Iraldi, A. and Zieher, L.M. (1963), Isolation of synaptic vesicles and structural organization of the acetylcholine system within brain nerve endings. *J. Neurochem.*, **10**, 225–235.

DeVivo, D.D., Leckie, M.P. and Agrawal, H.C. (1975), D-β-hydroxybutyrate: a major precursor of amino acids in developing rat brain. *J. Neurochem.*, **25**, 161–170.

DeVivo, D.C., Fujimoto, K., Leckie, M.P. and Agrawal, H.C. (1976), Subcellular distribution of ketone body metabolizing enzymes in the rat brain. *J. Neurochem.*, **26**, 635–637.

Diamond, I. (1971), Choline metabolism in brain. The role of choline transport and the effects of phenobarbital. *Archs. Neurol.*, **24**, 333–339.

Diamond, I. and Kennedy, E.P. (1968), A sensitive radiochemical assay for choline acetylase. *Analyt. Biochem.*, **24**, 90–95.

Diamond, I. and Kennedy, E.P. (1969), Carrier-mediated transport of choline into synaptic nerve endings. *J. biol. Chem.*, **244**, 3258–3263.

Diamond, I. and Milfay, D. (1972), Uptake of (^{3}H-methyl)choline by microsomal, synaptosomal, mitochondrial and synaptic vesicle fractions of rat brain. *J. Neurochem.*, **19**, 1899–1909.

Diamond, I., Franklin, G.M. and Milfay, D. (1974), The relationship of choline acetyltransferase activity at the neuromuscular junction to changes in muscle mass and function. *J. Physiol.* (Lond.), **236**, 247–257.

Dibner, M.D., Mytilineou, C. and Black, I.B. (1977), Target organ regulation of sympathetic neuron development. *Brain Res.*, **123**, 301–310.

Dieterich, H.A., Kaffei, H., Kilbinger, H. and Löffelholz, K. (1976), The effects of physostigmine on cholinesterase activity, storage and release of acetylcholine in the isolated chicken heart. *J. Pharmac. exp. Ther.*, **199**, 236–246.

Di Giamberardino, L., Bennett, G., Koenig, H.L. and Droz, B. (1973), Axonal migration of protein and glycoprotein to nerve endings. III. Cell fraction analysis of chicken ciliary ganglion after intracerebral injection of labelled precursors of proteins and glycoproteins. *Brain Res.*, **60**, 147–159.

Doležalová, H., Giacobini, E., Giacobini, G., Rossi, A. and Toschi, C. (1974), Developmental variations of choline acetyl-transferase, dopamine-β-hydroxylase and monoamineoxidase in chicken embryo and chicken sympathetic ganglia. *Brain Res.*, **73**, 309–320.

Donat, J.R. and Wiśniewski, H.M. (1973), The spatio-temporal pattern of Wallerian degeneration in mammalian peripheral nerves. *Brain Res.*, **53**, 41–53.

Dowdall, M.J. (1975), Synthesis and storage of acetylcholine in cholinergic nerve terminals. In: *Metabolic Compartmentation and Neurotransmission* (Berl, S., Clarke, D.D. and Schneider, D., eds), pp. 585–607, Plenum Publishing Corporation, New York.

Dowdall, M.J. and Simon, E.J. (1973), Comparative studies on synaptosomes: Uptake of (*N*-Me^{3}H)choline by synaptosomes from squid optic lobes. *J. Neurochem.*, **21**, 969–982.

Dowdall, M.J. and Zimmermann, H. (1974), Evidence for heterogenous pools of acetylcholine in isolated cholinergic synaptic vesicles. *Brain Res.*, **71**, 160–166.

Dowdall, M.J., Boyne, A.F. and Whittaker, V.P. (1974), Adenosine triphosphate; a constituent of cholinergic synaptic vesicles. *Biochem. J.*, **140**, 1–12.

Dowdall, M.J., Fox, G., Wächtler, K., Whittaker, V.P. and Zimmermann, H. (1976), Recent studies on the comparative biochemistry of the cholinergic neuron. *Cold Spring Harb. Symp. Quant. Biol.*, **40**, 65–81.

Drahota, Z., Hahn, P., Mourek, J. and Trojanová, M. (1965), The effect of aceto-acetate on oxygen consumption of brain slices from infant and adult rats. *Physiol. bohemoslov.*, **14**, 134–136.

Dreyfus, P. (1975), Identification de l'acétate comme précurseur du radical acétyle de l'acétylcholine des jonctions neuro-muscularires du rat. *C. r. Acad. Sci.* D **280**, 1893–1894.

Dross, K. (1975), Effects of di-isopropylfluorophosphate on the metabolism of choline and phosphatidylcholine in rat brain. *J. Neurochem.*, **24**, 701–706.

Dross, K. and Kewitz, H. (1972), Concentration and origin of choline in the rat brain. *Naunyn-Schmiedeberg's Arch. Pharmakol.*, **274**, 91–106.

Droz, B. (1973), Renewal of synaptic proteins. *Brain Res.*, **62**, 383–394.

Droz, B., Koenig, H.L. and Di Giamberardino, L. (1973), Axonal migration of protein and glycoprotein to nerve endings. I. Radioautographic analysis of the renewal of protein in nerve endings of chicken ciliary ganglion after intracerebral injection of [^{3}H]lysine. *Brain Res.*, **60**, 93–127.

Droz, B., Rambourg, A. and Koenig, H.L. (1975), The smooth endoplasmic reticulum: Structure and role in the renewal of axonal membrane and synaptic vesicles by fast axonal transport. *Brain Res.*, **93**, 1–13.

Dunant, Y., Gautron, J., Israël, M., Lesbats, B. and Manaranche, R. (1972), Les compartiments d'acétylcholine de l'organe électrique de la Torpille et leurs modifications par la stimulation. *J. Neurochem.*, **19**, 1987–2002.

Dunant, Y., Gautron, J., Israël, M., Lesbats, B. and Manaranche, R. (1974a), Evolution de la décharge de l'organe électrique de la Torpille et variations simultanées de l'acétylcholine au cours de la stimulation. *J. Neurochem.*, **23**, 635–643.

Dunant, Y., Jirounek, P., Israël, M., Lesbats, B. and Manaranche, R. (1974b), Sustained oscillations of acetylcholine during nerve stimulation. *Nature* (Lond.), **252**, 485–486.

Dunant, Y., Israël, M., Lesbats, B., Manaranche, R. and Mastour, P. (1975), Variations périodiques du taux d'acétylcholine durant la stimulation de l'organe électrique de la Torpille. *C. r. Acad. Sci.*, D **280**, 641–643.

Dunant, Y., Israël, M., Lesbats, B. and Manaranche, R. (1976), Loss of vesicular acetylcholine in the *Torpedo* electric organ on discharge against high external resistance. *J. Neurochem.*, **27**, 975–977.

Dunant, Y., Israël, M., Lesbats, B. and Manaranche, R. (1977), Oscillation of acetyl-choline during nerve activity in the *Torpedo* electric organ. *Brain Res.*, **125**, 123–140.

Dziegielewska, K.M., Saunders, N.R., Evans, C.A.N., Skacel, P.O., Häggendal, C.J., Heiwall, P.-O. and Dahlström, A.B. (1976), Effects of colchicine and vinblastine on axonal transport of choline acetyltransferase in rat sciatic nerve. *Acta physiol. scand.*, **96**, 486–494.

Eade, I., Hebb, C. and Mann, S.P. (1973), Free choline levels in the rat brain. *J. Neurochem.,* **20**, 1499–1502.

Ebel, A., Massarelli, R., Sensenbrenner, M. and Mandel, P. (1974), Choline acetyltransferase and acetylcholinesterase activities in chicken brain hemispheres *in vivo* and in cell culture. *Brain Res.,* **76**, 461–472.

Edström, A. and Hanson, M. (1973), Retrograde axonal transport of proteins *in vitro* in frog sciatic nerves. *Brain Res.,* **61**, 311–320.

Edwards, Y.H., Chase, J.F.A., Edwards, M.R. and Tubbs, P.K. (1974), Carnitine acetyltransferase: the question of multiple forms. *Eur. J. Biochem.,* **46**, 209–215.

Eggerer, H. (1965), Zum Mechanismus der biologischen Umwandlung von Citronensäure. VI. Citrat-synthase ist eine Acetyl–CoA-Enolase. *Biochem. Z.* **343**, 111–138.

Ehinger, B., Falck, B., Persson, H., Rosengren, A.-M. and Rosengren, E. (1966), Choline acetylase activity in the normal and denervated cat iris. *Life Sci.,* **5**, 481–483.

Ehinger, B., Falck, B., Persson, H., Rosengren, A.-M. and Sporrong, B. (1970), Acetylcholine in adrenergic terminals of the cat iris. *J. Physiol.* (Lond.), **209**, 557–565.

Eisenstadt, M.L. and Schwartz, J.H. (1975), Metabolism of acetylcholine in the nervous system of *Aplysia californica.* III. Studies of an identified cholinergic neuron. *J. gen. Physiol.,* **65**, 293–313.

Eisenstadt, M., Goldman, J.E., Kandel, E.R., Koike, H., Koester, J. and Schwartz, J.H. (1973), Intrasomatic injection of radioactive precursors for studying transmitter synthesis in identified neurons of *Aplysia californica. Proc. natn. Acad. Sci. U.S.A.,* **70**, 3371–3375.

Eisenstadt, M.L., Treistman, S.N. and Schwartz, J.H. (1975), Metabolism of acetylcholine in the nervous system of *Aplysia californica.* II. Regional localization and characterization of choline uptake. *J. gen. Physiol.,* **65**, 275–291.

Ekström, J. (1972), Choline acetyltransferase in salivary glands after surgical and chemical sympathectomy. *Acta physiol. scand.,* **86**, 539–545.

Ekström, J. (1973), Choline acetyltransferase and secretory responses of the rat's salivary glands after liquid diet. *Q. J. expl Physiol.,* **58**, 171–179.

Ekström, J. (1974), Choline acetyltransferase activity in rat salivary glands after cellulose rich diet or treatment with an atropine-like drug. *Q. J. expl Physiol.,* **59**, 191–199.

Ekström, J. (1975), Compensatory increase in choline acetyltransferase activity in salivary glands and diaphragm muscle of the rat. *Acta physiol. scand.,* **93**, 525–530.

Ekström, J. (1976), Choline acetyltransferase activity and weight of salivary glands in rats at different ages. *Acta physiol. scand.* **98**, 185–191.

Ekström, J. (1977a), The effect of teeth amputations on the choline acetyltransferase activity of rat submaxillary glands. *Acta physiol. scand.,* **99**, 48–52.

Ekström, J. (1977b), Choline acetyltransferase activity in parotid glands of rats after prolonged treatment with pilocarpine. *Acta physiol. scand.,* **99**, 110–112.

Ekström, J. and Emmelin, N. (1971), Movement of choline acetyltransferase in axons disconnected from their cell bodies. *J. Physiol.* (Lond.), **216**, 247–256.

Ekström, J. and Emmelin, N. (1974), Reinnervation of the denervated parotid gland of the cat. *Q. J. expl Physiol.,* **59**, 1–9.

Ekström, J. and Holmberg, J. (1972a), Choline acetyltransferase in the normal and parasympathetically denervated parotid gland of the dog. *Acta physiol. scand.*, **86**, 353–358.

Ekström, J. and Holmberg, J. (1972b), Effect of decentralization on the choline acetyltransferase of the canine parotid gland. *J. Physiol.* (Lond.), **222**, 93P–94P.

Emmelin, N., Nordenfelt, I. and Perec, C. (1966), Rate of fall in choline acetyltransferase activity in denervated diaphragms as dependent on the length of the degenerating nerve. *Experientia* (Basel), **22**, 725–726.

Emson, P.C. and Fonnum, F. (1974), Choline acetyltransferase, acetylcholinesterase and aromatic L-amino acid decarboxylase in single identified nerve cell bodies from snail *Helix aspersa*. *J. Neurochem.*, **22**, 1079–1088.

Emson, P.C., Malthe-Sørenssen, D. and Fonnum, F. (1974), Purification and properties of choline acetyltransferase from the nervous system of different invertebrates. *J. Neurochem.*, **22**, 1089–1098.

Endröczi, E., Hartmann, G. and Lissák, K. (1967), Maturation of the acetylcholine-cholinesterase system of the brain stem in the newborn rat. *Acta physiol., hung.*, **32**, 307–315.

Eng, L.F., Uyeda, C.T., Chao, L.P. and Wolfgram, F. (1974), Antibody to bovine choline acetyltransferase and immunofluorescent localisation of the enzyme in neurons. *Nature* (Lond.), **250**, 243–245.

Euler, U.S. v. (1972), Synthesis, uptake and storage of catecholamines in adrenergic nerves, the effect of drugs. In: *Catecholamines* (Blaschko, H. and Muscholl, E., eds), *Handbook of Experimental Pharmacology*, New Series, Vol. 32, pp. 186–230, Springer Verlag, Berlin.

Evans, C.A.N. and Saunders, N.R. (1967), The distribution of acetylcholine in normal and in regenerating nerves. *J. Physiol.* (Lond.), **192**, 79–92.

Fahn, S. and Côté, L.J. (1968), Regional distribution of choline acetylase in the brain of the rhesus monkey. *Brain Res.*, **7**, 323–325.

Fahn, S. and Côté, L.J. (1976), Stability of enzymes in post-mortem rat brain. *J. Neurochem.*, **26**, 1039–1042.

Fardeau, M., Israël, M. and Manaranche, R. (eds, (1973), *La transmission cholinergique de l'excitation.* Editions INSERM, Paris.

Fatt, P. and Katz, B. (1952), Spontaneous subthreshold activity at motor nerve terminals. *J. Physiol.* (Lond.), **117**, 109–128.

Feldberg, W. (1943), Synthesis of acetylcholine in sympathetic ganglia and cholinergic nerves. *J. Physiol.* (Lond.), **101**, 432–445.

Feldberg, W. and Hebb, C. (1947), The effects of magnesium ions and of creatine phosphate on the synthesis of acetylcholine. *J. Physiol.* (Lond.), **106**, 8–17.

Feldberg, W. and Lin, R.C.Y. (1960), Synthesis of acetylcholine in the wall of the digestive tract. *J. Physiol.*, (Lond.), **111**, 96–118.

Feldberg, W. and Mann, T. (1945), Formation of acetylcholine in cell-free extracts from brain. *J. Physiol.*, (Lond.), **104**, 8–20.

Feldberg, W. and Mann, T. (1946), Properties and distribution of the enzyme system which synthesizes acetylcholine in nervous tissue. *J. Physiol.* (Lond.), **104**, 411–425.

Filogamo, G. and Marchisio, P.C. (1970), Choline acetyltransferase activity of rabbit ileum wall. The effects of extrinsic and intrinsic denervation and of combined experimental hypertrophy. *Arch. int. Physiol.*, **78**, 141–152.

Filogamo, G. and Marchisio, P.C. (1971), Acetylcholine system and neural development. *Neurosciences Res.*, **4**, 29–64.

Fitzgerald, G.G. and Cooper, J.R. (1967), Studies on acetylcholine in the corneal epithelium. *Fedn. Proc. Fedn. Am. Socs. exp. Biol.*, **26**, 651.

Fitzgerald, G.G. and Cooper, J.R. (1971), Acetylcholine as a possible sensory mediator in rabbit corneal epithelium. *Biochem. Pharmac.*, **20**, 2741–2748.

Fletcher, P. and Forrester, T. (1975), The effect of curare on the release of acetylcholine from mammalian motor nerve terminals and an estimate of quantum content. *J. Physiol.* (Lond.), **251**, 131–144.

Flood, P.R., Fonnum, F. and Storm-Mathisen, J. (1970), Choline acetyltransferase and acetylcholinesterase in myo–tendinous and neuro–muscular junctions of mouse skeletal muscle. *Experientia* (Basel), **26**, 964–965.

Fonnum, F. (1967), The 'compartmentation' of choline acetyltransferase within the synaptosome. *Biochem. J.*, **103**, 262–270.

Fonnum, F. (1968), Choline acetyltransferase binding to and release from membranes. *Biochem. J.* **109**, 389–398.

Fonnum, F. (1969a), Isolation of choline esters from aqueous solution by extraction with sodium tetraphenylboron in organic solvents. *Biochem. J.* **113**, 291–298.

Fonnum, F. (1969b), Radiochemical microassays for the determination of choline acetyltransferase and acetylcholinesterase activities. *Biochem. J.* **115**, 465–472.

Fonnum, F. (1970a), Topographical and subcellular localization of choline acetyltransferase in rat hippocampal region. *J. Neurochem.*, **17**, 1029–1037.

Fonnum, F. (1970b), Surface charge of choline acetyltransferase from different species. *J. Neurochem.*, **17**, 1095–1100.

Fonnum, F. (1975), A rapid radiochemical method for the determination of choline acetyltransferase. *J. Neurochem.*, **24**, 407–409.

Fonnum, F. (1976), Radiochemical assays for choline acetyltransferase and acetylcholinesterase. In: *Research Methods in Neurochemistry* (Marks, N. and Rodnight, R., eds), Vol. 3, pp. 253–275, Plenum Publishing Co. New York.

Fonnum, F. and Guttormsen, D.M. (1969), Changes in acetylcholine content of rat brain by toxic doses of di-isopropyl phosphorofluoridate. *Experientia* (Basel), **25**, 505–506.

Fonnum, F. and Malthe-Sørenssen, D. (1972), Molecular properties of choline acetyltransferase and their importance for the compartmentation of acetylcholine synthesis. In: *Biochemical and Pharmacological Mechanisms Underlying Behaviour* (Bradley, P.B. and Brimblecombe, R.W., eds), *Progress in Brain Res.*, Vol. 36, pp. 13–27, Elsevier, Amsterdam.

Fonnum, F. and Malthe-Sørenssen, D. (1973), Membrane affinities and subcellular distribution of the different molecular forms of choline acetyltransferase from rat. *J. Neurochem.*, **20**, 1351–1359.

Fonnum, F., Frizell, M. and Sjöstrand, J. (1973), Transport, turnover and distribution of choline acetyltransferase and acetylcholinesterase in the vagus and hypoglossal nerves of the rabbit. *J. Neurochem.*, **21**, 1109–1120.

Fonnum, F., Frizell, M. and Sjöstrand, J. (1976), Redistribution of choline acetyltransferase and acetylcholinesterase in an isolated nerve segment of the rabbit vagus nerve. *J. Neurochem.*, **26**, 427–429.

Freeman, J.J. and Jenden, D.J. (1976), The source of choline for acetylcholine synthesis in brain. *Life Sci.*, **19**, 949–962.

Freeman, J.J., Choi, R.L. and Jenden, D.J. (1975a), Plasma choline: its turnover and exchange with brain choline. *J. Neurochem.*, **24**, 729–734.

Freeman, J.J., Choi, R.L. and Jenden, D.J. (1975b), The effect of hemicholinium on behavior and on brain acetylcholine and choline in the rat. *Psychopharmacol. Commun.*, **1**, 15–27.

Friesen, A.J.D. and Khatter, J.C. (1971), The effect of preganglionic stimulation on the acetylcholine and choline content of a sympathetic ganglion. *Can. J. Physiol. Pharmac.*, **49**, 375–381.

Fritz, I.B. and Yue, K.T.N. (1964), Effect of carnitine on acetyl–CoA oxidation by heart muscle mitochondria. *Amer. J. Physiol.*, **206**, 531–535.

Frizell, M. and Sjöstrand, J. (1974a), The axonal transport of slowly migrating [^{3}H]leucine labelled proteins and the regeneration rate in regenerating hypoglossal and vagus nerves of the rabbit. *Brain Res.*, **81**, 267–283.

Frizell, M. and Sjöstrand, J. (1974b), Transport of proteins, glycoproteins and cholinergic enzymes in regenerating hypoglossal neurons. *J. Neurochem.*, **22**, 845–850.

Frizell, M. and Sjöstrand, J. (1974c), Retrograde axonal transport of rapidly migrating proteins in the vagus and hypoglossal nerves of the rabbit. *J. Neurochem.*, **23**, 651–657.

Frizell, M., Hasselgren, P.O. and Sjöstrand, J. (1970), Axoplasmic transport of acetylcholinesterase and choline acetyltransferase in the vagus and hypoglossal nerve of the rabbit. *Expl. Brain Res.*, **10**, 526–531.

Frizell, M., McLean, W.G. and Sjöstrand, J. (1975), Slow axonal transport of proteins: blockade by interruption of contact between cell body and axon. *Brain Res.*, **86**, 67–73.

Furshpan, E.J., MacLeish, P.R., O'Lague, P.H. and Potter, D.D. (1976), Chemical transmission between rat sympathetic neurons and cardiac myocytes developing in microcultures: evidence for cholinergic, adrenergic, and dual-function neurons. *Proc. natn. Acad. Sci. U.S.A.*, **73**, 4225–4229.

Gaitonde, M.K., Dahl, D.R. and Elliott, K.A.C. (1965), Entry of glucose carbon into amino acids of rat brain and liver *in vivo* after an injection of uniformly ^{14}C labelled glucose. *Biochem. J.* **94**, 345–352.

Gardiner, J.E. and Domer, F.R. (1968), Movement of choline between the blood and cerebrospinal fluid in the cat. *Archs. int. Pharmacodyn. Thér.*, **175**, 482–496.

Gardiner, J.E. and Paton, W.D.M. (1972), The control of the plasma choline concentration in the cat. *J. Physiol.* (Lond.), **227**, 71–86.

Gardiner, J.E. and Whittaker, V.P. (1954), The identification of propionylcholine as a constituent of ox spleen. *Biochem. J.* **58**, 24–31.

Garland, P.B. and Yates, D.W. (1967), Fatty-acid oxidation and mitochondrial structure and compartmentation. In: *Mitochondrial Structure and Compartmentation* (Quagliariello, E., Papa, S., Slater, E.C. and Tager, J.M., eds), pp. 385–399, Adriatica Editrice, Bari.

Garland, P.B., Shepherd, D. and Yates, D.W. (1965), Steady-state concentrations of coenzyme A, acetyl–coenzyme A and long-chain fatty acyl–coenzyme A in rat-liver mitochondria oxidizing palmitate. *Biochem. J.* **97**, 587–594.

Gehring, U. and Lynen, F. (1972), Thiolase. In: *The Enzymes* (Boyer, P.D., ed.), 3rd edn., Vol. 7, pp. 391–405, Academic Press, New York.

Gerstein, J. and Jencks, W.P. (1964), Equilibria and rates for acetyl transfer among substituted phenyl acetates, acetylimidazole, *O*-acylhydroxamic acids, and thiol esters. *J. Am. chem. Soc.*, **86**, 4655–4663.

Giacobini, G. (1972), Embryonic and postnatal development of choline acetyltransferase activity in muscles and sciatic nerve of the chick. *J. Neurochem.*, **19**, 1401–1403.

Giacobini-Robecchi, M.G., Giacobini, G., Filogamo, G. and Changeux, J.-P. (1975), Effects of the type A toxin from *Clostridium botulinum* on the development of skeletal muscles and of their innervation in chick embryo. *Brain Res.*, **83**, 107–121.

Giarman, N.J. and Pepeu, G. (1962), Drug-induced changes in brain acetylcholine. *Brit. J. Pharmac.*, **19**, 226–234.

Gibson, G.E. and Blass, J.P. (1976), Impaired synthesis of acetylcholine in brain accompanying mild hypoxia and hypoglycemia. *J. Neurochem.*, **27**, 37–42.

Gibson, G.E., Jope, R. and Blass, J.P. (1975), Decreased synthesis of acetylcholine accompanying impaired oxidation of pyruvic acid in rat brain minces. *Biochem. J.* **148**, 17–23.

Gibson, K.D., Wilson, J.D. and Udenfried, S. (1961), The enzymatic conversion of phospholipid ethanolamine to phospholipid choline in rat liver. *J. biol. Chem.*, **236**, 673–679.

Giller, E. and Schwartz, J.H. (1971), Choline acetyltransferase in identified neurons of abdominal ganglion of *Aplysia californica*. *J. Neurophysiol.*, **34**, 93–107.

Giller, E.L., Schrier, B.K., Shainberg, A., Fisk, H.R. and Nelson, P.G. (1973), Choline acetyltransferase activity is increased in combined cultures of spinal cord and muscle cells from mice. *Science* **182**, 588–589.

Glover, V. and Green, D.P.L. (1972), A simple quick microassay for choline acetyltransferase. *J. Neurochem.*, **19**, 2465–2466.

Glover, V.A.S. and Potter, L.T. (1971), Purification and properties of choline acetyltransferase from ox brain striate nuclei. *J. Neurochem.*, **18**, 571–580.

Gnädinger, M.C., Heimann, R. and Markstein, R. (1973), Choline acetyltransferase in corneal epithelium. *Expl. Eye Res.*, **15**, 395–399.

Godfrey, D.A. and Matschinsky, F.M. (1975), Enzymes of the cholinergic system in islets of Langerhans. *J. Histochem. Cytochem.*, **23**, 645–651.

Goldberg, A.M. and Hanin, I. (eds), (1976), *Biology of Cholinergic Function.* Raven Press, New York.

Goldberg, A.M. and Welch, B.L. (1972), Adaptation of the adrenal medulla: Sustained increase in choline acetyltransferase by psychosocial stimulation. *Science* **178**, 319–320.

Goldberg, A.M., Kaita, A.A. and McCaman, R.E. (1969), Microdetermination of choline acetyltransferase. A comparison of reinecke vs. periodide precipitation. *J. Neurochem.*, **16**, 823–824.

Goldstein, F.B. (1969), The enzymatic synthesis of *N*-acetyl-L-aspartic acid by subcellular preparations of rat brain. *J. biol. Chem.*, **244**, 4257–4260.

Grafstein, B. (1969), Axonal transport: communication between soma and synapse. In: *Advances in Biochemical Psychopharmacology* (Costa, E. and Greengard, P., eds), Vol. 1, pp. 11–25, Raven Press, New York.

Grafstein, B., McEwen, B.S. and Shelanski, M.L. (1970), Axonal transport of neurotubule protein. *Nature* (Lond.), **227**, 289–290.

Grafstein, B., Forman, D.S. and McEwen, B.S. (1972), Effects of temperature on axonal transport and turnover of protein in goldfish optic system. *Expl. Neurol.*, **34**, 158–170.

Gray, E.G. and Whittaker, V.P. (1962), The isolation of nerve endings from brain: an electronmicroscopic study of cell fragments derived by homogenization and centrifugation. *J. Anat.*, **96**, 79–87.

Green, D.E., Loomis, W.F. and Auerbach, V.H. (1948), Studies on the cyclophorase system. I. The complete oxidation of pyruvic acid to carbon dioxide and water. *J. biol. Chem.*, **172**, 389–403.

Greene, L.A. and Rein, G. (1977), Synthesis, storage and release of acetylcholine by a noradrenergic pheochromocytoma cell line. *Nature* (Lond.), **268**, 349–351.

Greville, G.D. (1969), Intracellular compartmentation and the citric acid cycle. In: *Citric Acid Cycle* (Lowenstein, J.M. ed.), pp. 1–136, M. Dekker, New York.

Greville, G.D. and Tubbs, P.K. (1968), The catabolism of long chain fatty acids in mammalian tissues. In: *Essays in Biochemistry* (Campbell, P.N. and Greville, G.D., eds), Vol. 4, pp. 155–212, Academic Press, London.

Grewaal, D.S. and Quastel, J.H. (1973), Control of synthesis and release of radioactive acetylcholine in brain slices from the rat. *Biochem. J.* **132**, 1–14.

Griffin, J.W., Price, D.L., Drachman, D.B. and Engel, W.K. (1976), Axonal transport to and from the motor nerve endings. *Ann. N.Y. Acad. Sci.*, **274**, 31–45.

Groot, P.H.E., Scholte, H.R. and Hülsmann, W.C. (1976), Fatty acid activation: specificity, localization, and function. In: *Advances in Lipid Research* (Paoletti, R. and Kritchevsky, D., eds), Vol. 14, pp. 75–126, Academic Press, New York.

Gross, G.W. (1975), The microstream concept of axoplasmic and dendritic transport. In: *Advances in Neurology*, (Kreutzberg, G.W., ed.) Vol 12., pp. 283–296. Raven Press, New York.

Growdon, J.H., Cohen, E.L. and Wurtman, R.J. (1977), Effects of oral choline administration on serum and CSF choline levels in patients with Huntington's disease. *J. Neurochem.*, **28**, 229–231.

Grubić, Z., Kiauta, T. and Brzin, M. (1976), A radiometric method for the determination of choline acetylase activity based on thin-layer chromatography. *Analyt. Biochem.*, **74**, 354–358.

Guth, P.S. (1969), Acetylcholine binding by isolated synaptic vesicles *in vitro* *Nature* **224**, 384–385.

Gutmann, E. and Holubář, J. (1950), The degeneration of peripheral nerve fibres. *J. Neurol. Neurosurg. Psychiat.*, **13**, 89–105.

Gutmann, E. and Sanders, F.K. (1943), Recovery of fibre numbers and diameters in the regeneration of peripheral nerves. *J. Physiol.*, (Lond.), **101**, 489–518.

Gutmann, E., Vodička, Z. and Zelená, J. (1955), Changes in the cross-striated muscle after transection of the nerve in dependence on the length of the peripheral nerve stump (Russ.). *Physiol. bohemoslov.* **4**, 200–204.

Gutmann, E., Tuček, S. and Hanzlíková, V. (1969), Changes in the choline acetyltransferase and cholinesterase activities in the levator ani muscle of rats following castration. *Physiol. bohemoslov.* **18**, 195–203.

Gutmann, E., Schiaffino, S. and Hanzlíková, V. (1971), Mechanism of compensatory hypertrophy in skeletal muscle of the rat. *Expl. Neurol.*, **31**, 451–464.

Guyenet, P., Lefresne, P., Rossier, J., Beaujouan, J.-C. and Glowinski, J. (1973a) Effect of sodium, hemicholinium-3 and antiparkinson drugs on [^{14}C]acetylcholine synthesis and [^{3}H]choline uptake in rat striatal synaptosomes. *Brain Res.*, **62**, 523–529.

Guyenet, P., Lefresne, P., Rossier, J., Beaujouan, J.C. and Glowinski, J. (1973b) Inhibition by hemicholinium-3 of [^{14}C]acetylcholine synthesis and [^{3}H]choline high-affinity uptake in rat striatal synaptosomes. *Molec. Pharmac.*, **9**, 630–639.

Guyenet, P.G., Lefresne, P., Beaujouan, J.C. and Glowinski, J. (1975), The role of newly taken up choline in the synthesis of acetylcholine in rat striatal synaptosomes. In: *Cholinergic Mechanisms* (Waser, P.G., ed.), pp. 137–144, Raven Press, New York.

Guynn, R.W. (1976), Effect of ethanol on brain CoA and acetyl–CoA. *J. Neurochem.*, **27**, 303–304.

Guynn, R.W. and Veech, R.L. (1975), Enzymatic determination of acetate. In: *Meth. Enzymol.*, Vol. 35B (Lowenstein, J.M. ed.), pp. 302–307. Academic Press, New York.

Guynn, R.W., Gelberg, H.J. and Veech, R.L. (1973), Equilibrium constants of the malate dehydrogenase, citrate synthase, citrate lyase, and acetyl coenzyme A hydrolysis reactions under physiological conditions. *J. biol. Chem.*, **248**, 6957–6965.

Haak, R.A., Kleinhans, F.W. and Ochs, S. (1976), The viscosity of mammalian nerve axoplasm measured by electron spin resonance. *J. Physiol.* (Lond.), **263**, 115–137.

Haga, T. (1971), Synthesis and release of [^{14}C]acetylcholine in synaptosomes. *J. Neurochem.*, **18**, 781–798.

Haga, T. and Noda, H. (1973), Choline uptake systems of rat brain synaptosomes. *Biochim. biophys. Acta* **291**, 564–575.

Häggendal, C.J., Saunders, N.R. and Dahlström, A.B. (1971), Rapid accumulation of acetylcholine in nerve above a crush. *J. Pharm. Pharmac.*, **23**, 552–555.

Häggendal, C.J., Dahlström, A.B. and Saunders, N.R. (1973), Axonal transport and acetylcholine in rat preganglionic neurones. *Brain Res.*, **58**, 494–499.

Hamburger, V. (1955), Trends in experimental neuroembryology. In: *Biochemistry of the Developing Nervous System* (Waelsch, H., ed.), pp. 52–71, Academic Press, New York.

Hanin, I. (ed.), (1974), *Choline and acetylcholine: Handbook of chemical assay methods*, Raven Press, New York.

Hanin, I. and Costa, E. (1976), Approaches used to estimate brain acetylcholine turnover rate *in vivo*; effects of drugs on brain acetylcholine turnover rate. In: *Biology of Cholinergic Function* (Goldberg, A.M. and Hanin, I., eds), pp. 355–377, Raven Press, New York.

Hanin, I. and Schuberth, J. (1974), Labelling of acetylcholine in the brain of mice fed on a diet containing deuterium labelled choline: studies utilizing gas chromatography – mass spectrometry. *J. Neurochem.*, **23**, 819–824.

Hanin, I., Massarelli, R. and Costa, E. (1970), Environmental and technical preconditions influencing choline and acetylcholine concentrations in rat brain. In: *Drugs and Cholinergic Mechanisms in the CNS* (Heilbronn, E. and Winter, A., eds), pp. 33–54, Almqvist and Wiksell, Stockholm.

Hanley, M.R., Cottrell, G.A., Emson, P.C. and Fonnum, F. (1974), Enzymatic synthesis of acetylcholine by a serotonin-containing neurone from *Helix*. *Nature* (Lond.), **251**, 631–633.

Hardegg, W. (1966), Cholinacylasen. In: *Handbuch der physiologisch- und pathologisch-chemischen Analyse,* 10th edn (Lang, K., Lehnartz, O., Hoffman-Ostenhof, O. and Siebert, G., eds), Vol. VI/B, pp. 861–871. Springer Verlag, Berlin.

Harpur, R.P. and Quastel, J.H. (1949), Relations between acetylcholine synthesis and metabolism of carbohydrates and D-glucosamine in the central nervous system. *Nature* (Lond.), **164**, 779–782.

Hattori, T., Singh, V.K., McGeer, E.G. and McGeer, P.L. (1976), Immunohistochemical localization of choline acetyltransferase containing neostriatal neurons and their relationship with dopaminergic synapses. *Brain Res.*, **102**, 164–173.

Haubrich, D.R. (1976), Choline acetyltransferase and its inhibitors. In: *Biology of Cholinergic Function* (Goldberg, A.M. and Hanin, I., eds), pp. 239–268, Raven Press, New York.

Haubrich, D.R. and Wang, P.F.L. (1976), Inhibition of acetylcholine synthesis by juglone and 4-(1-naphtylvinyl)pyridine. *Biochem. Pharmac.*, **25**, 669–672.

Haubrich, D.R., Reid, W.D. and Gillette, J.R. (1972), Acetylcholine formation in mouse brain and effect of cholinergic drugs. *Nature New Biol.*, **238**, 88–89.

Haubrich, D.R., Wedeking, P.W. and Wang, P.F.L. (1974), Increase in tissue concentration of acetylcholine in guinea pigs *in vivo* induced by administration of choline. *Life Sci.*, **14**, 921–927.

Haubrich, D.R., Wang, P.F.L. and Wedeking, P.W. (1975a), Distribution and metabolism of intravenously administered choline (methyl-^{3}H) and synthesis *in vivo* of acetylcholine in various tissues of guinea pigs. *J. Pharmac. exp. Ther.*, **193**, 246–255.

Haubrich, D.R., Wang, P.F.L., Herman, R.L. and Clody, D.E. (1975b) Acetylcholine synthesis in rat brain: dissimilar effects of clozapine and chlorpromazine. *Life Sci.*, **17**, 739–748.

Haubrich, D.R., Wang, P.F.L., Clody, D.E. and Wedeking, P.W. (1975c) Increase in rat brain acetylcholine induced by choline or deanol. *Life Sci.*, **17**, 975–980.

Haubrich, D.R., Wang, P.F.L., Chippendale, T. and Proctor, E. (1976), Choline and acetylcholine in rats: effect of dietary choline. *J. Neurochem.*, **27**, 1305–1313.

Hawkins, R.A., Williamson, D.H. and Krebs, H.A. (1971), Ketone-body utilization by adult and suckling rat brain *in vivo. Biochem. J.* **122**, 13–18.

Hebb, C.O. (1956), Choline acetylase in the developing nervous system of the rabbit and guinea-pig. *J. Physiol.* (Lond.), **133**, 566–570.

Hebb, C.O. (1962), Acetylcholine content of the rabbit plantaris muscle after denervation. *J. Physiol.* (Lond.), **163**, 294–306.

Hebb, C. (1963), Formation, storage, and liberation of acetylcholine. In: *Cholinesterases and Anticholinesterase Agents* (Koelle, G.B., ed.), *Handbuch d. exper. Pharmakologie, Ergänzungswerk,* Vol. **15**, pp. 55–88, Springer Verlag, Berlin.

Hebb, C. (1972), Biosynthesis of acetylcholine in nervous tissue. *Physiol. Rev.,* **52**, 918–957.

Hebb, C.O. and Ratković, D. (1962), Choline acetylase in the placenta of man and other species. *J. Physiol.* (Lond.), **163**, 307–313.

Hebb, C.O. and Silver, A. (1956), Choline acetylase in the central nervous system of man and some other mammals. *J. Physiol.* (Lond.), **134**, 718–728.

Hebb, C.O. and Silver, A. (1961), Gradient of choline acetylase activity. *Nature* (Lond.), **189**, 123–125.

Hebb, C.O. and Silver, A. (1963), The effect of transection on the level of choline acetylase in the goat's sciatic nerve. *J. Physiol.* (Lond.), **169**, 41P–42P.

Hebb, C. and Silver, A. (1970), Biochemical parameters of central cholinergic nerves, mapping the distribution of acetylcholine and the enzymes which control its metabolism in the brain. In: *Neuropathology: Methods and Diagnosis* (Tedeschi, C.G., ed.), pp. 665–690, Little, Brown and Co., Boston.

Hebb, C.O. and Waites, G.M. (1956), Choline acetylase in antero- and retrograde degeneration of a cholinergic neuron. *J. Physiol.* (Lond.), **132**, 667–671.

Hebb, C.O. and Whittaker, V.P. (1958), Intracellular distribution of acetylcholine and choline acetylase. *J. Physiol.* (Lond.), **142**, 187–196.

Hebb, C.O., Krnjević, K. and Silver, A. (1963), Effect of undercutting on the acetylcholinesterase and choline acetyltransferase activity in the cat's cerebral cortex. *Nature* (Lond.), **198**, 692.

Hebb, C.O., Krnjević, K. and Silver, A. (1964a), Acetylcholine and choline acetyltransferase in the diaphragm of the rat. *J. Physiol.* (Lond.), **171**, 504–513.

Hebb, C.O., Ling, G.M., McGeer, E.G., McGeer, P.L. and Perkins, D. (1964b) Effect of locally applied hemicholinium on the acetylcholine content of the caudate nucleus. *Nature* (Lond.), **204**, 1309–1311.

Hebb, C., Mann, S.P. and Mead, J. (1975), Measurement and activation of choline acetyltransferase. *Biochem. Pharmac.,* **24**, 1007–1011.

Heilbronn, E. (1969), The effect of phospholipases on the uptake of atropine and acetylcholine by slices of mouse brain cortex. *J. Neurochem.,* **16**, 627–635.

Heilbronn, E. (1970), Further experiments on the uptake of acetylcholine and atropine and the release of acetylcholine from mouse brain cortex slices after treatment with phospholipases. *J. Neurochem.,* **17**, 381–389.

Heilbronn, E. and Pettersson, H. (1973), Acetylcholine and related enzymes in normal and ligated cholinergic nerves from *Torpedo marmorata. Acta physiol. scand.,* **88**, 590–592.

Heilbronn, E. and Winter, A. (eds), (1970), *Drugs and Cholinergic Mechanisms in the CNS.* Almqvist and Wiksell, Stockholm.

Heinrich, C.P., Stadler, H. and Weiser, H. (1973), The effect of thiamine deficiency on the acetylcoenzyme A and acetylcholine levels in the rat brain. *J. Neurochem.,* **21**, 1273–1281.

Heiwall, P.-O., Saunders, N.R., Dahlström, A. and Häggendal, J. (1976), The effect of local application of vinblastine or colchicine on acetylcholine accumulation in rat sciatic nerve. *Acta physiol. scand.,* **96**, 478–485.

Hellauer, H. and Umrath, K. (1939), Über Azetylcholin und Cholinesterase in degenerierenden. *Nerven. Z. Biol.,* **99**, 624–632.

Hemsworth, B.A. (1976), The pharmacological actions of some polymethylene-bis-(hydroethyl)-dimethyl-ammonium compounds on cholinergic transmission. *Eur. J. Pharmac.,* **35**, 127–134.

Hemsworth, B.A. and Morris, D. (1964), A comparison of the *N*-alkyl group specificity of choline acetyltransferase from different species. *J. Neurochem.,* **11**, 793–803.

Hemsworth, B.A. and Smith, J.C. (1970), The enzymic acetylation of choline analogues. *J. Neurochem.,* **17**, 171–177.

Hendrickson, A.E. (1972), Electron microscopic distribution of axoplasmic transport. *J. comp. Neurol.,* **144**, 381–398.

Hendry, I.A. (1976), Effects of axotomy on the trans-synaptic regulation of enzyme activity in adult rat superior cervical ganglia. *Brain Res.,* **107**, 105–116.

Henn, F.A., Anderson, D.J. and Rustad, D.G. (1976), Glial contamination of synaptosomal fractions. *Brain Res.,* **101**, 341–344.

Heslop, J.P. (1975), Axonal flow and fast transport in nerves. In: *Adv. Comp. Physiol. Biochem.,* (Lowenstein, O., ed.), Vol. **6**, pp. 75–163, Academic Press, New York.

Heuser, J. and Lennon, A. (1973), Morphological evidence for exocytosis of acetylcholine during formation of synaptosomes from *Torpedo* electric organ. *J. Physiol.* (Lond.), **233**, 39P–41P.

Heuser, J.E. and Reese, T.S. (1973), Evidence for recycling of synaptic vesicle membrane during transmitter release at the frog neuromuscular junction. *J. cell Biol.,* **57**, 315–344.

Higgins, J.A. and Barrnett, R.J. (1970), Cytochemical localization of transferase activities: Carnitine acetyltransferase. *J. cell Sci.,* **6**, 29–51.

Hildebrand, J.G., Townsel, J.G. and Kravitz, E.A. (1974), Distribution of acetylcholine, choline, choline acetyltransferase and acetylcholinesterase in regions and single identified axons of the lobster nervous system. *J. Neurochem.,* **23**, 951–963.

Hirsch, M.J., Growdon, J.H. and Wurtman, R.J. (1977), Increase in hippocampal acetylcholine after choline administration. *Brain Res.,* **125**, 383–385.

Hodgkin, A.L., and Martin, K. (1965), Choline uptake by giant axons of *Loligo. J. Physiol.* (Lond.), **179**, 26P–27P.

Hoffman, P.N. and Lasek, R.J. (1975), The slow component of axonal transport. Identification of major structural polypeptides of the axon and their generality among mammalian neurons. *J. cell Biol.,* **66**, 351–366.

Holden, J.T., Rossier, J., Beaujouan, J.C., Guyenet, P. and Glowinski, J. (1975), Inhibition of high-affinity choline transport in rat striatal synaptosomes by alkyl bisquaternary ammonium compounds. *Molec. Pharmac.*, **11**, 19–27.

Holldorf, A.W. (1964), Gleichgewichtskonstanten, freie Energien und Redoxpotentiale biologisch wichtiger Reaktionen. In: *Biochemisches Taschenbuch* (Rauen, H.M., ed.), Vol. 2, p. 134, Springer Verlag, Berlin.

Holmstedt, B., Härkönen, M., Lundgren, O. and Sundwall, A. (1967), Relationship between acetylcholine and cholinesterase activity in the brain following an organophosphorus cholinesterase inhibitor. *Biochem. Pharmac.*, **16**, 404–406.

Holtzman, E., Freeman, A.R. and Kashner, L.A. (1971), Stimulation-dependent alterations in peroxidase uptake at lobster neuromuscular junctions. *Science* **173**, 733–736.

Honegger, P. and Richelson, E. (1976), Biochemical differentiation of mechanically dissociated mammalian brain in aggregating cell culture. *Brain Res.*, **109**, 335–354.

Hubbard, J.I. (1970), Mechanism of transmitter release. *Progr. Biophys. molec. Biol.*, **21**, 33–124.

Hubbard, J.I. and Kwanbunbumpen, S. (1968), Evidence for the vesicle hypothesis. *J. Physiol.* (Lond.), **194**, 407–421.

Hubbard, J.I., Llinás, R. and Quastel, D.M.J. (1969), *Electrophysiological Analysis of Synaptic Transmission.* Arnold, London.

Husain, S.S. and Mautner, H.G. (1973), The purification of choline acetyltransferase of squid-head ganglia. *Proc. natn. Acad. Sci. U.S.A.*, **70**, 3749–3753.

Hutchinson, M., Kosterlitz, H.W. and Gilbert, J.C. (1976), Effects of physostigmine and electrical stimulation on the acetylcholine content of the guinea pig ileum. *Eur. J. Pharmac.*, **39**, 221–235.

Hüther, C. and Luppa, H. (1976), The histochemical demonstration of choline acetyltransferase by semipermeable membrane technique. *Histochemistry* **49**, 303–307.

Illingworth, D.R. and Portman, O.W. (1972), The uptake and metabolism of plasma lysophosphatidylcholine *in vivo* by the brain of squirrel monkeys. *Biochem. J.*, **130**, 557–567.

Ilson, D., Collier, B. and Boksa, P. (1977), Acetyltriethylcholine: a cholinergic false transmitter in cat superior cervical ganglion and rat cerebral cortex. *J. Neurochem.*, **28**, 371–381.

Israël, M. (1970), Localisation de l'acétylcholine des synapses myoneurales et nerf-électroplaque. *Archs. Anat. microsc. Morph. exp.*, **59**, 67–98.

Israël, M. and Dunant, Y. (1975), Dynamics of acetylcholine compartments at rest and during nerve activity. In: *Metabolic Compartmentation and Neurotransmission* (Berl, S., Clarke, D.D. and Schneider, D., eds), pp. 621–639, Plenum Publishing Corporation, New York.

Israël, M. and Tuček, S. (1974), Utilization of acetate and pyruvate for the synthesis of 'total', 'bound' and 'free' acetylcholine in the electric organ of *Torpedo. J. Neurochem.*, **22**, 487–491.

Israël, M., Gautron, J. and Lesbats, B. (1970), Fractionnement de l'organe électrique de la Torpille: localisation subcellulaire de l'acétylcholine. *J. Neurochem.*, **17**, 1441–1450.

Israël, M., Lesbats, B. and Manaranche, R. (1972), Variations d'acétylcholine en relation avec l'évolution de la décharge, pendant la stimulation de l'organe électrique de la Torpille. *C. r. Acad. Sci.*, D **275**, 2957–2960.

Israël, M., Hirt, L. and Mastour-Frachon, P. (1973), Métabolisme et échanges d'acétylcholine dans les terminaisons nerveuses de l'organe électrique de la Torpille. *C. r. Acad. Sci.*, D **276**, 2725–2728.

Israël, M., Lesbats, B., Marsal, J. and Meunier, F.-M. (1975), Oscillations des taux tissulaires d'acétylcholine et d'adénosine triphosphate au cours de la stimulation de l'organe électrique de la Torpille. *C. r. Acad. Sci.*, D **280**, 905–908.

Israël, M., Lesbats, B., Manaranche, R., Marsal, J., Mastour-Frachon, P. and Meunier, F.M. (1977), Related changes in amounts of ACh and ATP in resting and active *Torpedo* nerve electroplaque synapses. *J. Neurochem.*, **28**, 1259–1267.

Itoh, T. and Quastel, J.H. (1970), Acetoacetate metabolism in infant and adult rat brain *in vitro. Biochem. J.* **116**, 641–655.

Iversen, L.L. (1971), Role of transmitter uptake mechanisms in synaptic neurotransmission. *Brit. J. Pharmac.*, **41**, 571–591.

Jablecki, C. and Brimijoin, S. (1974), Reduced axoplasmic transport of choline acetyltransferase activity in dystrophic mice. *Nature* (Lond.), **250**, 151–154.

Jablecki, C. and Brimijoin, S. (1975), Axoplasmic transport of choline acetyltransferase activity in mice: effect of age and neurotomy. *J. Neurochem.*, **25**, 583–593.

Jaenicke, L. and Lynen, F. (1960), Coenzyme A. In: *The Enzymes,* 2nd edn. (Boyer, P.D., Hardy, H. and Myrbäck, K., eds), Vol. **3**, pp. 3–103. Academic Press, New York.

Jakoubek, B., Semiginovský, B., Bass, A. and Scott, D. (1970), The transport of proteins in Mauthner axon in fish as studied by autoradiography and interference microscopy. *J. Neurobiol.*, **1**, 263–274.

Jankowska, E., Lubińska, L. and Niemierko, S. (1969), Translocation of AChE-containing particles in the axoplasm during nerve activity. *Comp. Biochem. Physiol.*, **28**, 907–913.

Jeffrey, P.L. and Austin, L. (1973), Axoplasmic transport. In: *Progress in Neurobiology* (Kerkut, G.A. and Phillis, J.W., eds), Vol. **2**, part 3, pp. 205–255, Pergamon Press, Oxford.

Jencks, W.P., Cordes, S. and Carriuolo, J. (1960), The free energy of thiol ester hydrolysis, *J. biol. Chem.*, **235**, 3608–3614.

Jenden, D.J., Booth, R.A. and Roch, M. (1977), Simultaneous microestimation of choline and acetylcholine by gas chromatography. *Analyt. Chem.*, **44**, 1879–1881.

Jenden, D.J., Choi, L., Silverman, R.W., Steinborn, J.A., Roch, M. and Booth, R.A. (1974), Acetylcholine turnover estimation in brain by gas chromatography/ mass spectrometry. *Life Sci.*, **14**, 55–63.

Jenden, D.J., Jope, R.S. and Weiler, M.H. (1976), Regulation of acetylcholine synthesis: does cytoplasmic acetylcholine control high affinity choline uptake? *Science* **194**, 635–637.

Johnson, M., Ross, D., Mayers, M., Rees, R., Bunge, R., Wakshull, E. and Burton, H. (1976), Synaptic vesicle cytochemistry changes when cultured sympathetic neurones develop cholinergic interactions. *Nature* (Lond.), **262**, 308–310.

Johnson, W.J. and Quastel, J.H. (1953), Narcotics and biological acetylations. *Nature* (Lond.), **171**, 602–605.

Jones, S.F. and Kwanbunbumpen, S. (1968), On the role of synaptic vesicles in transmitter release. *Life Sci.,* **7**, 1251–1255.

Jönsson, L-E., Schuberth, J. and Sundwall, A. (1969), Amphetamine effect on the choline concentration of human cerebrospinal fluid. *Life Sci.,* **8**, 977–981.

Jope, R. (1978), Pyruvate utilization, choline transport and acetylcholine synthesis. In: *Cholinergic Mechanisms and Psychopharmacology* (Jenden, D., ed.), Plenum Press, New York, (in press).

Jope, R. and Blass, J.P. (1975), A comparison of the regulation of pyruvate dehydrogenase in mitochondria from rat brain and liver. *Biochem. J.* **150**, 397–403.

Jope, R. and Blass, J.P. (1976), The regulation of pyruvate dehydrogenase in brain *in vivo. J. Neurochem.,* **26**, 709–714.

Joseph, B.S. (1973), Somatofugal events in Wallerian degeneration: a conceptual overview. *Brain Res.,* **59**, 1–18.

Jung, I. and Baulieu, E.-E. (1972), Testosterone cytosol 'receptor' in the rat levator ani muscle. *Nature New Biol.,* **237**, 24–26.

Kahlson, G. and MacIntosh, F.C. (1939), Acetylcholine synthesis in a sympathetic ganglion. *J. Physiol.* (Lond.), **96**, 277–292.

Kaita, A.A. and Goldberg, A.M. (1969), Control of acetylcholine synthesis – the inhibition of choline acetyltransferase by acetylcholine. *J. Neurochem.,* **16**, 1185–1191.

Kaita-Ritchie, A. and Goldberg, A.M. (1970), Vesicular and synaptoplasmic synthesis of acetylcholine. *Science* **169**, 489–490.

Kanfer, J.N. (1972), Base exchange reactions of the phospholipids in rat brain particles. *J. Lipid Res.,* **13**, 468–476.

Kapeller, K. and Mayor, D. (1969a), An electron microscopic study of the early changes proximal to a constriction in sympathetic nerves. *Proc. R. Soc.* B, **172**, 39–51.

Kapeller, K. and Mayor, D. (1969b), An electron microscopic study of the early changes distal to a constriction in sympathetic nerves. *Proc. R. Soc.* B. **172**, 53–63.

Kaplan, N.O. and Lipman, F. (1948), The assay and distribution of coenzyme A. *J. biol. Chem.,* **174**, 37–44.

Karlsson, J.O. and Sjöstrand, J. (1971), Synthesis, migration and turnover of protein in retinal ganglion cells. *J. Neurochem.,* **18**, 749–767.

Karlström, L. and Dahlström, A. (1973), The effect of different types of axonal trauma on the synthesis and transport of amine storage granules in rat sciatic nerves. *J. Neurobiol.,* **4**, 191–200.

Kása, P. (1968), Acetylcholinesterase transport in the central and peripheral nervous tissue: The role of tubules in the enzyme transport. *Nature* (Lond.), **218**, 1265–1267.

Kása, P. (1971), Ultrastructural localization of choline acetyltransferase and acetylcholinesterase in central and peripheral nervous tissue. In: *Histochemistry of Nervous Transmission* (Eränkö, O., ed.), *Progress in Brain Res.,* Vol. **34**, pp. 337–344, Elsevier, Amsterdam.

Kása, P. (1975), Histochemistry of choline acetyltransferase. In: *Cholinergic Mechanisms* (Waser, P.G., ed.), pp. 271–281, Raven Press, New York.

Kása, P. (1978), Development of the spinal cord and the acetylcholine system. In: *Recent Developments of Neurobiology in Hungary* (Lissak, K., ed.), Vol. 1. Akadémiai Kiadó, Budapest, (in press).

Kása, P., Mann, S.P. and Hebb, C. (1970), Localization of choline acetyltransferase. *Nature* (Lond.), **226**, 812–816.

Kása, P., Mann, S., Karcus, S., Tóth, L. and Jordan, S. (1973), Transport of choline acetyltransferase and acetylcholinesterase in the rat sciatic nerve: a biochemical and electronhistochemical study. *J. Neurochem.*, **21**, 431–436.

Kataoka, K., Nakamura, Y. and Hassler, R. (1973), Habenulo-interpeduncular tract: a possible cholinergic neuron in rat brain. *Brain Res.*, **62**, 264–267.

Kato, J. (1960), Choline acetylase of human placenta. *J. Biochem.* (Tokyo), **48**, 768–771.

Kato, T. (1975), CoA cycling: An enzymatic amplification method for determination of CoASH and acetyl CoA. *Analyt. Biochem.*, **66**, 372–392.

Katz, B. (1969), *The Release of Neural Transmitter Substances* Liverpool University Press, Liverpool.

Katz, B. (1971), Quantal mechanism of neural transmitter release. *Science* **173**, 123–126.

Katz, B. and Miledi, R. (1977), Transmitter leakage from motor nerve endings. *Proc. R. Soc.* B, **196**, 59–72.

Katz, H.S., Salehmoghaddam, S. and Collier, B. (1973), The accumulation of radioactive acetylcholine by a sympathetic ganglion and by brain: failure to label endogenous stores. *J. Neurochem.*, **20**, 569–579.

Kerkut, G.A. (1975), Axoplasmic transport. *Comp. Biochem. Physiol.*, **51A**, 701–704.

Kewitz, H. and Pleul, O. (1976), Synthesis of choline from ethanolamine in rat brain. *Proc. natn. Acad. Sci. U.S.A.*, **73**, 2181–2185.

Kewitz, H., Dross, K. and Pleul, O. (1974), Choline and its metabolic successors in brain. In: *Central Nervous System* (Genazzani, E. and Herken, H., eds), pp. 21–32, Springer Verlag, Berlin.

Kewitz, H., Pleul, O., Dross, K. and Schwartzkopff, T. (1975), The supply of choline in rat brain. In: *Cholinergic Mechanisms* (Waser, P.G., ed.), pp. 131–135, Raven Press, New York.

Kimes, B., Tarikas, H. and Schubert, D. (1974), Neurotransmitter synthesis by two clonal nerve cell lines: changes with culture growth and morphological differentiation. *Brain Res.*, **79**, 291–295.

Klingenberg, M. (1970), Mitochondria metabolite transport. *FEBS Letters* **6**, 145–154.

Knappe, J. (1957), Dissertation. München 1957. Quoted by K. Decker, 1959.

Knowles, S.E., Jarrett, I.G., Filsell, O.H. and Ballard, F.J. (1974), Production and utilization of acetate in mammals. *Biochem. J.* **142**, 401–411.

Ko, C.-P., Burton, H., Johnson, M.I. and Bunge, R.P. (1976), Synaptic transmission between rat superior cervical ganglion neurons in dissociated cell cultures. *Brain Res.*, **117**, 461–485.

Kobayashi, R.M., Brownstein, M., Saavedra, J.M. and Palkovits, M. (1975), Choline acetyltransferase content in discrete regions of the rat brain stem. *J. Neurochem.*, **24**, 637–640.

Kobayashi, T., Kobayashi, T., Kato, J. and Minaguchi, H. (1963), Fluctuations in choline acetylase activity in hypothalamus of rat during estrous cycle and after castration. *Endocrinol. Japon.* **10**, 175–182.

Koelle, G.B. (1963), Cytological distribution and physiological functions of cholinesterases. In: *Cholinesterases and Anticholinesterase Agents* (Koelle, G.B., ed), *Handbuch d. exper. Pharmakologie, Ergänzungswerk,* Vol. **15**, pp. 187–298, Springer Verlag, Berlin.

Koenig, E. (1969), Nucleic acid and protein metabolism of the axon. In: *Handbook of Neurochemistry* (Lajtha, A., ed.), Vol. 2, pp. 423–434, Plenum Press, New York.

Koike, H., Eisenstadt, M. and Schwartz, J.H. (1972), Axonal transport of newly synthesized acetylcholine in an identified neuron of *Aplysia. Brain Res.,* **37**, 152–159.

Komiya, Y. and Austin, L. (1974), Axoplasmic flow of protein in the sciatic nerve of normal and dystrophic mice. *Exp. Neurol.,* **43**, 1–12.

Kopin, I.J., Breese, G.R., Krauss, K.R. and Weise, V.K. (1968), Selective release of newly synthesized noradrenaline from cat spleen during sympathetic nerve stimulation. *J. Pharmac. expl. Ther.* **161**, 271–278.

Korey, S.R., de Braganza, B. and Nachmansohn, D. (1951), Choline acetylase. V. Esterifications and transacetylations. *J. biol. Chem.,* **189**, 705–715.

Korkes, S., del Campillo, A., Korey, S.R., Stern, J.R., Nachmansohn, D. and Ochoa, S (1952), Coupling of acetyl donor systems with choline acetylase. *J. biol. Chem.,* **198**, 215–220.

Kornacker, M.S. and Lowenstein, J.M. (1965), Citrate and the conversion of carbohydrate into fat. The activities of citrate-cleavage enzyme and acetate thiokinase in livers of starved and re-fed rats. *Biochem. J.* **94**, 209–215.

Kovachich, G.B. and Haugaard, N. (1977), Pyruvate dehydrogenase activation in rat brain cortical slices by elevated concentrations of external potassium ions. *J. Neurochem.,* **28**, 923–927.

Kristensson, K. and Olsson, Y. (1971), Retrograde axonal transport of protein. *Brain Res.,* **29**, 363–365.

Kristensson, K. and Sjöstrand, J. (1972), Retrograde transport of protein tracer in the rabbit hypoglossal nerve during regeneration. *Brain Res.,* **45**, 175–181.

Krnjević, K. and Straughan, D.W. (1964), The release of acetylcholine from the denervated rat diaphragm. *J. Physiol.* (Lond.), **170**, 371–378.

Księżak, H. (1976), Effect of hypoxia, ischemia and barbiturate anesthesia on interconversion of pyruvate dehydrogenase in guinea pig brain. *FEBS Letters* **63**, 149–153.

Kuczenski, R., Segal, D.S. and Mandell, A.J. (1975), Regional and subcellular distribution and kinetic properties of rat brain choline acetyltransferase – some functional considerations. *J. Neurochem.,* **24**, 39–45.

Kuhar, M.J. and Simon, J.R. (1974), Acetylcholine uptake: lack of association with cholinergic neurons. *J. Neurochem.,* **22**, 1135–1137.

Kuhar, M.J., Sethy, V.H., Roth, R.H. and Aghajanian, G.K. (1975), Choline: selective accumulation by central cholinergic neurons. *J. Neurochem.,* **20**, 581–593.

Kuhar, M.J., DeHaven, R.N., Yamamura, H.I., Rommelspacher, H. and Simon, J.R. (1975), Further evidence for cholinergic habenulo–interpeduncular neurons: pharmacologic and functional characteristics. *Brain Res.*, **97**, 265–275.

Kumar, S. (1971), Glutamic acid as a precursor of acetylcholine synthesis in rat brain *in vivo*. Observations on the compartmentalization. *Brain Res.*, **33**, 578–580.

Kuno, M. (1971), Quantum aspects of central and ganglionic synaptic transmission in vertebrates. *Physiol. Rev.*, **51**, 647–678.

Kuno, M., Turkanis, S.A. and Weakly, J.N. (1971), Correlation between nerve terminal size and transmitter release at the neuromuscular junction of the frog. *J. Physiol.* (Lond.), **213**, 545–556.

Kuntscherová, J. (1971), Ein Beitrag zur Klarstellung der Acetylcholinumsatzstörung in den Geweben weisser Ratten mit partieller Pankreatektomie. *Acta physiol. hung.*, **39**, 57–61.

Kuntscherová, J. (1972), Effect of short-term starvation and choline on the acetylcholine content of organs of albino rats. *Physiol. bohemoslov.*, **21**, 655–660.

Kuntscherová, J. and Vlk, J. (1968), Über die Bedeutung der Cholin- und Glukosezufuhr für die Normalisierung der durch Hungern herabgesetzten Acetylcholinvorräte in den Geweben. *Plzeň. lék. Sborn.* **31**, 5–12.

Kuntscherová, J. and Vlk, J. (1970), Influence of alloxan diabetes on acetylcholine synthesis in tissues of the albino rat. *Physiol. bohemoslov.* **19**, 431–434.

Kuntscherová, J., Vitouš, J. and Mertl, F. (1974), Utilization of injected choline by the brain and ileum of albino rats. *Physiol. bohemoslov.* **23**, 461–465.

Kuriyama, K., Roberts, E. and Vos, J. (1968), Some characteristics of binding of γ-aminobutyric acid and acetylcholine to a synaptic vesicle fraction from mouse brain. *Brain Res.*, **9**, 231–252.

Kurokawa, M., Machiyama, Y. and Kato, M. (1963), Distribution of acetylcholine in the brain during various states of activity. *J. Neurochem.*, **10**, 341–348.

Kvist, U. and Sjöstrand, N.O. (1976), A further contribution to the question of trophic and hormonal influences on the noradrenaline content of the male reproductive tract: effect of combined androgen and estrogen treatment of prepuberally castrated rats. *Acta physiol. scand.*, **98**, 339–346.

Ladinsky, H., Consolo, S., Peri, G. and Garattini, S. (1972a), Acetylcholine, choline and choline acetyltransferase activity in the developing brain of normal and hypothyroid rats. *J. Neurochem.*, **19**, 1947–1952.

Ladinsky, H., Consolo, S. and Bareggi, S.R. (1972b), A simple method for detecting overlap of nanogram quantities of choline onto the acetylcholine band in paper electrophoresis. *Analyt. Biochem.*, **50**, 460–466.

Lam, D.M.K. (1972), Biosynthesis of acetylcholine in turtle photoreceptors. *Proc. natn. Acad. Sci. U.S.A.*, **69**, 1987–1991.

Landriscina, C., Papa, S., Coratelli, P., Mazzarella, L. and Quagliariello, E. (1970), Enzymatic activities of the matrix and inner membrane of pigeon-liver mitochondria. *Biochim. biophys. Acta*, **205**, 136–147.

Lanks, K., Somers, L., Papirmeister, B. and Yamamura, H. (1974), Choline transport by neuroblastoma cells in tissue culture. *Nature* (Lond.), **252**, 476–478.

Lasek, R.J. (1967), Bidirectional transport of radioactively labelled axoplasmic components. *Nature* (Lond.), **216**, 1212–1214.

Lasek, R.J. (1970), Protein transport in neurons. *Int. Rev. Neurobiol.*, **13**, 289–324.

Lasek, R.J. (1975), Axonal transport and the use of intracellular markers in neuroanatomical investigations. *Fedn. Proc. Fedn. Am. Socs. exp. Biol.*, **34**, 1603–1611.

LaVail, J.H. (1975), The retrograde transport method. *Fedn. Proc. Fedn. Am. Socs. exp. Biol.*, **34**, 1618–1624.

Lefresne, P. (1974), Contribution à l'étude du métabolisme de l'acétylcholine dans les terminaisons nerveuses du neostriatum chez le rat. Thèse de Doctorat. Université Paris VI, Paris.

Lefresne, P., Guyenet, P. and Glowinski, J. (1973), Acetylcholine synthesis from [2-^{14}C] pyruvate in rat striatal slices. *J. Neurochem.*, **20**, 1083–1097.

Lefresne, P., Guyenet, P., Beaujouan, J.C. and Glowinski, J. (1975), The subcellular localization of ACh synthesis in rat striatal synaptosomes investigated with the use of Triton X-100. *J. Neurochem.*, **25**, 415–422.

Lehninger, A.L. (1964), *The Mitochondrion,* Benjamin, New York.

Liang, C.C. and Quastel, J.H. (1969a), Uptake of acetylcholine in rat brain cortex slices. *Biochem. Pharmac.*, **18**, 1169–1185.

Liang, C.C. and Quastel, J.H. (1969b), Effects of drugs on the uptake of acetylcholine in rat brain cortex slices. *Biochem. Pharmac.*, **18**, 1187–1194.

Libertun, C., Timiras, P.S. and Kragt, C.L. (1973), Sexual differences in the hypothalamic cholinergic system before and after puberty: inductory effect of testosterone. *Neuroendocrinology,* **12**, 73–85.

Linn, T.C., Pettit, F.H. and Reed, L.J. (1969a), α-keto acid dehydrogenase complexes, X. Regulation of the activity of the pyruvate dehydrogenase complex from beef kidney mitochondria by phosphorylation and dephosphorylation. *Proc. natn. Acad. Sci. U.S.A.*, **62**, 234–241.

Linn, T.C., Pettit, F.H., Hucho, F. and Reed, L.J. (1969b), α-keto acid dehydrogenase complexes, XI. Comparative studies of regulatory properties of the pyruvate dehydrogenase complexes from kidney, heart, and liver mitochondria. *Proc. natn. Acad. Sci. U.S.A.*, **64**, 227–234.

Lipmann, F. (1954), Development of the acetylation problem, a personal account. *Science* **120**, 855–865.

Livett, B.G., Geffen, L.B. and Austin, L. (1968), Proximo–distal transport of [^{14}C] noradrenaline and protein in sympathetic nerves. *J. Neurochem.*, **15**, *International Review of Physiology,* Vol. **10**, pp. 37–124. University Park Press, Baltimore.

Livett, B.G., Geffen, L.B. and Austin, (1968), Proximo–distal transport of [^{14}C] noradrenaline and protein in sympathetic nerves. *J. Neurochem.*, **15**, 931–939.

Llinás, R., Blinks, J.R. and Nicholson, C. (1972), Calcium transient in presynaptic terminal of squid giant synapse: detection with aequorin. *Science* **176**, 1127–1129.

Lowenstein, J.M. (1964), The regulation of carbohydrate utilization. In: *Oxygen in the Animal Organism,* (Dickens, F. and Neil, E., eds), pp. 163–177, Pergamon Press, Oxford.

Lowenstein, J.M. (1968), Citrate and the conversion of carbohydrate into fat. In: *The Metabolic Roles of Citrate* (Goodwin, T.W., ed.), pp. 61–86, Academic Press, London.

Lubińska, L. (1964), Axoplasmic streaming in regenerating and in normal nerve fibres. In: *Mechanisms of Neural Regeneration* (Singer, M. and Schadé, J.P., eds), *Progress in Brain Res.*, Vol. **13**, pp. 1–66, Elsevier, Amsterdam.

Lubińska, L. (1975), On axoplasmic flow. *Int. Rev. Neurobiol.*, **17**, 241–296.

Lubińska, L. (1977), Early course of Wallerian degeneration in myelinated fibres of the rat phrenic nerve. *Brain Res.*, **130**, 47–63.

Lubińska, L. and Niemierko, S. (1971), Velocity and intensity of bidirectional migration of acetylcholinesterase in transected nerves. *Brain Res.*, **27**, 329–342.

Lubińska, L., Niemierko, S., Oderfeld, B., Szwarc, L. and Zelená, J. (1963a), Bidirectional movements of axoplasm in peripheral nerve fibres. *Acta Biol. exp.*, (Vars.) **23**, 239–247.

Lubińska, L., Niemierko, S., Oderfeld, B. and Szwarc, L. (1963b), The distribution of acetylcholinesterase in peripheral nerves. *J. Neurochem.*, **10**, 25–41.

Lubińska, L., Niemierko, S., Oderfeld-Nowak, B. and Szwarc, L. (1964), Behaviour of acetylcholinesterase in isolated nerve segments. *J. Neurochem.*, **11**, 493–503.

Luco, J.V. and Eyzaguirre, C. (1965), Fibrillation and hypersensitivity to ACh in denervated muscle: effect of length of degenerating nerve fibres. *J. Neurophysiol.*, **18**, 65–73.

Lux, H.D., Schubert, P., Kreutzberg, G.W. and Globus, A. (1970), Excitation and axonal flow: autoradiographic study on motoneurons intracellularly injected with a ^{3}H-amino acid. *Expl. Brain Res.*, **10**, 197–204.

Macková, E. and Hník, P. (1973), Compensatory muscle hypertrophy induced by tenotomy of synergists is not true working hypertrophy. *Physiol. bohemoslov.* **22**, 43–49.

MacIntosh, F.C. (1938), L'effet de la section des fibres préganglionnaires sur la teneur en acétylcholine du ganglion sympathique. *Archs. int. Physiol.*, **47**, 321–324.

MacIntosh, F.C. (1941), The distribution of acetylcholine in the peripheral and the central nervous system. *J. Physiol.*, (Lond.), **99**, 436–442.

MacIntosh, F.C. (1963), Synthesis and storage of acetylcholine in nervous tissue. *Can. J. Biochem. Physiol.*, **41**, 2555–2571.

MacIntosh, F.C. and Collier, B. (1976), Neurochemistry of cholinergic terminals. In: *Neuromuscular Junction* (Zaimis, E., ed.), *Handbook of Experimental Pharmacology,* New Series, Vol. **42**, pp. 99–228, Springer Verlag, Berlin.

MacIntosh, F.C. and Perry, W.L.M. (1950), Biological estimation of acetylcholine. In: *Methods in Medical Research,* (Gerard, R.W., ed.), Vol. **3**, pp. 78–92, The Year Book Publishers, Chicago.

Mahler, H.R. and Cordes, E.H. (1966), *Biological Chemistry,* Harper and Row, New York.

Mahoney, K., Vogel, W.H., Salvenmoser, F. and Boehme, D.H. (1971), Activity of choline acetyltransferase in various human adult and fetal tissues. *J. Neurochem.*, **18**, 1357–1359.

Main, A.R. (1976), Structure and inhibitors of cholinesterase. In: *Biology of Cholinergic Function,* (Goldberg, A.M. and Hanin, I., eds), pp. 269–353, Raven Press, New York.

Makita, T., Kiwaki, S. and Sandborn, E.B. (1973), Scanning electron microscopy and cytochemical localization of carnitine acetyltransferase activity in normal and dystrophic muscle of mice. *Histochem. J.* **5**, 335–342.

Maletta, G.J. and Timiras, P.S. (1968), Choline acetyltransferase activity and total protein content in selected optic areas of the rat after complete light-deprivation during CNS development. *J. Neurochem.*, **15**, 787–793.

Maloshevskii, S.G., Lenkov, D.N. and Bragina, T.A. (1975), Changes of synaptic vesicles in axonal terminals in the motor cortex of the cat after stimulation (Russ.). *Neirofiziologiya* (Kiev), **7**, 639–646.

Malthe-Sørenssen, D. (1975), Heterogeneity of choline acetyltransferase. In: *Cholinergic Mechanisms* (Waser, P.G., ed.), pp. 257–261, Raven Press, New York.

Malthe-Sørenssen, D. (1976a), Molecular properties of choline acetyltransferase from different species investigated by isoelectric focusing and ion exchange adosrption. *J. Neurochem.*, **26**, 861–865.

Malthe-Sørenssen, D. (1976b), Choline acetyltransferase – evidence for acetyl transfer by a histidine residue. *J. Neurochem.*, **27**, 873–881.

Malthe-Sørenssen, D. and Fonnum, F. (1972), Multiple forms of choline acetyltransferase in several species demonstrated by isoelectric focusing. *Biochem. J.* **127**, 229–236.

Malthe-Sørenssen, D., Eskeland, T. and Fonnum, F. (1973), Purification of rat brain choline acetyltransferase; some immunochemical properties of a highly purified preparation. *Brain Res.*, **62**, 517–522.

Mann, P.J.G. and Quastel, J.H. (1940), Vitamin B_1 and acetylcholine formation in isolated brain. *Nature* (Lond.), **145**, 856–857.

Mann, P.J.G., Tennenbaum, M. and Quastel, J.H. (1938), On the mechanism of acetylcholine formation in brain *in vitro*. *Biochem. J.* **32**, 243–261.

Mann, P.J.G., Tennenbaum, M. and Quastel, J.H. (1939), Acetylcholine metabolism in the central nervous system. The effects of potassium and other cations on acetylcholine liberation. *Biochem. J.* **33**, 822–835.

Mann, S.P. (1976), An investigation of choline levels in living nervous tissue and of the source of choline utilized as substrate in the synthesis of acetylcholine. Ph. D. Thesis. A.R.C. Institute of Animal Physiology, Babraham, Cambridge.

Mann, S.P. and Hebb, C. (1975), Inhibition of choline acetyltransferase bu quaternary ammonium analogues of choline. *Biochem. Pharmac.* **24**, 1013–1017.

Mann, S.P. and Hebb, C. (1977), Free choline in the brain of the rat. *J. Neurochem.*, **28**, 241–244.

Mannervik, B. and Sörbo, B. (1970), Inhibition of choline acetyltransferase from bovine caudate nucleus by sulfhydryl reagents and reactivation of the inhibited enzyme. *Biochem. Pharmac.* **19**, 2509–2516.

Marchbanks, R.M. (1968a), Exchangeability of radioactive acetylcholine with the bound acetylcholine of synaptosomes and synaptic vesicles. *Biochem J.* **106**, 87–95.

Marchbanks, R.M. (1968b), The uptake of [^{14}C]choline into synaptosomes *in vitro. Biochem. J.* **110**, 533–541.

Marchbanks, R.M. (1973), Problems concerning the compartmentation of acetylcholine in the synaptic region. In: *Metabolic Compartmentation in the Brain* (Balázs, R. and Cremer, J.E., eds), pp. 21–33, Macmillan Press, London.

Marchbanks, R.M. (1975a), The subcellular origin of the acetylcholine released at synapses. *Int. J. Biochem.*, **6**, 303–312.

Marchbanks, R.M. (1975b), Biochemistry of cholinergic neurons. In: *Handbook of Psychopharmacology* (Iversen, L.L., Iversen, S.D. and Snyder, S.H., eds), Vol. **3**, *Biochemistry of Biogenic Amines*, pp. 247–326, Plenum Press, New York.

Marchbanks, R.M. and Israël, M. (1971), Aspects of acetylcholine metabolism in the electric organ of *Torpedo marmorata*. *J. Neurochem.*, **18**, 439–448.

Marchisio, P.C. (1969), Choline acetyltransferase (ChAc) activity in developing chick optical centres and the effects of monolateral removal of retina at an early embryonic stage and at hatching. *J. Neurochem.*, **16**, 665–671.

Marchisio, P.C. and Consolo, S. (1968), Developmental changes of choline acetyltransferase (ChAc) activity in chick embryo spinal and sympathetic ganglia. *J. Neurochem.*, **15**, 759–764.

Marchisio, P.C. and Giacobini, G. (1969), Choline acetyltransferase activity in the central nervous system of the developing chick. *Brain Res.*, **15**, 301–304.

Marder, E. (1976), Cholinergic motor neurones in the stomatogastric system of the lobster. *J. Physiol.* (Lond.), **257**, 63–86.

Markov, D., Rambourg, A. and Droz, B. (1976), Smooth endoplasmic reticulum and fast axonal transport of glycoproteins, an electron microscope radioautographic study of thick sections after heavy metals impregnation. *J. Microscopie Biol. cell*, **25**, 57–60.

Marquis, N.R. and Fritz, I.B. (1965), The distribution of carnitine, acetylcarnitine, and carnitine acetyltransferase in rat tissues. *J. biol. Chem.*, **240**, 2193–2196.

Marshall, E.F., Chojnacki, T. and Ansell, G.B. (1965), The methylation of [^{32}P] phosphatidylmonomethylaminoethanol by S-adenosyl-L-[Me-^{14}C] methionine in liver preparations. *Biochem. J.* **95**, 30P–31P.

Martin, A.R. (1966), Quantal nature of synaptic transmission. *Physiol. Rev.*, **46**, 51–66.

Martin. B.R. and Denton, R.M. (1970), Intracellular localization of enzymes in white-adipose-tissue fat cells and permeability properties of fat-cell mitochondria. Transfer of acetyl units and reducing power between mitochondria and cytoplasm. *Biochem. J.* **117**, 861–877.

Masland, R.H. and Livingstone, C.J. (1976), Effect of stimulation with light on synthesis and release of acetylcholine by an isolated mammalian retina. *J. Neurophysiol.*, **39**, 1210–1219.

Massarelli, R. and Mandel, P. (1976), On the uptake mechanism of choline in nerve cell cultures. In: *Transport Phenomena in the Nervous System* (Levi, G., Battistin, L. and Lajtha, A., eds), pp. 199–209, Plenum Publishing Corporation, New York.

Massarelli, R., Sensenbrenner, M., Ebel, A. and Mandel, P. (1974a), Choline uptake in nerve cell cultures. *Neurobiology*, **4**, 293–300.

Massarelli, R., Ciesielski-Treska, J., Ebel, A. and Mandel, P. (1974b), Choline uptake in glial cell cultures. *Brain Res.*, **81**, 361–363.

Massarelli, R., Ciesielski-Treska, J., Ebel, A. and Mandel, P. (1974c) Kinetics of choline uptake in neurblastoma clones. *Biochem. Pharmac.*, **23**, 2857–2865.

Massarelli, R., Stefanovic, V. and Mandel, P. (1976), Cholinesterase activity and choline uptake in intact nerve cell cultures. *Brain Res.*, **112**, 103–112.

Mattson, M.E. and O'Brien, R.D. (1976), The binding of acetylcholine to synaptic vesicles from *Torpedo californica* electroplax. *J. Neurochem.*, **27**, 867–872.

McCaman, M.W. (1966), Biochemical effects of denervation on normal and dystrophic muscle: acetylcholinesterase and choline acetyltransferase. *Life Sci.*, **5**, 1459–1465.

McCaman, M.W. and McCaman, R.E. (1965), Effects of denervation on normal and dystrophic muscle: DNA and nucleotide enzymes. *Am. J. Physiol.*, **209**, 495–500.

McCaman, M.W., Stafford, M.L. and Skinner, E.C. (1967), Choline acetyltransferase and cholinesterase activities in muscle of dystrophic mice. *Am. J. Physiol.*, **212**, 228–232.

McCaman, R.E. and Aprison, M.H. (1964), The synthetic and catabolic enzyme system for acetylcholine and serotonin in several discrete areas of the developing rabbit brain. In: *The Developing Brain* (Himwich, W.A. and Himwich, H.E., eds), *Progress in Brain Res.*, Vol. **9**, pp. 220–233, Elsevier, Amsterdam.

McCaman, R.E. and Dewhurst, S.A. (1970), Choline acetyltransferase in individual neurons of *Aplysia californica. J. Neurochem.*, **17**, 1421–1426.

McCaman, R.E. and Hunt, J.M. (1965), Microdetermination of choline acetylase in nervous tissue. *J. Neurochem.*, **12**, 253–259.

McCaman, R.E. and McCaman, M.W. (1976), Biology of individual cholinergic neurons in the invertebrate CNS. In: *Biology of Cholinergic Function* (Goldberg, A.M. and Hanin, I., eds), pp. 485–513, Raven Press, New York.

McCaman, R.E., Rodríguez de Lores Arnaiz, G. and De Robertis, E. (1965), Species differences in subcellular distribution of choline acetylase in the CNS. *J. Neurochem.*, **12**, 927–935.

McCaman, R.E., McCaman, M.W. and Stafford, M.L. (1966), Carnitine acetyltransferase in nervous tissue. *J. biol. Chem.*, **241**, 930–934.

McClure, W.O. (1972), Effect of drugs upon axoplasmic transport. *Adv. Pharmac. Chemother.*, **10**, 185–220.

McEwen, B.S. and Grafstein, B. (1968), Fast and slow components in axonal transport of proteins. *J. cell Biol.*, **38**, 494–508.

McEwen, B.S., Forman, D.S. and Grafstein, B. (1971), Components of fast and slow axonal transport in the goldfish optic nerve. *J. Neurobiol.*, **2**, 361–377.

McGarry, J.D. and Foster, D.W. (1969), Ketogenesis and cholesterol synthesis in normal and neoplastic tissues of the rat. *J. biol. Chem.*, **244**, 4251–4256.

McGeer, E.G. and McGeer, P.L. (1975), Age changes in the human for some enzymes associated with metabolism of catecholamines, GABA and acetylcholine. *Adv. behav. Biol.*, **16**, 287–305.

McGeer, E.G., Fibiger, H.C., McGeer, P.L. and Wickson, V. (1971a), Aging and brain enzymes. *Exp. Geront.*, **6**, 391–396.

McGeer, E.G., Fibiger, H.C. and Wickson, V. (1971b), Differential development of caudate enzymes in the neonatal rat. *Brain Res.*, **32**, 433–440.

McGeer, P.L. and McGeer, E.G. (1973), Neurotransmitter synthetic enzymes. *Progress in Neurobiology* (Kerkut, G.A. and Phillis, J.W., eds), Vol. **2**, part 1, pp. 69–117, Pergamon, Press, Oxford.

McGeer, P.L. and McGeer, E.G. (1976), Enzymes associated with the metabolism of catecholamines, acetylcholine and GABA in human controls and patients with Parkinson's disease and Huntington's chorea. *J. Neurochem.*, **26**, 65–76.

McGeer, P.L., McGeer, E.G., Singh, V.K. and Chase, W.H. (1974), Choline acetyltransferase localization in the central nervous system by immunohistochemistry. *Brain Res.*, **81**, 373–379.

McIlwain, H. and Bachelard, H.S. (1971), *Biochemistry and the Central Nervous System*, 4th edn., Churchill Livingstone, London.

McLaughlin, J., Case, K.R. and Bosmann, B.H. (1973), Electrokinetic properties of isolated cerebral-cortex synaptic vesicles. *Biochem J.* **136**, 919–926.

McLean, W.G., Frizell, M. and Sjöstrand, J. (1976), Slow axonal transport of labelled proteins in sensory fibres of rabbit vagus nerve. *J. Neurochem.*, **26**, 1213–1216.

McLennan, H. and Elliott, K.A.C. (1950), Factors affecting the synthesis of acetylcholine by brain slices. *Am. J. Physiol.*, **163**, 605–613.

McLennan, H. and Elliott, K.A.C. (1951), Effects of convulsant and narcotic drugs on acetylcholine synthesis. *J. Pharmacol. exp. Ther.*, **103**, 35–43.

Megazzini, P., Bernardi, G. and Ballotti, P. (1965), Regional changes of the cholinergic system in the guinea pig's brain after physostigmine. *Experientia* (Basel), **21**, 406–408.

Mezentsev, A.N. and Messinova, O.V. (1971), Transport of the axoplasm and biosynthetic processes in the axon (Russ.). *Usp. sovr. biol.*, **72**, 62–76.

Michelson, M.J. and Zeimal, E.V. (1973), *Acetylcholine*, Pergamon Press, Oxford.

Middleton, B. (1973a), The oxoacyl–coenzyme A thiolases of animal tissues. *Biochem. J.* **132**, 717–730.

Middleton, B. (1973b), The acetoacetyl–coenzyme A thiolases of rat brain and their relative activities during postnatal development. *Biochem. J.* **132**, 731–737.

Miledi, R. (1960), Properties of regenerating neuromuscular synapses in the frog. *J. Physiol.*, (Lond.), **154**, 190–205.

Miledi, R. and Slater, C.R. (1968), Electrophysiology and electron-microscopy of rat neuromuscular junctions after nerve degeneration. *Proc. R. Soc.* B, **169**, 289–306.

Miledi, R. and Slater, C.R. (1970), On the degeneration of rat neuromuscular junctions after nerve section. *J. Physiol.*, (Lond.), **207**, 507–528.

Miledi, R. and Stefani, E. (1970), Miniature potentials in denervated slow muscle fibres of the frog. *J. Physiol.*, (Lond.), **209**, 179–186.

Miledi, R., Molenaar, P.C. and Polak, R.L. (1977), An analysis of acetylcholine in frog muscle by mass fragmentography. *Proc. R. Soc. Lond.* B. **197**, 285–297.

Mitchell, J.F. and Silver, A. (1963), The spontaneous release of acetylcholine from the denervated hemidiaphragm of the rat. *J. Physiol.*, (Lond.), **165**, 117–129.

Modak, A.T., Stavinoha, W.B. and Weintraub, S.T. (1975), Dichlorvos and the cholinergic system: effects on cholinesterase and acetylcholine contents of rat tissues. *Archs. int. Pharmacodyn. Ther.*, **217**, 293–301.

Molenaar, P.C. and Polak, R.L. (1973), Newly formed acetylcholine in synaptic vesicles in brain tissue. *Brain Res.*, **62**, 537–542.

Molenaar, P.C. and Polak, R.L. (1976), Analysis of the preferential release of newly synthesized acetylcholine by cortical slices from rat brain with the aid of two different labelled precursors. *J. Neurochem.*, **26**, 95–99.

Molenaar, P.C., Nickolson, V.J. and Polak, R.L. (1973a), Preferential release of newly synthesized ^{3}H-acetylcholine from rat cerebral cortex slices *in vitro*. *Brit. J. Pharmac.*, **47**, 97–108.

Molenaar, P.C., Polak, R.L. and Nickolson, V.J. (1973b), Subcellular localization of newly-formed [^{3}H] acetylcholine in rat cerebral cortex *in vitro*. *J. Neurochem.*, **21**, 667–678.

Morel, N. (1975), Incorporation d'acetate dans l'acetylcholine de l'organe electrique de *Torpille*: effets des concentrations d'acetate et de choline. *C. r. Acad. Sci.* D. **280**, 999–1001.

Morel, N. (1976), Effect of choline on the rates of synthesis and of release of acetylcholine in the electric organ of *Torpedo*. *J. Neurochem.*, **27**, 779–784.

Morgan, I.G. (1976), Synaptosomes and cell separation. *Neuroscience* **1**, 159–165.

Morris, D. (1966), The choline acetyltransferase of human placenta. *Biochem. J.* **98**, 754–762.

Morris, D. (1967), The effect of sulphydryl and other disulphide reducing agents on choline acetyltransferase activity estimated with synthetic acetyl–CoA. *J. Neurochem.*, **14**, 19–27.

Morris, D. and Grewaal, D.S. (1971), Human placental choline acetyltransferase. *Eur. J. Biochem.*, **22**, 563–572.

Morris, D. and Tuček, S. (1966), The influence of inorganic cations on the activities of choline acetyltransferase, phosphate acetyltransferase and acetylphosphatase. *J. Neurochem.*, **13**, 333–345.

Morris, D., Maneckjee, A. and Hebb, C. (1971), The kinetic properties of human placental choline acetyltransferase. *Biochem. J.* **125**, 857–863.

Morris, J.G. (1968), *A Biologist's Physical Chemistry*, pp. 165–219, 261–299, Addison-Wesley, Reading.

Mulder, A.H., Yamamura, H.I., Kuhar, M.J. and Snyder, S.H. (1974), Release of acetylcholine from hippocampal slices by potassium depolarization: dependence on high affinity choline uptake. *Brain Res.*, **70**, 372–376.

Muralt, A.v. and Schulthess, G.v. (1944), Ueber den Acetylcholingehalt des peripheren Nerven während der Degeneration. *Helv. physiol. Acta* **2**, 435–443.

Murrin, L.C. and Kuhar, M.J. (1976), Activation of high-affinity choline uptake *in vitro* by depolarizing agents. *Molec. Pharmac.*, **12**, 1082–1090.

Nachmansohn, D. (1959), *Chemical and Molecular Basis of Nerve Activity* Academic Press, New York.

Nachmansohn, D. and Berman, M. (1946), Studies on choline acetylase. III. On the preparation of the coenzyme and its effect on the enzyme. *J. biol. Chem.*, **165**, 551–563.

Nachmansohn, D. and Machado, A.L. (1943), The formation of acetylcholine A new enzyme: 'Choline acetylase', *J. Neurophysiol.*, **6**, 397–403.

Nachmansohn, D., John, H.M. and Berman, M. (1946), Studies on choline acetylase. II. The formation of acetylcholine in the nerve axon. *J. biol. Chem.*, **163**, 475–480.

Nadler, J.V., Matthews, D.A., Cotman, C.W. and Lynch, G.S. (1974), Development of cholinergic innervation in the hippocampal formation of the rat. II. Quantitative changes in choline acetyltransferase and acetylcholinesterase activities. *Develop. Biol.,* **36**, 142–154.

Nakamura, R. and Cheng, S.-C. (1969), Evidence for the metabolic compartmentalization of acetyl–coenzyme A in rat brain slices and its relation to the syntheses of acetylcholine and glutamate. *Life Sci.,* **8**, 657–662.

Nakamura, R., Cheng, S.-C. and Naruse, H. (1970), A study on the precursors of the acetyl moiety of acetylcholine in brain slices. *Biochem. J.* **118**, 443–450.

Neal, M.J. and Gilroy, J. (1975), High-affinity choline transport in the isolated retina. *Brain Res.,* **93**, 548–551.

Neidle, A., Van den Berg, C.J. and Grynbaum, A. (1969), The heterogeneity of rat brain mitochondria isolated on continuous sucrose gradients. *J. Neurochem.,* **16**, 225–234.

Nicklas, W.J., Clark, J.B. and Williamson, J.R. (1971), Metabolism of rat brain mitochondria. *Biochem. J.* **123**, 83–95.

Niemierko, S. and Lubińska, L. (1967), Two fractions of axonal acetylcholinesterase exhibiting different behaviour in severed nerves. *J. Neurochem.,* **14**, 761–769.

Nordberg, A. and Sundwall, A. (1975), Effect of pentobarbital on endogenous acetylcholine and biotransformation of radioactive choline in different brain regions. In: *Cholinergic Mechanisms* (Waser, P.G., ed.), pp. 229–239, Raven Press, New York.

Nordberg, A. and Sundwall, A. (1976), Biosynthesis of acetylcholine in different brain regions *in vivo* following alternative methods of sacrifice by microwave irradiation. *Acta physiol. scand.,* **98**, 307–317.

Nordenfelt, I. (1963), Choline acetylase in normal and denervated salivary glands. *Q. J. exp. Physiol.,* **48**, 67–79.

Nordenfelt, I. (1965), Choline acetylase in salivary glands of the cat after sympathetic denervation. *Q. J. exp. Physiol.,* **50**, 57–61.

Nordenfelt, I. (1967), Metabolism of transmitter substances in salivary glands. In: *Secretory Mechanisms of Salivary Glands* (Schneyer, L.H. and Schneyer, C.A., eds), pp. 142–154, Academic Press, New York.

Norum, K.R. and Bremer, J. (1967), The localization of acyl coenzyme A carnitine acyltransferases in rat liver cells. *J. biol. Chem.,* **242**, 407–411.

Nurse, C.A. and O'Lague, P.H. (1975), Formation of cholinergic synapses between dissociated sympathetic neurons and skeletal myotubes of the rat in cell culture. *Proc. natn. Acad. Sci. U.S.A.,* 1955–1959.

Ochs, S. (1971), Characteristics and a model for fast axoplasmic transport in nerve. *J. Neurobiol.,* **2**, 331–345.

Ochs, S. (1972a), Fast transport of materials in mammalian nerve fibers. *Science* **176**, 252–260.

Ochs, S. (1972b), Fast axoplasmic transport of materials in mammalian nerve and its integrative role. *Ann. N.Y. Acad. Sci.,* **193**, 43–58.

Ochs, S. (1972c), Rate of fast axoplasmic transport in mammalian nerve fibres. *J. Physiol.,* (Lond.), **227**, 627–645.

Ochs, S. (1974a), Systems of material transport in nerve fibers (axoplasmic transport) related to nerve function and trophic control. *Ann. N.Y. Acad. Sci.,* **228**, 202–223.

Ochs, S. (1974b), Energy metabolism and supply of NP to the fast axoplasmic transport mechanism in nerve. *Fedn. Proc. Fedn. Am. Socs. exp. Biol.*, **33**, 1049–1058.

Ochs, S. (1974c), Axoplasmic transport – energy metabolism and mechanism. In: *The Peripheral Nervous System* (Hubbard, J.I., ed), pp. 47–72, Plenum Press, New York.

Ochs, S. (1975), Retention and redistribution of proteins in mammalian nerve fibres by axoplasmic transport. *J. Physiol.*, (Lond.), **253**, 459–475.

Ochs, S. and Hollingsworth, D. (1971), Dependence of fast axoplasmic transport in nerve on oxidative metabolism. *J. Neurochem.*, **18**, 107–114.

Ochs, S. and Ranish, N. (1970), Metabolic dependence of fast axoplasmic transport in nerve. *Science* **167**, 878–879.

Oderfeld-Nowak, B., Narkiewicz, O., Dabrowska, J., Wieraszko, A. and Gradkowska, M. (1973), Acetylcholinesterase and choline acetyltransferase in hippocampus after various septal lesions in rats. In: *Central Nervous System,* (Genazzani, E. and Herken, H., eds), pp. 158–163, Springer Verlag, Berlin.

Oderfeld-Nowak, B., Narkiewicz, O., Biaowas, J., Dąbrowska, J., Wieraszko, A. and Grądkowska, M. (1974), The influence of septal nuclei lesions on activity of acetylcholinesterase and choline acetyltransferase in the hippocampus of the rat. *Acta Neurobiol. exp.*, **34**, 583–601.

Oesch, F. (1974), Trans-synaptic induction of choline acetyltransferase in the preganglionic neuron of the peripheral sympathetic nervous system. *J. Pharmac. exp. Ther.*, **188**, 439–446.

Oesch, F. and Thoenen, H. (1973), Increased activity of the peripheral sympathetic nervous system: induction of choline acetyltransferase in the preganglionic cholinergic neurone. *Nature,* (Lond.), **242**, 536–537.

Oesch, F., Otten, U. and Thoenen, H. (1973), Relationship between the rate of axoplasmic transport and subcellular distribution of enzymes involved in the synthesis of norepinephrine. *J. Neurochem.*, **20**, 1691–1706.

Osborne, N.N. (1976), The uptake of [^{3}H] choline by snail (*Helix pomatia*) nervous tissue *in vitro. J. Neurochem.*, **27**, 517–522.

Page, M.A., Krebs, H.A. and Williamson, D.H. (1971), Activities of enzymes of ketone-body utilization in brain and other tissues of suckling rats. *Biochem. J.*, **121**, 49–53.

Palade, G.E. (1954), Electron microscope observations of interneuronal and neuromuscular synapses. *Anat. Rec.*, **118**, 335–336.

Palay, S.L. (1954), Electron microscope study of the cytoplasm of neurons. *Anat. Rec.*, **118**, 336.

Palay, S.L. (1956), Synapses in the central nervous system. *J. biophys. biochem. Cytol.*, Suppl. **2**, 193–202.

Palay, S.L. and Chan-Palay, V. (1973), The structural heterogeneity of central nervous tissue. In: *Metabolic Compartmentation in the Brain* (Balázs, R. and Cremer, J.E., eds), pp. 187–207, Macmillian Press, London.

Palkovits, M., Saavedra, J.M., Kobayashi, R.M. and Brownstein, M. (1974), Choline acetyltransferase content of limbic nuclei of the rat. *Brain Res.*, **79**, 443–450.

Partlow, L.M., Ross, C.D., Motwani, R. and McDougal, D.B. (1972), Transport of axonal enzymes in surviving segments of frog sciatic nerve. *J. gen. Physiol.*, **60**, 388–405.

Partridge, W.M. and Oldendorf, W.H. (1977), Transport of metabolic substrates through the blood–brain barrier. *J. Neurochem.*, **28**, 5–12.

Patel, M.S. and Owen, O.E. (1976), Lipogenesis from ketone bodies in rat brain. Evidence for conversion of acetoacetate into acetyl–coenzyme A in the cytosol. *Biochem. J.*, **156**, 603–607.

Paton, W.D.M. and Zar, M.A. (1968), The origin of acetylcholine released from guinea-pig intestine and longitudinal muscle strips. *J. Physiol.*, (Lond.), **194**, 13–33.

Patterson, P.H. and Chun, L.L.Y. (1974), The influence of non-neuronal cells on catecholamine and acetylcholine synthesis and accumulation in cultures of dissociated sympathetic neurons. *Proc. natn. Acad. Sci. U.S.A.*, **71**, 3607–3610.

Patterson, P.H., Reichardt, L.F. and Chun, L.L.Y. (1966), Biochemical studies on the development of primary sympathetic neurons in cell culture. *Cold Spring Harb. Symp. Quant. Biol.*, **40**, 389–397.

Peng, L.Y. (1976), Developmental changes in activity of choline acetyltransferase, acetyl-cholinesterase and glutamic acid decarboxylase in the central nervous system of the toad, *Xenopus laevis*. *J. Neurochem.*, **26**, 1303–1305.

Perri, V., Sacchi, O. and Casella, C. (1970a), Nervous transmission in the superior cervical ganglion of the thiamine-deficient rat. *Q. J. exp. Physiol.*, **55**, 25–35.

Perri, V., Sacchi, O. and Casella, C. (1970b), Action of oxythiamine and pyrithiamine on the isolated rat superior cervical ganglion. *Q. J. exp. Physiol.*, **56**, 36–43.

Perry, W.L.M. (1953), Acetylcholine release in the cat's superior cervical ganglion. *J. Physiol.*, (Lond.), **119**, 439–454.

Pert, C.B. and Snyder, S.H. (1974), High affinity transport of choline into the myenteric plexus of guinea-pig intestine. *J. Pharmac. exp. Ther.*, **191**, 102–108.

Peters, A., Palay, S.L. and Webster, H. de F. (1970), *The Fine Structure of the Nervous System*, Hoeber, New York.

Peterson, G.R., Webster, G.W. and Shuster, L. (1973), Characterisitics of choline acetyltransferase and cholinesterases in two types of cultured cells from embryonic chick brain. *Develop. Biol.*, **34**, 119–134.

Pilar, G., Jenden, D.J. and Campbell, B. (1973), Distribution of acetylcholine in the normal and denervated pigeon ciliary ganglion. *Brain Res.*, **49**, 245–256.

Polak, R.L. (1969), The influence of drugs on the uptake of acetylcholine by slices of rat cerebral cortex. *Brit. J. Pharmac.*, **36**, 144–152.

Polak, R.L. and Meeuws, M.M. (1966), The influence of atropine on the release and uptake of acetylcholine by the isolated cerebral cortex of the rat. *Biochem. Pharmac.*, **15**, 989–992.

Polak, R.L., Molenaar, P.C. and Van Gelder, M. (1977a), Acetylcholine metabolism and choline uptake in cortical slices. *J. Neurochem.*, **29**, 477–485.

Polak, R.L., Molenaar, P.C. and Braggaar-Schaap, P. (1977b), Regulation of acetylcholine synthesis in rat brain. In: *Cholinergic Mechanisms and Psychopharmacology*, (Jenden, D.J., ed), Plenum Press, New York, (in press).

Polsky, R. and Shuster, L. (1976a), Preparation and characterization of two isozymes of choline acetyltransferase from squid head ganglia. I. Purification and properties. *Biochim. biophys. Acta,* **445**, 25–42.

Polsky, R. and Shuster, L. (1976b), Preparation and characterization of two isozymes of choline acetyltransferase from squid head ganglia. II. Self-association, molecular weight determinations, and studies with inactivating antisera. *Biochim. biophys. Acta,* **445**, 43–66.

Potempska, A., Grądkowska, M. and Oderfeld-Nowak, B. (1975), Early changes in acetylcholine pools in the hippocampus of the rat brain after septal lesions. *J. Neurochem.*, **24**, 787–789.

Potter, L.R. (1968), Uptake of choline by nerve endings isolated from the rat cerebral cortex. In: *The Interaction of Drugs and Subcellular Components of Animal Cells,* (Campbell, P.N., ed.), pp. 293–304, Churchill, London.

Potter, L.T. (1970), Synthesis, storage and release of [^{14}C] acetylcholine in isolated rat diaphragm muscles. *J. Physiol.*, (Lond.), **206**, 145–166.

Potter, L.T. (1971), Microdetermination of acetylcholinesterase, choline acetyltransferase, and choline. In: *Meth. Enzymol.*, Vol. **17B**, (Tabor, H. and Tabor, C.W., eds), pp. 778–781, Academic Press, New York.

Potter, L.T. and Murphy, W. (1967), Electrophoresis of acetylcholine, choline and related compounds. *Biochem. Pharmac.*, **16**, 1386–1388.

Potter, L.T., Glover, V.A.S. and Saelens, J.K. (1968), Choline acetyltransferase from rat brain. *J. biol. Chem.*, **243**, 3864–3870.

Potter, L.T. and Glover, V.A.S. (1971), Choline acetyltransferase (mammalian brain). In: *Meth. Enzymol.*, Vol. **17B**, (Tabor, H. and Tabor, C.W., eds), pp. 798–801, Academic Press, New York.

Prajmovsky, M. and Welsh, J.H. (1948), Total and free acetylcholine in rat peripheral nerves. *J. Neurophysiol.*, **11**, 1–8.

Prasad, K.N., Mandal, B., Waymire, J.C., Lees, G.J., Vernadakis, A. and Weiner, N. (1973), Basal level of neurotransmitter synthesizing enzymes and the effect of cyclic AMP agents on the morphological differentiation of isolated neuroblastoma clones. *Nature New Biol.*, **21**, 117–119.

Prempeh, A.B.A., Prince, A.K. and Hide, E.G.J. (1972), The reaction of acetyl-coenzyme A with choline acetyltransferase. *Biochem J.*, **129**, 991–994.

Prenant, A. and Bouin, P. (1911), *Traité d'Histologie.* Masson, Paris.

Prestige, M.C. (1970), Differentiation, degeneration, and the role of the periphery: quantitative considerations. In: *The Neurosciences, Second Study Program,* (Schmitt, F.O., ed), pp. 73–82, The Rockefeller University Press, New York.

Price, D.L. (1974), The influence of the periphery on spinal motor neurons. *Ann. N.Y. Acad. Sci.*, **228**, 355–363.

Prince, A.K. (1967), Properties of choline acetyltransferase isolated from squid ganglia. *Proc. natn. Acad. Sci. U.S.A.*, **57**, 1117–1122.

Prince, A.K. (1971), Choline acetyltransferase. In: *Meth. Enzymol.*, Vol. **17B**, (Tabor, H. and Tabor, C.W., eds), pp. 788–797, Academic Press, New York.

Prince, A.K. and Hide, E.G.J. (1971), Activation of choline acetyltransferase by salts. *Nature,* (Lond.), **234**, 222–223.

Pysh, J.J. and Wiley, R.G. (1974), Synaptic vesicle depletion and recovery in cat sympathetic ganglia electrically stimulated *in vivo. J. cell Biol.*, **60**, 365–374.

Quastel, J.H. (1966), Molecular transport at cell membranes. *Proc. R. Soc.* B. **163**, 169–196.

Quastel, J.H., Tennenbaum, M. and Wheatley, A.H.M. (1936), Choline ester formation in, and choline esterase activities of, tissues *in vitro. Biochem. J.,* **30**, 1668–1681.

Racagni, G., Trabucchi, M. and Cheney, D.L. (1975), Steady-state concentrations of choline and acetylcholine in rat brain parts during a constant rate infusion of deuterated choline. *Naunyn-Schmiedebergs Arch. Pharmakol.,* **290**, 99–105.

Racagni, G., Cheney, D.L., Trabucchi, M. and Costa, E. (1976), *In vivo* actions of clozapine and haloperidol on the turnover rate of acetylcholine in rat striatum. *J. Pharmac. exp. Ther.,* **196**, 323–332.

Ranish, N. and Ochs, S. (1972), Fast axoplasmic transport of acetylcholinesterase in mammalian nerve fibres. *J. Neurochem.,* **19**, 2641–2649.

Rastogi, R.B., Hrdina, P.D., Dubas, T. and Singhal, R.L. (1977), Alterations of brain acetylcholine metabolism during neonatal hyperthyroidism. *Brain Res.,* **123**, 188–192.

Reed, L.J., Linn, T.C., Pettit, F.H., Oliver, R.M., Hucho, F., Pelley, J.W., Randall, D.D. and Roche, T.E. (1972), Pyruvate dehydrogenase complex: structure, function and regulation. In: *Energy Metabolism and the Regulation of Metabolic Processes in Mitochondria,* (Mehlman, M.A. and Hanson, R.W., eds), pp. 253–270, Academic Press, New York.

Reid, W.D., Haubrich, D.R. and Krishna, G. (1971), Enzymic radioassay for acetylcholine and choline in brain. *Analyt. Biochem.,* **42**, 390–397.

Reijnierse, G.L., Veldstra, H. and Van den Berg, C.J. (1975), Short-chain fatty acid synthases in brain. *Biochem. J.,* **152**, 477–484.

Rentsch, G. (1961), Die cholinacetylierenden Fermente des Meerschweinchenhirns. *Naturwissenschaften,* **48**, 308.

Reynolds, S.F. and Blass, J.P. (1975), Normal levels of acetyl coenzyme A and of acetylcholine in the brains of thiamin-deficient rats. *J. Neurochem.,* **24**, 185–186.

Richelson, E. and Thompson, E.J. (1973), Transport of neurotransmitter precursors into cultured cells. *Nature New Biol.,* **241**, 201–204.

Richter, D. and Crossland, J. (1949), Variation in acetylcholine content of the brain with physiological state. *Am. J. Physiol.,* **159**, 247–255.

Richter, J.A. (1976), Characteristics of acetylcholine release by superfused slices of rat brain. *J. Neurochem.,* **26**, 791–797.

Richter, J.A. and Marchbanks, R.M. (1971a), Synthesis of radioactive acetylcholine from [^{3}H] choline and its release from cerebral cortex slices *in vitro. J. Neurochem.,* **18**, 691–703.

Richter, J.A. and Marchbanks, R.M. (1971b), Isolation of [^{3}H]acetylcholine pools by subcellular fractionation of cerebral cortex slices incubated with [^{3}H]choline, *J. Neurochem.,* **18**, 705–712.

Rommelspacher, H. and Kuhar, M.J. (1975), Effects of drugs and axotomy on acetylcholine levels in central cholinergic neurons. *Naunyn-Schmiedeberg's Arch. Pharmak.,* **291**, 17–21.

Roodyn, D.B. (1965), The classification and partial tabulation of enzyme studies on subcellular fractions isolated by differential centrifuging. *Int. Rev. Cytol.*, **18**, 99–190.

Rosenberg, P., Mackey, E.A., Higman, H.B. and Dettbarn, W.-D. (1964), Choline acetylase and cholinersterase activity in denervated electroplax. *Biochim. biophys. Acta*, **82**, 266–275.

Rosenblueth, K., Lissák, K. and Lanari, A. (1939), An explanation of the five stages of neuromuscular and ganglionic synaptic transmission. *Am. J. Physiol.*, **128**, 31–44.

Roskoski, R. (1973), Choline acetyltransferase. Evidence for an acetylenzyme reaction intermediate. *Biochemistry*, **12**, 3709–3714.

Roskoski, R. (1974a), Choline acetyltransferase; inhibition by thiol reagents. *J. biol. Chem.*, **249**, 2156–2159.

Roskoski, R. (1974b), Choline acetyltransferase: reversible inhibition by bromoacetyl coenzyme A and bromoacetylcholine. *Biochemistry*, **13**, 2295–2298.

Roskoski, R. (1974c), Choline acetyltransferase and acetylcholinesterase: evidence for essential histidine residues. *Biochemistry*, **13**, 5141–5144.

Roskoski, R., Mayer, H.E. and Schmid, P.G. (1974), Choline acetyltransferase activity in guinea pig heart *in vitro*. *J. Neurochem.*, **23**, 1197–1200.

Ross, C.D. and McDougal, D.B. (1976), The distribution of choline acetyltransferase activity in vertebrate retina. *J. Neurochem.*, **26**, 521–526.

Rossier, J. (1975), Immunochistochemical localization of choline acetyltransferase: real or artefact? *Brain Res.*, **98**, 619–622.

Rossier, J. (1976a), Purification of rat brain choline acetyltransferase. *J. Neurochem.*, **26**, 543–548.

Rossier, J. (1976b), Immunological properties of rat brain choline acetyltransferase. *J. Neurochem.*, **26**, 549–553.

Rossier, J. (1976c), Biophysical properties of rat brain choline acetyltransferase. *J. Neurochem.*, **26**, 555–559.

Rossier, J. (1977a), Choline acetyltransferase: A review with special reference to its cellular and subcellular localization. *Int. Rev. Neurobiol.*, **20**, (in press).

Rossier, J. (1977b), Acetyl–coenzyme A and coenzyme A analogues: their effects on rat brain choline acetyltransferase. *Biochem. J.*, **165**, 321–326.

Rossier, J. and Benda, P. (1977), Activation of choline acetyltransferase by chloride: a possible regulatory mechanism. In: *Cholinergic Mechanism and Psychopharmacology* (Jenden, D.J., ed.), Plenum Press, New York, (in press).

Rossier, J., Bauman, A. and Benda, P. (1973a), Improved purification of rat brain choline acetyltransferase by using an immunoabsorbent, *FEBS Letters*, **32**, 231–234.

Rossier, J., Bauman, A. and Benda, P. (1973b), Antibodies to rat brain choline acetyltransferase: species and organ specificity. *FEBS Letters*, **36**, 43–48.

Rous, S. (1971), Role modeste du citrate comme transporteur d'acétyl–CoA chez l'animal vivant. *FEBS Letters*, **12**, 338–340.

Rous, S. (1973), Acetylaspartate as an extramitochondrial physiological carrier of acetyl CoA for fatty acid synthesis. *Life Sci.*, **13**, 1715–1724.

Rous, S. (1976), On the occurrence of enzymes of ketone-body metabolism in human adipose tissue. *Biochem. biophys. Res. Commun.*, **69**, 74–78.

Ruderman, N.B., Ross, P.S., Berger, M. and Goodman, M.N. (1974), Regulation of glucose and ketone-body metabolism in brain of anaesthetized rat. *Biochem. J.*, **138**, 1–10.

Ryan, R.L. and McClure, W.O. (1976), Purification and some properties of a choline acetylase from bovine caudate nucleus. *Fedn. Proc., Am. Socs. exp. Biol.*, **35**, 1647

Sabri, M.I. and Ochs, S. (1973), Characterization of fast and slow transported proteins in dorsal root and sciatic nerve of cat. *J. Neurobiol.*, **4**, 145–165.

Sacchi, O. and Perri, V. (1973), Quantal mechanism of transmitter release during progressive depletion of the presynaptic stores at a ganglionic synapse. *J. gen. Physiol.*, **61**, 342–360.

Saelens, J.K., Allen, M.P. and Simke, J.P. (1970), Determination of acetylcholine and choline by an enzymatic assay. *Archs. int. Pharmacodyn. Thér.*, **186**, 279–286.

Saelens, J.K., Simke, J.P., Allen, M.P. and Conroy, C.A. (1973), Some of the dynamics of choline and acetylcholine metabolism in rat brain. *Archs. int. Pharmacodyn. Thér.*, **203**, 305–312.

Saito, M. and Kanfer, J. (1973), Solubilization and properties of a membrane-bound enzyme from rat brain catalyzing a base-exchange reaction. *Biochem. biophys. Res. Commun.*, **53**, 391–398.

Salehmoghaddam, S.H. and Collier, B. (1976), The relationship between acetylcholine release from brain slices and the acetylcholine content of subcellular fractions prepared from brain. *J. Neurochem.*, **27**, 71–76.

Samson, F.E. (1971), Mechanism of axoplasmic transport. *J. Neurobiol.*, **2**, 347–360.

Sanadi, D.R. (1963), Pyruvate and α-ketoglutarate oxidation enzymes. In: *The Enzymes,* 2nd edn. (Boyer, P.D., Lardy, H. and Myrbäck, K., eds), Vol. **7**, pp. 307–344, Academic Press, New York.

Sastry, B.V.R. and Henderson, G.I. (1972), Kinetic mechanisms of human placental choline acetyltransferase. *Biochem. Pharmac.*, **21**, 787–802.

Sastry, B.V.R., Olubadewo, J., Harbison, R.D. and Schmidt, D.E. (1976), Human placental cholinergic system. Occurrence, distribution and variation with gestational age of acetylcholine in human placenta. *Biochem. Pharmac.*, **25**, 425–431.

Satake, M. (1972), Some aspects of protein metabolism of the neuron. *Int. Rev. Neurobiol.*, **15**, 189–213.

Sattin, A. (1966), The synthesis and storage of acetylcholine in the striatum. *J. Neurochem.*, **13**, 515–524.

Saunders, N.R., Dziegielewska, K., Häggendal, C.J. and Dahlström, A.B. (1973), Slow accumulation of choline acetyltransferase in crushed sciatic nerves of the rat. *J. Neurobiol.*, **4**, 95–103.

Schafer, R. (1973), Acetylcholine: fast axoplasmic transport in insect chemoreceptor fibers. *Science,* **180**, 315–317.

Schmidt, D.E. and Speth, R.C. (1975), Simultaneous analysis of choline and acetylcholine levels in rat brain by pyrolysis gas chromatography. *Analyt. Biochem.*, **67**, 353–357.

Schmidt, D.E., Szilagyi, P.I.A., Alkon, D.L. and Green, J.P. (1969), Acetylcholine: release from neural tissue and identification by pyrolysis – gas chromatography *Science,* **165**, 1370–1371.

Schmidt, R.E., Matschinsky, F.M., Godfrey, D.A., Williams, A.D. and McDougal, D.B. (1975), Fast and slow axoplasmic flow in sciatic nerve of diabetic rats. *Diabetes,* **24**, 1081–1085.

Schmitt, F.O. (1968), Fibrous proteins – neuronal organelles. *Proc. natn. Acad. Sci. U.S.A.,* **60**, 1092–1101.

Schnaitman, C. and Greenawalt, J.W. (1968), Enzymatic properties of the inner and outer membranes of rat liver mitochondria. *J. cell Biol.,* **38**, 158–175.

Scholte, H.R., Wit-Peeters, E.M. and Bakker, J.C. (1971), The intracellular and intramitochondrial distribution of short-chain acyl–CoA synthetases in guinea pig heart. *Biochim. biophys. Acta,* **231**, 479–486.

Schrier, B.K. and Shuster, L. (1967), A simplified radiochemical assay for choline acetyltransferase. *J. Neurochem.,* **14**, 977–985.

Schubert, D., Heinemann, S., Carlisle, W., Tarikas, H., Kimes, B., Patrick, J., Steinbach, J.H., Culp, W. and Brandt, B.L. (1974), Clonal cell lines from the rat central nervous system. *Nature,* (Lond.), **249**, 224–227.

Schuberth, J. (1963), Radiochemical determination of choline acetyltransferase. *Acta chem. scand.,* **17**, suppl. **1**, S233–S237.

Schuberth, J. (1965), On the biosynthesis of acetyl coenzyme A in the brain. I. The enzymic formation of acetyl coenzyme A from acetate, adenosine triphosphate and coenzyme A. *Biochim. biophys. Acta,* **98**, 1–7.

Schuberth, J. (1966), Choline acetyltransferase. Purification and effect of salts on the mechanism of the enzyme-catalyzed reaction. *Biochim. biophys. Acta,* **122**, 470–481.

Schuberth, J. and Jenden, D.J. (1975), Transport of choline from plasma to cerebrospinal fluid in the rabbit with reference to the origin of choline and to acetylcholine metabolism in brain. *Brain Res.,* **84**, 245–256.

Schuberth, J. and Sörbo, B. (1971), Measurement of choline acetylase. In: *Analysis of Biogenic Amines and Their Related Enzymes* (Glick, D., ed.), pp. 275–296, John Wiley and Sons, New York.

Schuberth, J. and Sundwall, A. (1967), Effects of some drugs on the uptake of acetylcholine in cortex slices of mouse brain. *J. Neurochem.,* **14**, 807–812.

Schuberth, J. and Sundwall, A. (1971), A method for the determination of choline in biological materials. *Acta pharmac.,* **29**, Suppl. **4**, 51.

Schuberth, J., Sollenberg, J., Sundwall, A. and Sörbo, B. (1965), Determination of acetylcoenzyme A in brain. *J. Neurochem.,* **12**, 451–454.

Schuberth, J., Sundwall, A., Sörbo, B. and Lindell, J.-O. (1966a), Uptake of choline by mouse brain slices. *J. Neurochem.,* **13**, 347–352.

Schuberth, J., Sollenberg, J., Sundwall, A. and Sörbo, B. (1966b), Acetylcoenzyme A in brain. The effect of centrally active drugs, insulin coma and hypoxia. *J. Neurochem.,* **13**, 819–822.

Schuberth, J., Sparf, B. and Sundwall, A. (1969), A technique for the study of acetylcholine turnover in mouse brain *in vivo. J. Neurochem.,* **16**, 695–700.

Schuberth, J., Sparf, B. and Sundwall, A. (1970a), Determinations of choline. In: *Drugs and Cholinergic Mechanisms in the CNS* (Heilbronn, E. and Winter, A., eds), pp. 15–26, Almqvist and Wiksell, Stockholm.

Schuberth, J., Sparf, B. and Sundwall, A. (1970b), On the turnover of acetylcholine in nerve endings of mouse brain *in vivo. J. Neurochem.,* **17**, 461–468.

Schwartz, J.H., Eisenstadt, M.L. and Cedar, H. (1975), Metabolism of acetylcholine in the nervous system of *Aplysia californica.* I. Source of choline and its uptake by intact nervous tissue. *J. gen. Physiol.,* **65**, 255–273.

Scott, F.H. (1906), On the relation of nerve cells to fatigue of their nerve fibres. *J. Physiol.,* (Lond.), **34**, 145–162.

Sethy, V.H., Kuhar, M.J., Roth, R.G., Van Woert, M.H. and Aghajanian, G.K. (1973), Cholinergic neurons: effect of acute septal lesion on acetylcholine and choline content of rat hippocampus. *Brain Res.,* **55**, 481–484.

Sethy, V.H. and Van Woert, M.H. (1973), Effect of L-dopa on brain acetylcholine and choline in rats. *Neuropharmacology,* **12**, 27–31.

Sethy, V.H., Roth, H.R., Kuhar, M.J. and Van Woert, M.H. (1973), Choline–acetylcholine regional distribution and effect of degeneration of cholinergic nerve terminals in the rat hippocampus. *Neuropharmacology,* **12**, 819–823.

Severin, S.E. and Artenie, V. (1967), Extraction, partial purification and some properties of choline acetyltransferase from rabbit brain (Russ.). *Biokhimiya,* **32**, 125–132.

Severin, S.E. and Artenie, V. (1968), Influence of imidazole and cysteine on the activity and stability of choline acetyltransferase (Russ.). *Vopr. med. khim.,* **14**, 89–94.

Severin, S.E. and Lu S.-S. (1962), Biosynthesis of acetylcholine in the nerve and muscle tissues of insects (Russ.). *Biokhimiya,* **27**, 1085–1091.

Severin, S.E. and Popova, I.A. (1965), Participation of imidazole, adenylic acid, CoA and of their acetylated derivatives in the synthesis and biosynthesis of acetylcholine (Russ.). *Biokhimiya,* **30**, 970–979.

Sharkawi, M. (1972), Effects of some centrally acting drugs on acetylcholine synthesis by rat cerebral cortex slices. *Brit. J. Pharmac.,* **46**, 473–479.

Sharkawi, M. and Schulman, M.P. (1969a), Relationship between acetylcholine synthesis and its concentration in rat cerebral cortex. *Brit. J. Pharmac.,* **36**, 373–379.

Sharkawi, M. and Schulman, M.P. (1969b), Inhibition by morphine of the release of [^{14}C]acetylcholine from rat brain cortex slices. *J. Pharm. Pharmac.,* **21**, 546–547.

Sharkova, E.V. (1968), Acetyl–CoA synthetase reaction (Russ.). *Usp. biol. khim.,* **9**, 245–252.

Shea, P.A. and Aprison, M.H. (1973), An enzymatic method for measuring picomole quantities of acetylcholine and choline in CNS tissue. *Analyt. Biochem.,* **56**, 165–177.

Shea, P.A. and Aprison, M.H. (1977), The distribution of acetyl–CoA in specific areas of the CNS of the rat as measured by a modification of a radio-enzymatic assay for acetylcholine and choline. *J. Neurochem.,* **28**, 51–58.

Sheridan, M.N., Whittaker, V.P. and Israël, M. (1966), The subcellular fractionation of the electric organ of *Torpedo. Z. Zellforsch.,* **74**, 291–307.

Shuster, L. and O'Toole, C. (1974), Inactivation of choline acetyltransferases by an antiserum to the enzyme from mouse brain. *Life Sci.,* **15**, 645–656.

Silver, A. (1974), *The Biology of Cholinesterases.* North-Holland Publishing Company, Amsterdam.

Simon, J.R. and Kuhar, M.J. (1975), Impulse-flow regulation of high affinity choline uptake in brain cholinergic nerve terminals. *Nature,* (Lond.), **255**, 162–163.

Simon, J.R. and Kuhar, M.J. (1976), High affinity choline uptake: ionic and energy requirements. *J. Neurochem.,* **27**, 93–99.

Simon, J.R., Mittag, T.W. and Kuhar, M.J. (1975), Inhibition of synaptosomal uptake of choline by various choline analogs. *Biochem. Pharmac.,* **24**, 1139–1142.

Simon, J.R., Atweh, S. and Kuhar, M.J. (1976), Sodium-dependent high affinity choline uptake: a regulatory step in the synthesis of acetylcholine. *J. Neurochem.,* **26**, 909–922.

Singer, G., Ho, A. and Gershon, S. (1971), Changes in activity of choline acetylase in central nervous system of rat after intraventricular administration of noradrenaline. *Nature New Biol.,* **230**, 152–153.

Singh, V.K. and McGeer, P.L. (1974a) Antibody production to choline acetyltransferase purified from human brain. *Life Sci.,* **15**, 901–913.

Singh, V.K. and McGeer, P.L. (1974b) Cross-immunity of antibodies to human choline acetyltransferase in various vertebrate species. *Brain Res.,* **82**, 356–359.

Singh, V.K. and McGeer, E.G. (1977a), Choline acetyltransferase in developing rat brain and spinal cord. *Brain Res.,* **127**, 159–163.

Singh, V.K. and McGeer, P.L. (1977b), Studies on choline acetyltansferase purified from human brain. *Neurochem. Res.,* **2**, 281–291.

Singh, V.K., Fibiger, H.C., McGeer, E.G. and McGeer, P.L. (1974), Analysis of proteins undergoing axonal transport in nigro-striatal neurons of the rat. *J. Neurochem.,* **22**, 119–124.

Singh, V.K., McGeer, E.G. and McGeer, P.L. (1975), Two immunologically different choline acetyltransferases in human neostriatum. *Brain Res.,* **96**, 187–191.

Sjöstrand, N.O. and Swedin, G. (1976), Influence of age, growth, castration and testosterone treatment on the noradrenaline levels of the ductus deferens and the auxiliary male reproductive glands of the rat. *Acta physiol. scand.,* **98**, 323–338.

Sjöstrand, J., Frizell, M. and Hasselgren, P.-O. (1970), Effects of colchicine on axonal transport in peripheral nerves. *J. Neurochem.,* **17**, 1563–1570.

Škarda, J. and Bílek, J. (1973), Glycidový metabolismus přežvýkavců I. *Čs. fysiol.,* **22**, 419–447.

Smith, A.D. (1972), Cellular control of the uptake, storage and release of noradrenaline in sympathetic nerves. *Biochem. Soc. Symp.,* **36**, 103–131.

Smith, B.H. and Kreutzberg, G.W. (1976), Neuron-target cell interaction. *Neurosciences Res. Programm Bull.,* **14**, 211–453.

Smith, J.E., Lane, J.D., Shea, P.A., McBride, W.J. and Aprison, M.H. (1975), A method for concurrent measurement of picomole quantities of acetylcholine, choline, dopamine, norepinephrine, serotonin, 5-hydroxytryptophan, 5-hydroxyindoleacetic acid, tryptophan, tyrosine, glycine, aspartate, glutamate, alanine and gamma-aminobutyric acid in single tissue samples from different areas of rat central nervous system. *Analyt. Biochem.,* **64**, 149–169.

Snoswell, A.M. and Koundakjian, P.P. (1972), Relationships between carnitine and coenzyme A esters in tissues of normal and alloxan-diabetic sheep. *Biochem , J.,* **127**, 133–141.

Snyder, D.H., Rifenberick, D.H. and Max, S.R. (1973), Effects of neuromuscular activity on choline acetyltransferase and acetylcholinesterase. *Expl. Neurol.*, **40**, 36–42.

Sollenberg, J. and Sörbo, B. (1970), On the origin of the acetyl moiety of acetylcholine in brain studied with a differential labelling technique using ^{3}H-^{14}C-mixed labelled glucose and acetate. *J. Neurochem.*, **17**, 201–207.

Sorimachi, M. and Kataoka, K. (1974a), Developmental change of choline acetyltransferase and acetylcholinesterase in the ciliary and the superior cervical ganglion of the chick. *Brain Res.*, **70**, 123–130.

Sorimachi, N. and Kataoka, K. (1974b), Choline uptake by nerve terminals: a sensitive and a specific marker of cholinergic innervation *Brain Res.*, **72**, 350–353.

Sorimachi, M. and Kataoka, K. (1975), High affinity choline uptake: an early index of cholinergic innervation in rat brain. *Brain Res.*, **94**, 325–336.

Sorimachi, M., Miyamoto, K. and Kataoka, K. (1974), Postnatal development of choline uptake by cholinergic terminals in rat brain. *Brain Res.*, **79**, 343–346.

Spanner, S., Hall, R.C. and Ansell, B. (1976), Arterio-venous differences of choline and choline lipids across the brain of rat and rabbit. *Biochem. J.*, **154**, 133–140.

Spantidakis, Y., Rossier, J. and Benda, P. (1976), Influence des ions chlore sur les paramètres cinétiques de la choline acétyltransférase du cerveau de Rat. *C. r. Acad. Sci.* (Paris), D **282**, 1621–1624.

Sparf, B. (1973), On the turnover of acetylcholine in the brain. An experimental study using intravenously injected radioactive choline. *Acta physiol. scand.*, suppl. **397**, 1–47.

Spector, L.B. (1972), Citrate cleavage and related enzymes. In: *The Enzymes* (Boyer, P.D., ed.), 3rd. edn., Vol. **7**, pp. 357–389, Academic Press, New York.

Spencer, P.S. (1972), Reappraisal of the model for 'bulk axoplasmic flow'. *Nature New Biol.*, **240**, 283–285.

Srere, P.A. (1959), The citrate cleavage enzyme. I. Distribution and purification. *J. biol. Chem.*, **234**, 2544–2547.

Srere, P.A. (1965), The molecular physiology of citrate. *Nature,* (Lond.), **205**, 766–770.

Srere, P.A. (1967), A magnetic resonance study of the citrate synthase reaction. *Biochem. biophys. Res. Commun.*, **26**, 609–614.

Srere, P.A. (1972), The citrate enzymes: their structures, mechanisms, and biological functions. In: *Current Topics in Cellular Regulation* (Horecker, B.L. and Stadtman, E.R., eds), pp. 228–283, Academic Press, New York.

Srere, P.A. (1975), The enzymology of the formation and breakdown of citrate. *Adv. Enzymol.*, **43**, 57–101.

Stavinoha, W.B. and Weintraub, S.T. (1974a), Estimation of choline and acetylcholine in tissue by pyrolysis gas chromatography. *Analyt. Chem.*, **46**, 757–760.

Stavinoha, W.B. and Weintraub, S.T. (1974b), Choline content of rat brain. *Science,* **183**, 964–965.

Stavinoha, W.B., Weintraub, S.T. and Modak, A.T. (1974), Regional concentrations of choline and acetylcholine in the rat brain. *J. Neurochem.*, **23**, 885–886.

Stedman, E. and Stedman, E. (1937), The mechanism of the biological synthesis of acetylcholine. I. The isolation of acetylcholine produced by brain tissue *in vitro. Biochem. J.*, **31**, 817–827.

Stein, Y. and Stein, O. (1966), Metabolism of labeled lysolecithin. Lysophosphatidyl ethanolamine and lecithin in the rat. *Biochim. biophys. Acta,* **116**, 95–107.

Stephenson, M. and Rowatt, E. (1947), The production of acetylcholine by a strain of *Lactobacillus plantarum. J. gen. Microbiol.*, **1**, 279–298.

Stewart, D.M. and Martin, A.W. (1966), Acetylcholine and cholinesterase activity of the denervated hemidiaphragm of the rat. *Expl. Neurol.*, **16**, 299–306.

Sundwall, A. (1973), Effect of pentobarbital on the turnover of acetylcholine in brain nerve terminals *in vivo. Brain Res.* **62**, 531–536.

Suszkiw, J.B. (1976), Acetylcholine translocation in synaptic vesicle ghosts *in vitro. J. Neurochem.*, **27**, 853–857.

Suszkiw, J.B. and Pilar, G. (1976), Selective localization of a high affinity choline uptake system and its role in ACh formation in cholinergic nerve terminals. *J. Neurochem.*, **26**, 1133–1138.

Suszkiw, J.B., Beach, R.L. and Pilar, G.R. (1976), Choline uptake by cholinergic neuron cell somas. *J. Neurochem.*, **26**, 1123–1131.

Svendgaard, N.-A., Björklund, A. and Stenevi, U. (1976), Regeneration of central cholinergic neurones in the adult rat brain. *Brain. Res.*, **102**, 1–22.

Swaiman, K.F. and Milstein, J.M. (1965), Oxidation of leucine, isoleucine and related ketoacids in developing rabbit brain. *J. Neurochem.*, **12**, 981–986.

Tauc, L., Hoffman, A., Tsuji, S., Hinzen, D.H. and Faille, L. (1974), Transmission abolished on a cholinergic synapse after injection of acetylcholinesterase into the presynaptic neurone. *Nature,* (Lond.), **250**, 496–498.

Tencati, J.R. and Rosenberg, R.N. (1973), A radioisotopic, chromatographic microassay for acetyl–coenzyme A synthetase and some preliminary studies on the rat brain enzyme. *Biochim. biophys. Acta,* **293**, 542–551.

Tewari, H.B. and Bourne, G.H. (1960), Biochemical localization of specific and non-specific cholinesterases, and simple esterase in myelinated nerves. *Expl. cell Res.*, **21**, 245–248.

Thoenen, H., Saner, A., Angeletti, P.U. and Levi-Montalcini, R. (1972), Increased activity of choline acetyltransferase in sympathetic ganglia after prolonged administration of nerve growth factor. *Nature,* (Lond.), **236**, 26–28.

Thomas, L.L., Radulovački, M. and Schulman, M.P. (1976), Inhibition of glucose utilization for acetylcholine synthesis by cerebrospinal fluid. *J. Neurochem.*, **26**, 531–536.

Thomitzek, W.-D. and Strack, E. (1964), Acetylcarnitin als Acetyldonator bei der enzymatischen Bildung von Acetylcholin. *Acta biol. med. germ.*, **13**, 110–125.

Thompson, G.A. (1973), Phospholipid metabolism in animal tissues. In: *Form and Function of Phospholipids* (Ansell, G.B., Dawson, R.M.C. and Hawthorne, J.N., eds), pp. 67–96, Elsevier, Amsterdam.

Tiegs, O.W. (1953), Innervation of voluntary muscle. *Physiol. Rev.*, **33**, 90–144.

Tochino, Y. and Schanker, L.S. (1965), Active transport of quaternary ammonium compounds by the choroid plexus *in vitro*. *Am. J. Physiol.*, **208**, 666–673.

Tonge, D.A., Gradidge, T.J. and Marchbanks, R.M. (1975), Effects of botulinum and tetanus toxins on choline acetyltransferase activity in skeletal muscle in the mouse. *J. Neurochem.*, **25**, 329–331.

Treistman, S.N. and Schwartz, J.H. (1977), Metabolism of acetylcholine in the nervous system of *Aplysia californica*. IV. Studies of an identified cholinergic axon. *J. gen. Physiol.*, **69**, 725–741.

Tubbs, P.K. and Garland, P.B. (1968), Membranes and fatty acid metabolism. *Brit. med. Bull.*, **24**, 158–164.

Tuček, S. (1965), Changes in choline acetyltransferase activity in the cardiac auricles of dogs during postnatal development. *Physiol. bohemoslov.*, **14**, 530–535.

Tuček, S. (1966a), Binding of choline acetyltransferase in the nerve ending particles of brain. *Nature*, (Lond.), **212**, 1247–1249.

Tuček, S. (1966b), On subcellular localization and binding of choline acetyltransferase in the cholinergic nerve endings of the brain. *J. Neurochem.*, **13**, 1317–1327.

Tuček, S. (1966c), On the question of the localization of choline acetyltransferase in synaptic vesicles. *J. Neurochem.*, **13**, 1329–1332.

Tuček, S. (1966d), The synthesis of acetyl–coenzyme A and acetylcholine from citrate and acetate in the nerve endings of mammalian brain. *Biochim. biophys. Acta*, **117**, 278–280.

Tuček, S. (1967a), Observations on the subcellular distribution of choline acetyltransferase in the brain tissue of mammals and comparisons of acetylcholine synthesis from acetate and citrate in homogenates and nerve-endings fractions. *J. Neurochem.*, **14**, 519–529.

Tuček, S.(1967b), Subcellular distribution of acetyl–CoA synthetase, ATP citrate lyase, citrate synthase, choline acetyltransferase, fumarate hydratase and lactate dehydrogenase in mammalian brain tissue. *J. Neurochem.*, **14**, 531–545.

Tuček, S. (1967c), The use of choline acetyltransferase for measuring the synthesis of acetyl–coenzyme A and its release from brain mitochondria. *Biochem. J.*, **104**, 749–756.

Tuček, S. (1967d), Activation of choline acetyltransferase in subcellular fractions of the brain by hyposomotic treatment and by ether. *Biochem. Pharmac.*, **16**, 109–113.

Tuček, S. (1968a), Motor nerve and the activity of choline acetyltransferase in the skeletal muscle. *Biochim. biophys. Acta*, **170**, 457–458.

Tuček, S. (1968b), Post-denervation changes of choline acetyltransferase activity in skeletal muscle of rats. *Physiol. bohemoslov.*, **17**, 496.

Tuček, S. (1970), Subcellular localization of enzymes generating acetyl–CoA and their possible relation to the biosynthesis of acetylcholine. In: *Drugs and Cholinergic Mechanisms in the CNS* (Heilbronn, E. and Winter, A., eds), pp. 117–131. Almqvist and Wiksell, Stockholm.

Tuček, S. (1972), Choline acetyitransferase activity in rat skeletal muscles during postnatal development. *Expl. Neurol.*, **36**, 378–388.

Tuček, S. (1973a), Choline acetyltransferase activity in skeletal muscles after denervation. *Expl. Neurol.*, **40**, 23–35.

Tuček, S. (1973b), Origin of acetyl groups in brain acetylcholine. In: *La Transmission Cholinergique de l'Excitation* (Fardeau, M., Israël, M. and Manaranche, R. eds), pp. 83–90, Editions INSERM, Paris.

Tuček, S. (1973c), An improved solvent system for liquid scintillation counting in choline acetyltransferase activity assays by Fonnum's method. *J. Neurochem.*, **20**, 901–903.

Tuček, S. (1974), Transport and changes of activity of choline acetyltransferase in the peripheral stump of an interrupted nerve. *Brain Res.*, **82**, 249–261.

Tuček, S. (1975), Transport of choline acetyltransferase and acetylcholinesterase in the central stump and isolated segments of a peripheral nerve. *Brain Res.*, **86**, 259–270.

Tuček, S. and Cheng, S.-C. (1970), Precursors of acetyl groups in acetylcholine in the brain *in vivo. Biochim. biophys. Acta,* **208**, 538–540.

Tuček, S. and Cheng, S.-C. (1974), Prevenance of the acetyl group of acetylcholine and compartmentation of acetyl–CoA and Krebs cycle intermediates in the brain *in vivo. J. Neurochem.*, **22**, 893–914.

Tuček, S. and Diepold, F. (1963), The metabolism of acetylcholine in the brain in experimental hyperthyroidism. *Physiol. bohemoslov.*, **12**, 258–262.

Tuček, S. and Gutmann, E. (1973), Choline acetyltransferase activity in muscles of old rats. *Expl. Neurol.*, **38**, 349–360.

Tuček, S. and Koudelková, Z. (1966), Choline acetyltransferase and acetylcholine in brain, heart atria, intestine, uterus and diaphragm of rats and guinea pigs. *Archs. int. Physiol. Biochem.*, **74**, 123–134.

Tuček, S. and Vlk, J. (1962), The effect of vagotomy on the acetylcholine content and cholinesterase activity in various regions of the rat heart atria. *Physiol. bohemoslov.*, **11**, 319–328.

Tuček, S., Koštířová, D. and Hanzlíková, V. (1975), Axonal transport of choline acetyltransferase and acetylcholinesterase in interrupted nerves and isolated nerve segments; effects of ischaemia on axonal transport and degeneration. In: *Abstracts of the 5th Meeting of International Society of Neurochemistry,* p. 257, Barcelona.

Tuček, S., Koštířová, D. and Gutmann, E. (1976a), Testosterone-induced changes of choline acetyltransferase and cholinesterase activities in rat levator ani muscle. *J. neurol. Sci.*, **27**, 353–362.

Tuček, S., Koštířová, D. and Gutmann, E. (1976b), Effects of castration, testosterone and immobilization on the activities of choline acetyltransferase and cholinesterase in rat limb muscles. *J. neurol. Sci.*, **27**, 363–372.

Tuček, S., Havránek, M. and Ge, I. (1978), Synthesis of [acetyl-^{14}C] carnitine and the use of tetraphenylboron for differential extraction of [acetyl-^{14}C] choline and [acetyl-^{14}C] carnitine. *Analyt. Biochem.*, (in press).

Tuček, S., Hanzlíková, V. and Stráníková, D. (1978b), Effect of ischemia on axonal transport of choline acetyltransferase and acetylcholinesterase and on ultrastructural changes of isolated segments of rabbit nerves *in situ. J. Neurol. Sci.*, **178**, (in press).

Ulus, I.H., Hirsch, M.J. and Wurtman, R.J. (1977), Trans-synaptic induction of adrenomedullary tyrosine hydroxylase activity by choline: evidence that choline administration can increase cholinergic transmission. *Proc. natn. Acad. Sci. U.S.A.*, **74**, 798–800.

Umrath, K., Bohn, H. and Klemencic, E. (1966), Nervöse Überträgersubstanzen bei der Nervendegeneration. *Z. Biol.*, **115**, 165–170.

Veldsema-Currie, R.D., Wolters, E.C.M.J. and Leeuwin, R.S. (1976), The effect of corticosteroids and hemicholinium-3 on choline uptake and incorporation into acetylcholine in rat diaphragm. *Eur. J. Pharmac.*, **35**, 399–402.

Verkhratsky, N.S. (1970), Acetylcholine metabolism peculiarities in aging. *Expl. Geront.*, **5**, 49–56.

Vial, J.D. (1955), The influence of axon length on the course of Wallerian degeneration of the motor end-plates. *Acta Physiol. latinoamer.*, **5**, 95–103.

Vlk, J. and Tuček, S. (1961), Distribution of acetylcholine in the auricles of the mammalian heart. *Physiol. bohemoslov.*, **10**, 65–71.

Vlk, J. and Tuček, S. (1964), The formation of acetylcholine in isolated heart auricles of white rats and guinea pigs. *Physiol. bohemoslov.*, **13**, 310–314.

Vos, J., Kuriyama, K. and Roberts, E. (1968), Electrophoretic mobilities of brain subcellular particles and binding of γ-aminobutyric acid, acetylcholine, norepinephrine, and 5-hydroxytryptamine. *Brain Res.*, **9**, 224–230.

Voskresenskii, O.N. and Maksimovich, Ya. B. (1967), Choline and its biological role (Russ.). *Usp. sovr. biol.*, **64**, 53–74.

Wakade, A.R. and Kirpekar, S.M. (1973), 'Trophic' influence on the sympathetic nerves of the vas deferens and seminal vesicle of the guinea pig. *J. Pharmac. exp. Ther.*, **186**, 528–536.

Wang, F.L. and Haubrich, D.R. (1975), A simple, sensitive, and specific assay for free choline in plasma. *Analyt. Biochem.*, **63**, 195–201.

Waser, P.G. (ed.) (1975), *Cholinergic Mechanisms*, Raven Press, New York.

Watson, W.E. (1968), Centripetal passage of labelled molecules along mammalian motor axons. *J. Physiol.*, (Lond.), **196**, 122P–123P.

Watson, W.E. (1974), Cellular responses to axotomy and to related procedures. *Brit. med. Bull.*, **30**, 112–115.

Weinreich, D., McCaman, M.W., McCaman, R.E. and Vaughn, J.E. (1973), Chemical, enzymatic and ultrastructural characterization of 5-hydroxytryptamine-containing neurons from the ganglia of *Aplysia californica* and *Tritonia diomedia. J. Neurochem.*, **20**, 969–976.

Weiss, P. (1963), Self-renewal and proximo–distal convection in nerve fibres. In: *The Effect of Use and Disuse on Neuromuscular Functions* (Gutmann, E. and Hník, P., eds), pp. 171–183, Nakladatelství ČSAV, Praha.

Weiss, P.A. (1970), Neuronal dynamics and neuroplasmic flow. In: *The Neurosciences, Second Study Program* (Schmitt, F.O. ed.), pp. 840–850, The Rockefeller University Press, New York.

Weiss, P.A. (1972a), Neuronal dynamics and axonal flow. V. The semisolid state of the moving axonal column. *Proc. natn. Acad. Sci. U.S.A.*, **69**, 620–623.

Weiss, P.A. (1972b), Neuronal dynamics and axonal flow: axonal peristalsis. *Proc. natn. Acad. Sci. U.S.A.*, **69**, 1309–1312.

Weiss, P. and Hiscoe, H.B. (1948), Experiments on the mechanism of nerve growth. *J. exp. Zool.*, **107**, 315–395.

Welch, B.L. and Goldberg, A.M. (1973), Adrenal choline acetyltransferase activity: sustained effects of chronic intermittent psychological and psychosocial stimulation. *Int. J. Neurosci.*, **5**, 95–99.

Welch, M.J., Markham, C.H. and Jenden, D.J. (1976), Acetylcholine and choline in cerebrospinal fluid of patients with Parkinson's disease and Huntington's chorea. *J. Neurol. Neurosurg. Psychiat.*, **39**, 367–374.

Welsch, F. (1977), The cholinergic system in tissues without innervation. Choline acetyltransferase, choline and acetylcholine in the placenta of the rhesus monkey (Macaca mulatta). *Biochem. Pharmac.*, **26**, 1281–1286.

Welsch, F. and Dettbarn, W.-D. (1970), The subcellular distribution of acetylcholine, choline acetyltransferase and cholinesterases in lobster walking leg nerves. *J. Neurochem.*, **17**, 927–940.

Welsh, J.H. (1943), Acetylcholine level of rat cerebral cortex under conditions of anoxia and hypoglycemia. J. Neurophysiol., **6**, 329–336.

Welsh, J.H. and Hyde, J.E. (1944a), The effects of potassium on the synthesis of acetylcholine in brain. *Am. J. Physiol.*, **142**, 512–518.

Welsh, J.H. and Hyde, J.E. (1944b), The distribution of acetylcholine in brains of rats of different ages. *J. Neurophysiol.*, **7**, 41–49.

Wenthold, R.J. and Mahler, H.R. (1975), Purification of rat brain choline acetyltransferase and an estimation of its half-life. *J. Neurochem.*, **24**, 963–967.

White, H.L. and Cavallito, C.J. (1970a), Choline acetyltransferase. Enzyme mechanism and mode of inhibition by a styrylpyridine analogue. *Biochim. biophys. Acta,* **206**, 343–358.

White, H.L. and Cavallito, C.J. (1970b), Inhibition of bacterial and mammalian choline acetyltransferase by styrylpyridine analogues. *J. Neurochem.*, **17**, 1579–1589.

White, H.L. and Wu, J.C. (1973a), Kinetics of choline acetyltransferases (E.C. 2.3.1.6) from human and other mammalian central and peripheral nervous tissues. *J. Neurochem.*, **20**, 297–307.

White, H.L. and Wu, J.C. (1973b), Separation of apparent multiple forms of human brain choline acetyltransferase by isoelectric focusing. *J. Neurochem.*, **21**, 939–947.

White, H.L. and Wu, J.C. (1973c), Choline and carnitine acetyltransferases of heart. *Biochemistry,* **12**, 841–846.

Whittaker, V.P. (1959), The isolation and characterization of acetylcholine-containing particles from brain. *Biochem. J.*, **72**, 694–706.

Whittaker, V.P. (1963), Identification of acetylcholine and related esters of biological origin. In: *Cholinesterases and Anticholinesterase Agents* (Koelle, G.B., ed.), *Handbuch d. exper. Pharmakologie, Ergänzungswerk,* Vol. **15**, pp. 2–39, Springer Verlag, Berlin.

Whittaker, V.P. (1965), The application of subcellular fractionation techniques to the study of brain function. *Progr. Biophys. molec. Biol.*, **15**, 39–96.

Whittaker, V.P. (1969a), The synaptosome. In: *Handbook of Neurochemistry* (Lajtha, A., ed.), Vol. 2, pp. 327–364, Plenum Press, New York.

Whittaker, V.P. (1969b), The nature of acetylcholine pools in brain tissue. In: *Mechanisms of Synaptic Transmission* (Akert, K. and Waser, P.G., eds), *Progress in Brain Res.,* Vol. **31**, pp. 211–222, Elsevier, Amsterdam.

Whittaker, V.P. (1972), The storage and release of acetylcholine. *Biochem. J.*, **128**, 73P–74P.

Whittaker, V.P. and Dowdall, M.J. (1975), Current state of research on cholinergic synapses. In: *Cholinergic Mechanisms* (Waser, P.G., ed.), pp. 23–42, Raven Press, New York.

Whittaker, V.P. and Sheridan, M.N. (1965), The morphology and acetylcholine content of isolated cerebral cortical synaptic vesicles. *J. Neurochem.*, **12**, 363–372.

Whittaker, V.P., Michaelson, I.A. and Kirkland, R.J.A. (1963), The separation of synaptic vesicles from disrupted nerve-ending particles. *Biochem. Pharmac.*, **12**, 300–302.

Whittaker, V.P., Michaelson, I.A. and Kirkland, R.J.A. (1964), The separation of synaptic vesicles from nerve-ending particles ('synaptosomes'). *Biochem. J.*, **90**, 293–303.

Whittaker, V.P., Dowdall, M.J. and Boyne, A.F. (1972), The storage and release of acetylcholine by cholinergic nerve terminals: recent results with non-mammalian preparations. *Biochem. Soc. Symp.*, **36**, 49–68.

Widlund, L. and Heilbronn, E. (1974), Uptake of acetylcholine and choline into rat brain cortical slices and synaptosomes as related to $^{32}P_i$ incorporation into their phospholipids. *J. Neurochem.*, **22**, 991–998.

Wilbur, D.O. and Patel, M.S. (1974), Development of mitochondrial pyruvate metabolism in rat brain. *J. Neurochem.*, **22**, 709–715.

Willard, M., Cowan, W.M. and Vagelos, P.R. (1974), The polypeptide composition of intra-axonally transported proteins: evidence for four transport velocities. *Proc. natn. Acad. Sci. U.S.A.*, **71**, 2183–2187.

Wilson, W.S., Schulz, R.A. and Cooper, J.R. (1973), The isolation of cholinergic synaptic vesicles from bovine superior cervical ganglion and estimation of their acetylcholine content. *J. Neurochem.*, **20**, 659–667.

Wit-Peeters, E.M., Scholte, H.R., Van Den Akker, F. and De Nie, I. (1971), Intra-mitochondrial localization of palmityl–CoA dehydrogenase, β-hydroxyacyl–CoA dehydrogenase and enoyl–CoA hydratase in guinea pig heart. *Biochim. biophys. Acta*, **231**, 23–31.

Wonnacott, S. and Marchbanks, R.M. (1976), Inhibition by botulinum toxin of depolarization-evoked release of [^{14}C]acetylcholine from synaptosomes *in vitro. Biochem., J.*, **156**, 701–712.

Wooten, G.F. and Coyle, J.T. (1973), Axonal transport of catecholamine synthesizing and metabolizing enzymes. *J. Neurochem.*, **20**, 1361–1371.

Wooten, G.F., Kopin, I.J. and Axelrod, J. (1975), Effects of colchicine and vinblastine on axonal transport and transmitter release in sympathetic nerves. *Ann. N.Y. Acad. Sci.*, **253**, 528–534.

Wykle, R.L. and Schremmer, J.M. (1974), A lysophospholipase D pathway in the metabolism of ether-linked lipids in brain microsomes. *J. biol. Chem.*, **249**, 1742–1746.

Yamamura, H.J. and Snyder, S.H. (1972), Choline: high-affinity uptake by rat brain synaptosomes. *Science*, **178**, 626–628.

Yamamura, H.I. and Snyder, S.H. (1973), High affinity transport of choline into synatosomes of rat brain. *J. Neurochem.*, **21**, 1355–1374.

Yamamura, H.I., Kuhar, M.J., Greenberg, D. and Snyder, S.H. (1974), Muscarinic cholinergic receptor binding: regional distribution in monkey brain. *Brain Res.*, **66**, 541–546.

Yates, D.W. and Garland, P.B. (1966), The partial latency and intramitochondrial distribution of carnitine-palmitoyltransferase (E.C. 2.3.1.-), and the CoASH and carnitine permeable space of rat liver mitochondria. *Biochem. biophys. Res. Commun.*, **23**, 460–465.

Zahniser, N.R., Chou, D. and Hanin, I. (1977), Is 2-dimethylaminoethanol (Deanol) indeed a precursor of brain acetylcholine? A gas chromatographic evaluation. *J. Pharmacol. exp. Ther.*, **200**, 545–559.

Zaimis, E. (ed.) (1976), *Neuromuscular Junction Handbook of Experimental Pharmacology*, New Series, Vol. **42**, Springer Verlag, Berlin.

Zelená, J. (1969), Bidirectional shift of mitochondria in axons after injury. *Symp. Int. Soc. cell Biol.*, **8**, 73–94.

Zelená, J. (1972), Ribosomes in myelinated axons of dorsal root ganglia. *Z. Zellforsch.* **124**, 217–229.

Zelená, J. and Lubínska, L. (1962), Early changes in the acetylcholinesterase activity near the lesion in crushed nerves. *Physiol. bohemoslov.*, **11**, 261–268.

Zelená, J., Lubínska, L. and Gutmann, E. (1968). Accumulation of organelles at the ends of interrupted axons. *Z. Zellforsch.*, **91**, 200–219.

Zhabotinskii, Yu. M. (1965), *Normal and Pathological Morphology of the Neuron* (Russ.), pp. 233–252, Meditsina, Leningrad.

Zimmermann, H. and Denston, C.R. (1977a), Recycling of synaptic vesicles in the cholinergic synapses of the *Torpedo* electric organ during induced transmitter release. *Neuroscience*, **2**, 695–715.

Zimmermann, H. and Denston, C.R. (1977b), Separation of synaptic vesicles of different functional states from the cholinergic synapses of the *Torpedo* electric organ. *Neuroscience*, **2**, 715–730.

Zimmermann, H. and Whittaker, V.P. (1974a), Effect of electrical stimulation on the yield and composition of synaptic vesicles from the cholinergic synapses of the electric organ of *Torpedo*: A combined biochemical, electrophysiological and morphological study. *J. Neurochem.*, **22**, 435–450.

Zimmermann, H. and Whittaker, V.P. (1974b), Different recovery rates of the electrophysiological, biochemical and morphological parameters in the cholinergic synapses of the *Torpedo* electric organ after stimulation. *J. Neurochem.*, **22**, 1109–1114.

Zimmermann, H. and Whittaker, V.P. (1977), Morphological and biochemical heterogeneity of cholinergic synaptic vesicles. *Nature*, (Lond.), **267**, 633–635.

Zsilla, G., Cheney, D.L. and Costa, E. (1976), Regional changes in the rate of turnover of acetylcholine in rat brain following diazepam or muscimol. *Naunyn-Schmiedeberg's Archs. Pharmak.*, **294**, 251–255.

Index